3RD EDITION

CRIMINALISTICS
An Introduction
to Forensic Science

RICHARD SAFERSTEIN, Ph.D.

Chief Forensic Chemist, New Jersey State Police
Lecturer, Trenton State College
Assistant Adjunct Professor of Science, Ocean County College

PRENTICE-HALL, INC. Englewood Cliffs, New Jersey 07632

Library of Congress Cataloging-in-Publication Data

Saferstein, Richard (date)
  Criminalistics: an introduction to forensic science.

  Bibliography
  Includes index.
  1. Criminal investigation.   2. Forensic ballistics.
3. Chemistry, Forensic.   I. Title.
HV8073.S2 1987   363.2'5   86-16941
ISBN 0-13-193269-1

Editorial/production supervision: Bernie Scheier and Mary Miller
Cover design: Lundgren Graphics
Manufacturing buyer: Harry P. Baisley

Printed in the United States of America

10 9 8 7 6 5 4 3 2 1

ISBN 0-13-193269-1 025

Prentice-Hall International (UK) Limited, *London*
Prentice-Hall of Australia Pty. Limited, *Sydney*
Prentice-Hall Canada, Inc., *Toronto*
Prentice-Hall Hispanoamericana, S.A., *Mexico*
Prentice-Hall of India Private Limited, *New Delhi*
Prentice-Hall of Japan, Inc., *Tokyo*
Prentice-Hall of Southeast Asia Pte. Ltd., *Singapore*
Editora Prentice-Hall do Brasil, Ltda., *Rio de Janeiro*

Contents

3

PHYSICAL EVIDENCE   *47*

4

PHYSICAL PROPERTIES: GLASS AND SOIL   *74*

5

ORGANIC ANALYSIS   *104*

6

INORGANIC ANALYSIS   *136*

7

THE MICROSCOPE *155*

8

HAIRS, FIBERS, AND PAINT *183*

9

DRUGS *221*

10

FORENSIC TOXICOLOGY   *253*

11

FORENSIC ASPECTS OF ARSON AND EXPLOSIVE INVESTIGATIONS   *283*

12

FORENSIC SEROLOGY   *312*

13

FINGERPRINTS   *347*

14

FIREARMS, TOOL MARKS, AND OTHER IMPRESSIONS   *369*

15

DOCUMENT AND VOICE EXAMINATION   *400*

16

THE FUTURE   *423*

CASE READINGS   *431*

GLOSSARY   *461*

APPENDICES   *470*

ANSWERS   *485*

INDEX   *489*

Preface

Making science relevant and pertinent to the interests and goals of the student is a desirable but often elusive goal pursued by educators. *Criminalistics* is written with such lofty objectives in mind. The third edition of *Criminalistics* retains the purpose and intent of its previous editions. First and foremost is a presentation of the techniques, skills, and limitations of the modern crime laboratory for a reader who has no background in the forensic sciences. The nature of physical evidence is emphasized along with the limitations that technology and knowledge impose on its individualization and characterization.

A major portion of the text centers on discussions of the common items of physical evidence encountered at crime scenes. These chapters include updated techniques describing forensic analysis as well as procedures and practices relating to the proper collection and preservation of evidence at crime scenes. Particular attention is paid to the meaning and role of probability in interpreting the evidential significance of scientifically evaluated evidence.

In selecting the subject matter for the book, I have drawn upon my experience both as an active forensic scientist and as an instructor of forensic science at the college level. No prior knowledge about scientific principles or techniques is assumed of the reader. He/she is introduced to those areas of chemistry and biology relating to the analysis of physical evidence with a minimum of scientific terminology and equations. It is not the intent of this book to make scientists or forensic experts of the reader. For this reason, the chemistry and biology discussed are limited to a minimum core of facts and principles that will make the subject matter comprehensible and meaningful to the nonscientist. Nevertheless, it will certainly be gratifying if this effort motivates some students to seek further scientific knowledge, and perhaps direct their education toward a career in forensic science.

Though *Criminalistics* is an outgrowth of a one-semester course offered as a part of a criminal justice program at many New Jersey colleges, its subject matter is not limited to the college student. Optimum utilization of crime laboratory services requires that criminal investigators have a knowledge of the techniques and capabilities of the laboratory that extends beyond any summary that may be gleaned from departmental brochures dealing with the collection and packaging of physical evidence. Only by combining a knowledge of the principles and techniques of forensic science with logic and common sense will the investigator gain a comprehensive insight into the meaning and significance of physical evidence and its role in criminal investigations. Forensic science begins at the crime scene. If the investigator cannot recognize, collect, and package evidence properly, no amount of equipment or expertise will salvage the situation.

Likewise, there is a dire need to bridge the "communication gap" that presently exists between lawyers, judges, and the forensic scientist. An intelligent evaluation of the scientist's data and any subsequent testimony that may follow will again depend on the familiarity of the underlying principles of forensic science. Too many practitioners of the law profess ignorance of the subject or at best attempt to gain a superficial understanding of its meaning and significance only minutes before meeting the expert witness. To this end, it is hoped that the book will provide a painless route to comprehending the nature of the science.

In order to merge theory with practice, a number of actual forensic case histories are included in the text. It is intended that these illustrations will remove forensic science from the domain of the abstract and make its applications relevant to the real world of criminal investigation.

I am indebted to many people for their assistance and advice in the preparation of this book. Many faculty members, colleagues, and friends have read and commented on various portions of the text. I want to particularly thank the following people for their critical reading and discussions of the manuscript:

Michael Camp, Jew-Ming Chao, James Chickos, Frank Creveling, Peter DeForest, Norman Demeter, Wayne Dunning, Robert Epstein, David Garin, John Lintott, Raymond Murray, Jay Siegel, Richard Tidey, and Charles Tindall.

I'm appreciative of the time and talent given by Peggy Cole and my production editors, Mary Miller and Bernie Scheier.

I would also like to give credit to John Bartek, Linda Jankowski, and the New Jersey State Police Photography Laboratory for the special photographic skills that they so generously gave to this book. In addition, I am indebted to the New Jersey State Police, as well as those law enforcement agencies, governmental agencies, private individuals, and equipment manufacturers cited in the text for contributing their photographs and illustrations. I particularly wish to express my appreciation to Major E.R. Leibe and Major V.P. O'Donoghue for their encouragement and their support of efforts to improve the quality of forensic science services.

Anyone who expects to write a textbook must be prepared to contribute countless hours to the task, often at the expense of family obligations. This effort was no exception. My efforts would have fallen well short of completion without the patience and encouragement of my wife Gail. Her typing and critical readings of the manuscript, as well as her strength of character under circumstances that were less than ideal, will always be remembered.

The views and opinions expressed in this book are those of the author and do not necessarily represent those of the New Jersey State Police or any other governmental agency.

Richard Saferstein, Ph.D.

To the Memory of Fran and Michael

1

Introduction

DEFINITION AND SCOPE OF FORENSIC SCIENCE

Forensic science in its broadest definition is the application of science to law. As our society has grown more complex, it has become more dependent on rules of law to regulate the activities of its members. Forensic science offers the knowledge and technology of science for the definition and enforcement of such laws.

Each year, as government finds it increasingly necessary to regulate those activities that most intimately influence our daily lives, science merges more closely with civil and criminal law. Consider, for example, the laws and agencies that regulate the quality of our food, the nature and potency of drugs, the extent of automobile emissions, the kind of fuel oil we burn, the purity of our drinking water, and the pesticides we use on our crops and plants. It would be difficult to conceive of any food and drug regulation or any environmental protection act that could be effectively monitored and enforced without the assistance of scientific technology and the skill of the scientific community.

In the arena of criminal justice, laws are continually being broadened and revised to counter the alarming increase in crime rates. In response to public concern, law enforcement agencies have expanded their patrol and investigative functions, hoping to stem the rising tide of crime. At the same time they are looking more and more to the scientific community for advice and technical support of their efforts. Can the technology that put man on

1

the moon, split the atom, and eradicated man's most dreaded diseases be enlisted in this critical battle? Unfortunately, science cannot offer final and authoritative solutions to problems that stem from a maze of social and psychological factors. However, as the contents of this book will attest, science does occupy an important and unique role in the criminal justice system—a role that relates to the scientist's ability to supply accurate and objective information that reflects the events that have occurred at a crime. It will also become apparent to the reader that a good deal of work remains to be done if the full potential of science as it is applied to criminal investigations is to be realized.

Considering the vast array of civil and criminal laws that regulate society, forensic science, in its broadest sense, has become so comprehensive a subject as to make a meaningful introductory textbook treatment of its role and techniques most difficult, if not overwhelming. For this reason, we must find practical limits that narrow the scope of the subject. Fortunately, common usage provides us with such a limited definition: **Forensic science is the application of science to those criminal and civil laws that are enforced by police agencies in a criminal justice system.**

Even within this limited definition we will restrict our discussion in this book to only those areas of chemistry, biology, physics, and geology that are useful for determining the evidential value of crime-scene and related evidence, omitting any references to the subject of medicine and the law. Forensic pathology, psychology, and odontology certainly encompass important and relevant areas of knowledge and practice in law enforcement, each being an integral part of the total forensic science service that is provided to any up-to-date criminal justice system. However, these subjects go beyond the intended range of the book, and the reader is referred elsewhere for discussions of their applications and techniques.[1] Instead, we will attempt to focus on the services of what has popularly become known as the *crime laboratory*. It is here that the principles and techniques of the physical and natural sciences are practiced and applied to the analysis of crime-scene evidence.

For many, the term *criminalistics* seems more descriptive for describing the services of a crime laboratory. However, it will serve no useful purpose to rationalize whether the subject matter included in this book can best be classified as criminalistics or forensic science, if indeed this distinction can be made at all. For all intents and purposes the two terms are taken to be one and the same and will be used interchangeably in the text. Regardless of title, criminalist or forensic scientist, the trend of events has made the scientist in the crime laboratory an active participant in the criminal justice system.

---

[1] Two excellent references are: André A. Moenssens, Fred E. Inbau, and James Starrs, *Scientific Evidence in Criminal Cases*, 3rd ed. (Mineola, N.Y.: The Foundation Press, Inc., 1986; and Werner U. Spitz and Russell S. Fisher, eds., *Medicolegal Investigation of Death*, 2nd ed. (Springfield, Ill.: Charles C Thomas, Publisher, 1980).

HISTORY AND DEVELOPMENT OF FORENSIC SCIENCE

Forensic science owes its origins first to those individuals who developed the principles and techniques needed to identify or compare physical evidence, and second to those who recognized the necessity of merging these principles into a coherent discipline that could be practically applied to a criminal justice system.

Today, many believe that Sir Arthur Conan Doyle had a considerable influence on popularizing scientific crime-detection methods through his fictional character Sherlock Holmes. It was Holmes who first applied the newly developing principles of serology, fingerprinting, firearm identification, and questioned-document examination long before their value was first recognized and accepted by real-life criminal investigators. Holmes's feats excited the imagination of an emerging generation of forensic scientists and criminal investigators. Even in the first Sherlock Holmes novel, *A Study in Scarlet*, published in 1887, we find examples of Doyle's uncanny ability to describe scientific methods of detection years before they were actually discovered and implemented. For instance, here Holmes is probing and recognizing the potential usefulness of forensic serology to criminal investigation:

> "I've found it. I've found it," he shouted to my companion, running towards us with a test tube in his hand. "I have found a reagent which is precipitated by hemoglobin and by nothing else. . . . Why, man, it is the most practical medico-legal discovery for years. Don't you see that it gives us an infallible test for blood stains? . . . The old gracium test was very clumsy and uncertain. So is the microscopic examination for blood corpuscles. The latter is valueless if the stains are a few hours old. Now, this appears to act as well whether the blood is old or new. Had this test been invented, there are hundreds of men now walking the earth who would long ago have paid the penalty of their crimes. . . . Criminal cases are continually hinging upon that one point. A man is suspected of a crime months perhaps after it has been committed. His linen or clothes are examined and brownish stains discovered upon them. Are they blood stains, or rust stains, or fruit stains, or what are they? That is a question which has puzzled many an expert, and why? Because there was no reliable test. Now we have the Sherlock Holmes test, and there will no longer be any difficulty."

There are many who can be cited for their specific contributions to the field of forensic science. The following is just a brief list of those who made the earliest contributions to formulating the disciplines that now constitute forensic science.

Mathieu Orfila (1787–1853). Orfila is considered the father of forensic toxicology. A native of Spain, he ultimately became a renowned teacher of medicine in France. In 1814, Orfila published the first scientific treatise on the detection of poisons and their effects on animals. This treatise established forensic toxicology as a legitimate scientific endeavor.

Alphonse Bertillon (1853-1914). The first scientific system of personal identification was devised by Alphonse Bertillon. In 1879, Bertillon began to develop the science of anthropometry, a systematic procedure of taking a series of body measurements as a means of distinguishing one individual from another. For nearly two decades this system was considered the most accurate method of personal identification. Although anthropometry was eventually replaced by fingerprinting in the early 1900s, Bertillon's early efforts have earned him the distinction of being known as the father of criminal identification.

Francis Galton (1822-1911). Galton undertook the first definitive study of fingerprints and developed a methodology of classifying them for filing. In 1892, he published a book entitled *Finger Prints*, which contained the first statistical proof supporting the uniqueness of his method of personal identification. His work went on to describe the basic principles that form the present system of identification by fingerprints.

Leone Lattes (1887-1954). In 1901, Dr. Karl Landsteiner discovered that blood can be grouped into different categories. These blood groups or types are now recognized as A, B, AB, and O. The possibility that blood grouping could be a useful characteristic for the identification of an individual intrigued Dr. Leone Lattes, a professor at the Institute of Forensic Medicine at the University of Turin in Italy. In 1915, he devised a relatively simple procedure for determining the blood group of a dried bloodstain, a technique that he immediately applied to criminal investigations. Even to this day Dr. Lattes's procedure is often utilized by forensic scientists.

Calvin Goddard (1891-1955). To determine whether or not a particular gun has fired a bullet requires a comparison of the bullet with one that has been test-fired from the suspect's weapon. Calvin Goddard, a U.S. Army colonel, refined the techniques of such an examination by utilizing the comparison microscope. Goddard's expertise established the comparison microscope as the indispensable tool of the modern firearms examiner.

Albert S. Osborn (1858-1946). Osborn's development of the fundamental principles of document examination was responsible for the acceptance of documents as scientific evidence by the courts. In 1910, Osborn authored the first significant text in this field, *Questioned Documents;* this book is still considered a primary reference for document examiners.

Hans Gross (1847-1915). The first treatise describing the application of scientific disciplines to the field of criminal investigation was written by Hans Gross in 1893. Gross, a public prosecutor and judge in Graz, Austria, spent many years studying and developing principles of criminal investigation. In his classic book, *Handbuch für Untersuchungsrichter* (later published in English under the title *Criminal Investigation*), he detailed the assistance that investigators could expect from the fields of microscopy, chemistry, physics, mineralogy, zoology, botany, anthropometry, and fingerprinting. He later introduced the forensic journal *Kriminologie*, which still serves as a medium for reporting improved methods of scientific crime detection.

Edmond Locard (1877–1966). Although Gross was a strong advocate of the use of the scientific method in criminal investigation, he did not make any specific technical contributions to this philosophy. It was left instead to a Frenchman, Edmond Locard, to demonstrate how the principles enunciated by Gross could be incorporated within a workable crime laboratory. Locard's formal education was in both medicine and law. In 1910, he persuaded the Police Department in Lyons to give him two attic rooms and two assistants to start a police laboratory.

During his first years of work, the only instruments available to Locard were a microscope and a rudimentary spectrometer. However, his enthusiasm quickly overcame the technical and monetary deficiencies he encountered. From these modest beginnings Locard's research and accomplishments became known throughout the world by forensic scientists and criminal investigators. Eventually he became the founder and director of the Institute of Criminalistics at the University of Lyons; this quickly developed into a leading international center for study and research in forensic science.

It was Locard's belief that when a criminal came in contact with an object or person, a cross-transfer of evidence occurs (Locard's Exchange Principle). Locard believed strongly that every criminal can be connected to his crime by dust particles carried from the crime scene. This concept was reinforced by a series of successful and well-publicized investigations. In one case, confronted with counterfeit coins and the names of three suspects, Locard urged the police to bring the suspects' clothing to his laboratory. Upon careful examination, he located small metallic particles in all the garments. Chemical analysis revealed that the particles and coins were composed of exactly the same metallic elements. Confronted with this evidence, the suspects were arrested and soon confessed to the crime. During the post-World War I period, Locard's successes served as an impetus for the formation of police laboratories in Vienna, Berlin, Sweden, Finland, and Holland.

It was in the United States that the most ambitious commitment to forensic science was undertaken. In 1932, the Federal Bureau of Investigation, under the directorship of J. Edgar Hoover, organized a national laboratory that aimed to offer forensic services to all law enforcement agencies in the country. During its formative stages, extensive consultations were made with businessmen, manufacturers, and scientists whose knowledge and experience were useful in guiding the new facility through its infancy. The FBI Laboratory is now the world's largest forensic laboratory, performing nearly one million examinations every year. Its accomplishments have earned it worldwide recognition, and its structure and organization have served as a model for newly formed forensic laboratories at the state and local levels in the United States as well as in other countries. Furthermore, the opening of the FBI's Forensic Science Research and Training Center in 1981 gave the United States, for the first time, a facility dedicated to conducting research to develop new and reliable scientific methods that can be applied to forensic science. This facility is also used to train crime laboratory personnel in the latest forensic science techniques and methods.

The oldest forensic laboratory in the United States is that of the Los Angeles Police Department, created in 1923 by August Vollmer, a police chief from Berkeley, California. In the 1930s, Vollmer headed the first U.S. university institute for criminology and criminalistics at the University of California at Berkeley. However, this institute lacked any official status in the university until 1948, when a school of criminology was formed. The famous criminalist Paul Kirk (Figure 1-1) was selected to head its criminalistics department. Many of the graduates of this school have gone on to become actively engaged in the development of forensic laboratories in other parts of the state and country.

Presently, California has numerous federal, state, county, and city crime laboratories located within its boundaries. Many of these facilities operate independently of one another. However, in 1972 the California Department of Justice embarked on an ambitious plan to create a network of state-operated crime laboratories. As a result, California has created a model system of integrated forensic laboratories consisting of eight regional

Figure 1-1. Paul Leland Kirk, 1902–1970. *Courtesy* Blackstone-Shelburne, N.Y.

and seven satellite facilities. An informal exchange of information and expertise is facilitated among California's criminalist community through a regional professional society, the California Association of Criminalists. This organization was the forerunner of a number of regional organizations that have developed throughout the United States to foster cooperation among the nation's growing community of criminalists.

Another important milestone marking the development of forensic science was the creation of the Central Research Establishment in Aldermaston, England, in 1966. This laboratory was the first of its kind in the world to be solely dedicated to performing basic research in forensic science. In contrast to the American system of independent local laboratories, Britain has developed a national system of regional laboratories under the direction of the government's Home Office. With the exception of London which is served by the Metropolitan Police Laboratory, England and Wales are serviced by six regional laboratories. The Central Research Establishment is the research arm of this national system.

Relieved of the necessity of performing routine analyses, the Central Research Establishment's staff is making substantial progress in developing new forensic procedures, gathering statistical data, and collecting and disseminating vital information relating to all facets of forensic science.

THE ORGANIZATION OF A CRIME LABORATORY

The development of crime laboratories in the United States has been characterized by rapid growth accompanied by a lack of national and regional planning and coordination. At present, there are approximately 319 public crime laboratories operating at various levels of government—federal, state, county, and municipal. This represents more than a threefold increase over the number of crime laboratories operating in 1966.

The size and diversity of crime laboratories make it impossible to select any one model that can best describe a typical crime laboratory. Although the majority of these facilities function as elements of police departments, others have been placed under the direction of the prosecutor's or district attorney's office, and some have had their functions combined with laboratories of the medical examiner or coroner. Far fewer are affiliated with universities or exist as independent agencies in government. Laboratory staff sizes may range from one person to over a hundred, and their services may be diverse or specialized, depending on the responsibilities of the agency that houses the laboratory.

For the most part, crime laboratories have been organized by those agencies that either foresaw their potential application to criminal investigation or were pressed by the increasing demands of casework. A number of reasons can rightfully be cited for explaining the unparalleled growth of crime laboratories during the past twenty years. There is little doubt that Supreme Court decisions in the 1960s were responsible for the police placing greater emphasis on securing scientifically evaluated evidence. The requirement to advise criminal suspects of their constitutional rights and their right of immediate access to counsel has all but eliminated confessions as a routine investigative tool. Today, successful prosecution of criminal cases requires a thorough and professional police investigation frequently incorporating the skills of forensic science experts. Fortuitously, modern technology has provided forensic scientists with many new skills and techniques to meet the challenges accompanying their increased participation in the criminal justice system.

Coinciding with changing judicial requirements has been the staggering increase in crime rates in the United States. This factor alone would probably have sufficed to account for the increased utilization of crime laboratory services by police agencies were it not for the fact that only a small percentage of police investigations generate evidence requiring scientific examination. There is, however, one important exception to this observation, and that is drug-related arrests. All illicit drug seizures must be sent to a forensic laboratory for confirmatory chemical analysis before the case can be adjudicated in court. Since the mid-1960s, drug abuse has accelerated to nearly uncontrollable levels and has resulted in crime laboratories being inundated with drug specimens.

The impact of this trend can be gauged by the experiences of the New Jersey State Police Laboratory. Since 1968, this organization has seen a significant rise in drug cases. For 1985, 18,000 drug-related cases were analyzed, which represents a 200 percent increase over 1968. To cope with this increase, and to adequately perform other casework as well, it has been necessary to add some 70 chemists to the laboratory's staff and to expand its facilities to include three new regional laboratories. The demand for laboratories to perform drug analyses has probably been the single most important factor in the recent expansion of forensic services in New Jersey and elsewhere in the United States.

Historically, a federal system of government, combined with a desire to retain local control, has produced a variety of independent laboratories in the United States, precluding the creation of a national system of crime laboratories. Crime laboratories to a large extent mirror the fragmented law enforcement structure that exists on the national, state, and local levels. The federal government has no single law enforcement or investigative agency that has unlimited jurisdiction. Four major federal crime laboratories have been created for the purpose of assisting in the investigation and enforcement of criminal laws that extend beyond the jurisdictional boundaries of state and local forces. The FBI (Department of Justice) maintains the largest crime laboratory in the world. Its expertise and technology support its broad investigative powers. The Drug Enforcement Administration Laboratories (Department of Justice) are responsible for the analysis of drugs seized in violation of federal laws regulating the production, sale, and transportation of drugs. The laboratories of the Bureau of Alcohol, Tobacco, and Firearms (Department of the Treasury) have responsibility for analyzing alcoholic beverages and documents relating to tax law enforcement, as well as for examining weapons, explosive devices, and related evidence received in conjunction with enforcement of the Gun Control Act of 1968 and the Organized Crime Control Act of 1970. The U.S. Postal Inspection Service maintains laboratories concerned with criminal investigations relating to the postal service. Each of these federal facilities will offer its expertise to any local agency that requests assistance in relevant investigative matters.

Most state governments maintain a crime laboratory to service state and local law enforcement agencies that do not have ready access to a laboratory. Some states, such as Alabama, California, Illinois, Michigan, New Jersey, Virginia, and Florida, have developed a comprehensive statewide system of regional or satellite laboratories. These operate under the direction of a central facility and provide forensic services to most areas of the state. The concept of a regional laboratory operating as part of a statewide system has successfully increased the accessibility of many local law enforcement agencies to a crime laboratory, while at the same time minimizing the duplication of services and assuring maximum interlaboratory cooperation through the sharing of expertise and equipment.

Local laboratories provide services to county and municipal agencies. Generally, these facilities operate independently of the state crime laboratory and are financed directly by local government. However, as costs have risen, some counties have found it desirable to combine resources and create multi-county laboratories to service their jurisdictions. At this time many of the larger cities in the United States maintain their own crime laboratories, usually under the direction of the local police department. Frequently, high population and high crime rates combine to make a municipal facility, such as New York City's or Chicago's, the largest crime laboratory in the state.

Like the United States, most countries in the world have created and now maintain forensic facilities. Reference has already been made to the British regional laboratory system. In Canada, forensic services are provided by three government-funded institutes: (1) eight Royal Canadian Mounted Police regional laboratories, (2) the Centre of Forensic Sciences in Toronto, and (3) the Institute of Legal Medicine and Police Science in Montreal. Altogether, 80 countries throughout the world are known to have at least one laboratory facility offering services in the field of forensic science.

SERVICES OF THE CRIME LABORATORY

Bearing in mind the independent development of crime laboratories in the United States, the wide variation in total services offered in different communities is not surprising. There are many reasons for this, among which are: (1) variations in local laws, (2) the different capabilities and functions of the organization to which a laboratory is attached, and (3) budgetary and manpower limitations.

In recent years, many local crime laboratories have been created solely for the purpose of processing drug specimens. Often these facilities were staffed with few personnel and operated under limited budgets. Although many have gone on to expand their forensic services, some are still engaged primarily in performing drug analyses. However, even among crime laboratories providing services beyond drug identification, the diversity and quality of services rendered will vary significantly. For the purposes of this text, I have taken the liberty of arbitrarily designating the units that should constitute a "full-service" crime laboratory, as discussed below.

BASIC SERVICES PROVIDED BY FULL-SERVICE CRIME LABORATORIES

Physical Science Unit. The physical science unit applies principles and techniques of chemistry, physics, and geology to the identification and comparison of crime-scene evidence. It is staffed by criminalists who have the expertise to utilize chemical tests and modern analytical instrumentation for the examination of items as diverse as drugs, glass, paint, explosives, and soil. In a laboratory that has a staff large enough to permit specialization, the responsibilities of this unit may be further subdivided into sections devoted to drug identification, soil and mineral analyses, and the examination of a variety of trace physical evidence (see Figure 1-2).

Biology Unit. The biology unit is staffed with biologists and serologists who apply their knowledge to the identification and grouping of dried bloodstains and other body fluids, the comparison of hairs and fibers, and the identification and comparison of botanical materials such as wood and plants.

Firearms Unit. The examination of firearms, discharged bullets, cartridge cases, shotgun shells, and ammunition of all types is conducted by the firearms unit. Garments and other objects are also examined in order to detect firearm discharge residues, and to approximate the distance from a target at which a weapon was fired. The basic principles of firearm examination are also applied here to the comparison of marks made by tools.

Document Examination Unit. The handwriting and typewriting on questioned documents are studied by the documentation unit to ascertain authenticity and/or source. Related responsibilities also include analysis of paper and ink, as well as examination of indented writings (the term usually applied to the partially visible depressions appearing on a sheet of paper underneath the one on which the visible writing appears), obliterations, erasures, and burned or charred documents.

Photography Unit. A complete photographic laboratory is maintained by the photography unit to examine and record physical evidence. Its pro-

Figure 1-2. Work area of the chemistry section of the Metropolitan Police Laboratory. *Courtesy* Metropolitan Police Laboratory, London, England.

cedures may require the use of highly specialized photographic techniques, such as infrared, ultraviolet, and X-ray photography, to make invisible information visible to the naked eye. This unit also aids in the preparation of photographic exhibits for courtroom presentation.

Toxicology Unit. Body fluids and organs are examined by the toxicology group to determine the presence or absence of drugs and poisons. Frequently, such functions are shared with or may be the sole responsibility of a separate laboratory facility placed under the direction of the medical examiner's or coroner's office.

In most jurisdictions, field instruments such as the Breathalyzer are used to determine the amount of alcoholic consumption of individuals. Often the toxicology section has the responsibility of training operators as well as maintaining and servicing these instruments.

Latent Fingerprint Unit. The responsibility for processing and examining evidence for latent fingerprints when they are submitted in conjunction with other laboratory examinations belongs to the latent fingerprint unit.

Polygraph Unit. The polygraph, or lie detector, has come to be recognized as an essential tool of the criminal investigator rather than the forensic scientist. However, during the formative years of polygraph technology many police agencies incorporated this unit into the laboratory's administrative structure, where it sometimes remains today. In any case, its functions are handled by people trained in the techniques of criminal investigation and interrogation.

Voiceprint Analysis Unit. In cases involving telephoned threats or tape-recorded messages, investigators may require the skills of the voiceprint analysis unit to tie the voice to a particular suspect. To this end, a good deal of casework has been performed by the sound spectrograph, an instrument that transforms speech into a visual graphic display called a *voiceprint*. The validity of this technique as a means of personal identification rests on the premise that the sound patterns produced in speech are unique to the individual and that the voiceprint displays this uniqueness.

Evidence Collection Unit. The concept of incorporating crime-scene evidence collection into the total forensic science service is slowly gaining recognition in the United States. This unit dispatches specially trained personnel (civilian and/or police) to the crime scene to collect and preserve physical evidence that will later be processed at the crime laboratory.

THE FUNCTIONS OF THE FORENSIC SCIENTIST

ANALYSIS OF PHYSICAL EVIDENCE

First and foremost the forensic scientist must be skilled in applying the principles and techniques of the physical and natural sciences to the analysis of the many types of evidence that may be recovered during crime investigation. However, in doing this the scientist must also be aware of the demands and constraints that are imposed by the judicial system. The procedures and techniques that are utilized in the laboratory must not only rest on a firm scientific foundation but must also satisfy the criteria of admissibility that have been established by the courts.

In rejecting the scientific validity of the lie detector (polygraph), the District of Columbia Circuit Court in 1923 set forth what has since become the standard guideline for determining the judicial admissibility of scientific examinations. In *Frye* v. *United States*[2] the court stated the following:

> Just when a scientific principle or discovery crosses the line between the experimental and demonstrable stages is difficult to define. Somewhere in this twilight zone the evidential force of the principle must be recognized, and while the courts will go a long way in admitting expert testimony deduced from a well-recognized scientific principle or discovery, the thing from which the deduction is made must be sufficiently established to have gained general acceptance in the particular field in which it belongs.

Courts have usually interpreted the "general acceptance" principle of *Frye* most liberally, and have allowed testimony by experts on a wide range of scientific principles and techniques, leaving it to the jury to weigh the conclusions that the expert derives from the data. It is only when a new technique is introduced into evidence that its relevancy to the criteria of *Frye* is questioned; thus, in some cases the courts have found it necessary to interpret and expand the meaning of *Frye*. For example, a California appellate court in *People* v. *Williams*,[3] when considering a new test for determining narcotic addiction (the Nalline test), weighed the argument that because most physicians had no knowledge of the test, this meant that it was not accepted by the *entire* medical profession and therefore did not meet the *Frye* definition of "general acceptance." In rejecting this argument, the court recognized the existence and need for specialization within a given field of endeavor; it concluded:

> All of the medical testimony points to the reliability of the test. It has been generally accepted by those who would be expected to be familiar with its use. In this age of specialization no more should be required.

If a court is confronted with a new or novel scientific technique whose admissibility is under challenge, then it is the ultimate responsibility of the presiding judge to decide the issue. Normally, each side will present expert witnesses to either support or refute contentions about the reliability of the

---

[2] 293 Fed. 1013 (1923).
[3] 164 Cal. App. 2d Supp. 848, 331 P.2d 251 (1958).

method at issue or the extent of its acceptance within the forensic science community. Furthermore, in determining whether a novel technique meets criteria for admissibility, courts have frequently taken note of books and papers written on the technique, as well as prior judicial decisions relating to the reliability and general acceptance of the technique. However, even with the above considerations, the trial judge still enjoys wide latitude in admitting scientific tests into evidence. A leading case which exemplifies this discretion is *Coppolino* v. *Florida.*[4] Here a medical examiner testified to his finding that the victim had died of an overdose of a drug known as succinylcholine chloride. This drug had never before been detected in the human body. The medical examiner's findings were dependent on a toxicological report that identified an abnormally high concentration of succinic acid, a breakdown product of the drug, in the victim's body. The defense argued that this test for the presence of succinylcholine chloride was new and the absence of corroborative experimental data by other scientists meant that it had not yet gained general acceptance in the toxicology profession. The court, in rejecting this argument, recognized the necessity that exists for devising new scientific tests to solve the special problems that are continually arising in the forensic laboratory. It emphasized, however, that although these tests may be new and unique, they are admissible only if they are based on scientifically valid principles and techniques:

> The tests by which the medical examiner sought to determine whether death was caused by succinylcholine chloride was novel and devised specifically for this case. This does not render the evidence inadmissible. Society need not tolerate homicide until there develops a body of medical literature about some particular lethal agent.

PROVISION OF EXPERT TESTIMONY

Because their work product may ultimately be a factor in determining a person's guilt or innocence, forensic scientists may be required to testify with respect to their methods and conclusions at a trial or hearing. Trial courts have broad discretion in accepting an individual as an *expert witness* on any particular subject. Generally, if a witness can establish to the satisfaction of a trial judge that he or she possesses a particular skill, or has knowledge in a trade or profession that will aid the court in determining the truth of the matter at issue, that individual will be accepted as an expert witness. Depending on the subject area in question the court will usually consider that knowledge acquired through experience, training, or educa-

---

[4] 223 So. 2d 68 (Fla. App. 1968), app. dismissed 234 So. 2d (Fla., 1969), cert. denied 399 U.S. 927.

tion or a combination is sufficient grounds for qualification as an expert witness.

In court, the qualifying questions that are asked of the expert by counsel are often directed toward demonstrating the witness's ability and competence pertaining to the matter at hand. Competency may be established by having him or her cite educational degrees, participation in special courses, membership in professional societies, and any professional articles or books published. Also important to the issue is the number of years of occupational experience in which the witness has engaged in areas related to the matter before the court.

Unfortunately, there are few schools that confer degrees in forensic science. Most chemists, biologists, geologists, or physicists usually prepare themselves for careers in forensic science by combining training under an experienced examiner with independent study. Of course, formal education provides the scientist with a firm foundation for learning and understanding the principles and techniques of forensic science. Nevertheless, for the most part, courts must rely on training and years of experience as a measurement of the knowledge and ability of the expert.

Before the judge rules on the witness's qualifications, the opposing attorney will be given the opportunity to cross-examine the witness and to point out weaknesses in background and knowledge. Most courts are very reluctant to disqualify an individual as an expert even when presented with someone whose background is only remotely associated with the issue at hand. The question of what credentials are suitable for qualification as an expert is one that is obviously ambiguous and highly subjective, and one that the courts wisely try to avoid. However, the weight that a judge or jury will assign to "expert" testimony in subsequent deliberations is quite another matter. Undoubtedly, education and experience are factors that have considerable bearing on the value assigned to the expert's opinions. Just as important may be the witness's demeanor and ability to explain scientific data and conclusions clearly, concisely, and logically to a judge and jury composed of nonscientists. The problem of sorting out the strengths and weaknesses of expert testimony falls to prosecution and defense counsels, who themselves must endeavor to prepare themselves adequately for this undertaking.

The ordinary or lay witness must give testimony on events or observations that arise from personal knowledge. This testimony must be factual and, with few exceptions, cannot contain the personal opinions of the witness. On the other hand, the expert witness is called upon to evaluate evidence which the court lacks the expertise to do. This expert will then express an opinion as to the significance of the findings. The views expressed are accepted only as representing the expert's opinion and may later be accepted or ignored in jury deliberations.

It must be recognized that it is not possible for the expert to render any view with absolute certainty. At best, one may only be able to offer an opinion that is based on a reasonable scientific certainty derived from training and experience. Obviously, the expert is expected to defend vigorously the techniques and conclusions of the analysis, but at the same time there must be no reluctance to discuss impartially those findings that could minimize the significance of the analysis. The forensic scientist should not be an advocate of one party's cause, but only an advocate of truth. An adversary system of justice must give the prosecutor and defense ample opportunity to offer expert opinions and to argue the merits of such testimony. Ultimately, it will be the duty of the judge or jury to weigh the pros and cons of all the information presented in deciding guilt or innocence.

FURNISHES TRAINING IN THE PROPER RECOGNITION, COLLECTION, AND PRESERVATION OF PHYSICAL EVIDENCE

The competence of a laboratory staff and the sophistication of its analytical equipment have little or no value if relevant evidence cannot be properly recognized, collected, and preserved at the site of a crime. For this reason, it is important that the forensic staff have responsibilities that will influence the conduct of the crime-scene investigation.

The most direct and effective response to this problem has been to dispatch specially trained evidence-collection technicians to the crime scene. A growing number of crime laboratories and the police agencies they service have recognized the necessity of having trained "evidence technicians" on 24-hour call to aid criminal investigators in retrieving evidence. These technicians are trained by the laboratory staff to recognize and gather pertinent physical evidence at the crime scene. They are administratively assigned to the laboratory to facilitate their continued exposure to forensic techniques and procedures. They have at their disposal all the proper tools and supplies that will make possible the proper collection and packaging of evidence for future scientific examination.

Unfortunately, many police forces have still not adopted this approach. Often a patrol officer or detective is charged with the responsibility of collecting the evidence. His (or her) effectiveness in this role will be dependent on the extent of his training and working relationship with the laboratory. If maximum utilization is to be made of the skills of the crime laboratory, training of the crime-scene investigator must go beyond superficial classroom lectures to involve extensive personal contact with the forensic scientist. Each must become aware of the other's problems, techniques, and limitations.

The training of police officers in evidence collection and their familiarization with the capabilities of a crime laboratory should not be restricted to a select group of personnel on the force. Every officer engaged in fieldwork, whether it be traffic, patrol, investigation, or juvenile control, will often have to process evidence for laboratory examination. Obviously, it would be a difficult and time-consuming operation to give everyone the in-depth training and attention that a qualified criminal investigator requires. However, a familiarity with crime laboratory services and capabilities can be facilitated through periodic lectures, laboratory tours, and the dissemination of manuals prepared by the laboratory staff that outline the proper methods for collecting and submitting physical evidence to the laboratory. Examples of such manuals are shown in Figure 1-3.

A brief outline describing the proper collection and packaging of common types of physical evidence is found in Appendix I. The procedures and information summarized in this guide will be discussed in greater detail in forthcoming chapters.

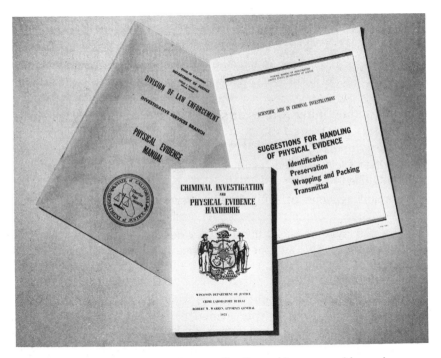

Figure 1-3.   Representative evidence collection guides prepared by various police agencies. *Courtesy* New Jersey State Police.

REVIEW QUESTIONS

1. The application of science to law describes _____.
2. The fictional exploits of _____ excited the imagination of an emerging generation of forensic scientists and criminal investigators.
3. A system of personal identification using a series of body measurements was first devised by _____.

4. _____ is responsible for developing the first statistical study proving the uniqueness of fingerprints.

5. The Italian scientist _____ devised the first workable procedure for typing dried bloodstains.

6. The comparison microscope became an indispensable tool of firearm examination through the efforts of _____.

7. Early efforts at applying scientific principles to document examination are associated with _____.

8. The application of science to criminal investigation was advocated by the Austrian magistrate _____.

9. One of the first functional crime laboratories to be formed existed in Lyons, France, under the direction of _____.

10. The first forensic laboratory in the United States was created in 1923 by the _____ Police Department.

11. The state of _____ is an excellent example of a geographical area in the United States that has created a system of integrated regional and satellite laboratories.

12. In contrast to the United States, Britain's crime laboratory system is characterized by a national system of _____ laboratories.

13. The increasing demand for _____ analyses has been the single most important factor in the recent expansion of crime laboratory services in the United States.

14. Four important agencies offering forensic service at the federal level are _____, _____, _____, and _____.

15. A decentralized system of crime laboratories presently exists in the United States under the auspices of various governmental agencies at the _____, _____, _____, and _____ levels of government.

16. The application of chemistry, physics, and geology to the identification and comparison of crime-scene evidence is the function of the _____ unit of a crime laboratory.

17. The examination of blood, hairs, fibers, and vegetative materials is conducted in the _____ unit of a crime laboratory.

18. The examination of bullets, cartridge cases, shotgun shells, and ammunition of all types is the responsibility of the _____ _____ unit.

19. The examination of body fluids and organs for drugs and poisons is a function belonging to the _____ unit.

20. The _____ unit dispatches trained personnel to the scene of a crime to retrieve evidence for laboratory examination.

21. The "general acceptance" principle, which serves as a criterion for the

judicial admissibility of scientific evidence, was set forth in the case of
_____.

22. In the case *People* v. *Williams* the court recognized the existence and need for _____ within a given field of endeavor in evaluating the admissibility of scientific evidence.

23. In the case of _____ new and unique test results were ruled admissible so long as they were based on scientifically valid principles and techniques.

24. An _____ is one who can demonstrate a particular skill, or has knowledge in a trade or profession that will assist the court in determining the truth of the matter at issue.

25. The expert witness's courtroom demeanor may play an important role in deciding what weight the court will assign to his testimony. (True, False)

26. The testimony of an expert witness incorporates his personal opinion relating to a matter he has either studied or examined. (True, False)

27. The ability of the investigator to recognize and collect crime-scene evidence properly is dependent on the amount of _____ received from the crime laboratory.

FURTHER REFERENCES

Berg, Stanton O., "Sherlock Holmes: Father of Scientific Crime Detection," *Journal of Criminal Law, Criminology and Police Science*, 61, no. 3 (1970), pp. 446–52.

Brunelle, Richard L., "Novel Techniques for the Examination of Physical Evidence," *Journal of the Association of Official Analytical Chemists*, 56 (1973), 1391.

Cohen, Stanley A., "The Role of the Forensic Expert in a Criminal Trial," *The Canadian Society of Forensic Science Journal*, 12 (1979), 75.

Conrad, Edwin, "Landmarks and Hallmarks in Scientific Evidence," in *Sourcebook in Criminalistics*, Carroll Hormachea, ed. Reston, Va.: Reston Publishing Company, 1974.

Doyle, Sir Arthur Conan, *The Complete Sherlock Holmes*, Vol. 1. New York: Doubleday, 1956.

Huber, R. A., "I Give You Yesterday," *The Canadian Society of Forensic Science Journal*, 8 (1975), 1.

Kagan, J. D., "On Being a Good Expert Witness in a Criminal Case," *Journal of Forensic Sciences*, 23 (1978), 190.

Kuzmack, Nicholas T., "Legal Aspects of Forensic Science," in *Forensic Science Handbook*, R. Saferstein, ed. Englewood Cliffs, N.J.: Prentice-Hall, Inc., 1982.

Peterson, J. L., S. Mihajlovic, and J. L. Bedrosian, "The Capabilities, Uses, and Effects of the Nation's Criminalistics Laboratories," *Journal of Forensic Sciences*, 30 (1985), 10.

Starrs, James E., "Montebanks among Forensic Scientists," in *Forensic Science Handbook*, Vol. 2, R. Saferstein, ed. Englewood Cliffs, N.J.: Prentice-Hall, Inc., 1987.

Thornton, John I., "Criminalistics—Past, Present, and Future," *Lex et Scientia, The International Journal of Law and Science*, 11 (1975), 1.

Thorwald, Jürgen, *Crime and Science*. New York: Harcourt, Brace & World, 1967.

——, *The Century of the Detective*. New York: Harcourt, Brace & World, 1964.

Walls, H. J., *Forensic Science*, 2nd ed. New York: Praeger, 1974.

——, "The Forensic Science Service in Great Britain: A Short History," *Journal of the Forensic Science Society*, 16 (1976), 273.

CASE READING

The case of *State* v. *Jascalevich* offers an excellent example of the legal and scientific issues involved in assessing the admissibility and value of scientific evidence in the courtroom. Dr. Jascalevich was accused of murdering a number of his patients by administering lethal doses of the drug curare. The issue of whether the curare was detected and identified in the exhumed bodies of the alleged murder victims was central to proving the state's case against the defendant. What ensued at the trial was a classic illustration of conflicting expert testimony on both sides of a scientific issue. Ultimately, it was the jury's task to weigh the data and arguments presented by both sides and to reach a verdict.

DETECTION OF CURARE IN THE JASCALEVICH MURDER TRIAL

Lawrence H. Hall

The Star-Ledger, *Newark, New Jersey*

Roland H. Hirsch

Chemistry Department, Seton Hall University, South Orange, New Jersey

The murder trial of Dr. Mario E. Jascalevich was one of the most complicated criminal proceedings ever tried in an American courtroom. The 34-week trial before a Superior Court judge in New Jersey resulted in a not-guilty verdict for the Englewood Cliffs, N.J., surgeon. The questions concerning analytical chemistry raised in the trial will continue to be discussed in years to come.

Not since the controversial trial of Dr. Carl Coppolino—convicted in a Florida courtroom in 1967 of murdering his wife with succinylcholine chloride—have so many forensic experts of national and international stature labored so long over the scientific questions at issue in the case:

What happens to human tissue, embalmed and interred for a decade?

Assuming lethal doses of a drug such as curare were given to hospital patients, would the drug have changed chemically or have been destroyed entirely over a 10-year period?

Assuming again that the drug had been injected, what analytical techniques could be employed to trace submicrogram amounts of it?

Could components of embalming fluids or bacteria in the earth react chemically, forming substances giving a false positive reading in the analytical procedures used?

Forensic scientists first grappled with these questions during the latter part of 1966. Two of Jascalevich's colleagues at Riverdell Hospital in Oradell, N.J.—Dr. Stanley Harris, a surgeon, and Dr. Allan Lans, an osteopathic physician—suspected him of murdering their patients with curare. There were no eyewitnesses to the alleged murders, but Drs. Harris and Lans discovered 18 vials of curare in Jascalevich's surgical locker after breaking into it.

They took their suspicions to the Bergen County Prosecutor's office in November 1966, and a brief but unpublicized investigation was launched. Items taken from the surgeon's locker, including the vials of curare and syringes, were sent for analysis at the New York City Medical Examiner's office.

In the interim, Jascalevich told authorities he used the muscle-relaxant drug in animal experiments at the Seton Hall Medical College. The surgeon presented the prosecutor his medical research papers and other documentation to support his contention. In addition, he reviewed the medical charts of the alleged murder victims and told the prosecutor there was no need for the operations the patients received. Malpractice and misdiagnosis were the causes of the deaths, Jascalevich stated at that time.

Dr. Milton Helpern, chief of the New York City Medical Examiner's office, and his staff in early 1967 concluded their testing on the items taken from Jascalevich's locker. Dog hair and animal blood were detected on the vials of curare and syringes.

The prosecutor's office terminated its investigation and stated there were more reasons to look into allegations of malpractice than murder at the small osteopathic hospital.

In January 1976 a series of articles about a "Doctor X" suspected of murdering patients at Riverdell Hospital appeared in the *New York Times*, and the Bergen County Prosecutor's office reopened its case.

A month prior to the case being officially reopened, however, New York Deputy Medical Examiner Dr. Michael Baden supplied an affidavit with the Superior Court in Bergen County stating that at least a score of patients who died at Riverdell in 1966 succumbed from other reasons than those stated on death certificates.

In his affidavit in support of exhumation of the patient's remains, Dr. Baden stated,

> It is my professional opinion that the majority of these cases reviewed are not explainable on the basis of natural causes and are consistent with having been caused by a respiratory depressant.
>
> [The deputy medical examiner continued] I am aware that because unexplainable respiratory arrests have been involved in many of these deaths, the possibility of poisoning by a curare-like substance (specifically *d*-tubocurarine) was considered and investigated at the time of the initial inquiry in 1966.
>
> The ability to identify *d*-tubocurarine, often referred to as curare, in human tissue was limited at the time of the initial investigation.
>
> It is my professional opinion that recent technological advances now permit the detection of very minute amounts of *d*-tubocurarine in tissues removed from dead bodies. This is because *d*-tubocurarine is a chemically stable compound that can exist unaltered for many years.
>
> Therefore, the aforementioned new techniques to detect curare-like compounds can be applied to tissues removed from bodies that have been interred for long periods of time.

A Superior Court judge signed the order in January 1976, granting the prosecutor's office the right to exhume the bodies of Nancy Savino, 4; Emma Arzt, 70; Frank Biggs, 59; Margaret Henderson, 27; and Carl Rohrbeck, 73.

All these patients entered Riverdell Hospital between December 1965 and September 1966 for routine surgical procedures and succumbed days afterward.

In mid-January 1976 the body of the Savino child was exhumed from a gravesite in Bergen County and taken to the medical examiner's office in New York City.

There, Dr. Baden, in the presence of New Jersey State Medical Examiner Dr. Edwin Albano and others, began performing the almost 4-h examination of the child's body, which was said to be well preserved.

Assisting Dr. Baden in the analytical studies carried out on the tissues were Dr. Leo Dal Cortivo, chief toxicologist for Suffolk County, N.Y., and Dr. Richard J. Coumbis, chief toxicologist for the New Jersey Medical Examiner's office. The defense experts, headed by former Westchester County (N.Y.) Medical Examiner Dr. Henry Siegel, were not permitted to be present at the reautopsies.

The state began its work. In March, a week before the grand jury met, a newspaper article declared that curare had been detected in the Savino child. However, in his grand jury testimony weeks later, Dr. Baden stated his experts could not be certain if curare could be detected: "We have to look and see whether or not we can develop adequate procedures."

On May 18, 1976, Dr. Jascalevich was indicted for five murders.

A little more than a year later, the state's forensic experts began using radioimmunoassay (RIA) and high-performance liquid chromatography (HPLC) on the tissue specimens. In the fall of 1977, the defense received from Drs. Baden and Dal Cortivo samples of tissues and embalming fluids of the alleged murder victims.

For the remainder of the year, both the defense and the state experts worked to develop analytical procedures to settle the question of detection of curare in human tissue.

In addition, there were numerous pretrial hearings at which time the defense, headed by Jersey City attorney Raymond Brown, requested medical slides, reports, and patient charts relating to the alleged murder victims, as well as the methodologies used in treating the specimens.

On February 28, 1978, a panel of 18 jurors was chosen for what was to become the second longest criminal trial in the nation's history. At the outset, the defense wanted a hearing to ascertain the validity of the scientific procedures employed by the state to reportedly detect curare.

The defense contended that RIA and HPLC were relatively new procedures and could not be used to detect curare in human tissue. RIA, for example, could only be used to detect drugs in blood and body fluids, according to defense experts.

The defense motion for a hearing outside of the presence of the jury was denied by Superior Court Judge William J. Arnold, who maintained the motion could be made later in the trial when the evidence obtained by the analytical techniques would actually be scheduled for presentation to the jury.

The trial got underway with testimony by osteopathic physicians, nurses, and other hospital personnel employed by Riverdell during the time the alleged murders were committed. The physicians told Assistant Prosecutor Sybil Moses that in each instance the patient had been recovering from surgery when he succumbed.

However, on cross-examination, the physicians admitted they had misdiagnosed their patients' conditions and that there was inferior postoperative care. For example, in the case of the Savino child, the defense experts held that the little girl died of acute diffuse peritonitis—the source of her abdominal pain when she was brought into Riverdell after having been diagnosed as having acute appendicitis.

After the prosecution completed presentation of the medical aspects of its case, the defense renewed its request for a special hearing on the admissibility of the evidence obtained by radioimmunoassay, liquid chromatography, and other analytical techniques. This request came as Dr. Baden took the witness stand to explain why he had recommended reautopsy of the bodies. The prosecution was opposed to a hearing:

> The techniques used by the State are not new toxicological methodologies, but are standard methods, used widely throughout the field. These methodologies include radioimmunoassay and high-pressure liquid chromatography. . . .
>
> Since the methodologies used to detect the curare are widely accepted in the scientific community, there is no necessity for the Court to conduct a hearing as to their reliability.

Nevertheless, Judge Arnold ruled that a hearing should be held. Arguments began, in the absence of the jury, on June 10. Both sides presented statements by their technical experts and affidavits from other scientists regarding the validity of the analytical methods. The prosecution cited various cases in support of its position:

> Practically every new scientific discovery has its detractors and unbelievers, but neither unanimity of opinion nor universal infallibility is required for judicial acceptance of generally recognized matters [*State* v. *Johnson*, 42 N.J. 146, 171 (1964)].
>
> The law in its efforts to enforce justice by demonstrating a fact in issue, will allow evidence of those scientific processes, which are the work of educated and skillful men in their various departments and apply them to the demonstration of a fact, leaving the weight and effect to be given to the effort and its results entirely to the consideration of the jury [*State* v. *Cerciello*, 86 N.J.L. 309, 314 (E&A 1914)].

The prosecution stated, "Federal courts have held that newness or lack of absolute certainty in a test does not require its inadmissibility." In one case involving neutron-activation analysis, a federal appellate court held in part:

> Every useful new development must have its first day in court. And court records are full of the conflicting opinions of doctors, engineers, and accountants to name just a few of the legions of expert witnesses [*United States* v. *Stifel*, 433 F. 2d. 431, 437, 438 (6th Cir. 1970)].

The prosecution noted,

> The Florida Appellate Court in *Coppolino* v. *State* . . . held that not only established techniques but methods developed specifically for that case could be used to detect a previously undetectable drug in the body of the decedent. . . .
>
> The tests by which the medical examiner sought to determine whether death

was caused by succinylcholine chloride were novel and devised specifically for this case. This does not render the evidence inadmissible. Society need not tolerate homicide until there develops a body of medical knowledge about some particular lethal agent. The expert witnesses were examined and cross-examined at great length and the jury could either believe or doubt the prosecution's testimony as it chose [*Coppolino* v. *State*, 223 So. 2d. 75 (Fla. App. 1968)].

Finally, the prosecution noted the following holding of the New Jersey Superior Court Appellate Division:

The general rule in New Jersey regarding the admissibility of scientific test results is that, if the equipment or the methodology used is proven to have a high degree of scientific reliability, and if the test is performed or administered by qualified persons, the results will be admissible at trial [*State* v. *Chatman*, 101 N.J.L.S. index 307, 308 (App. Div. 1973)].

The defense contended that

the methodologies of thin layer chromatography (TLC), high pressure liquid chromatography, ultraviolet spectrophotometry, and radioimmunoassay which have been utilized by the State do not meet the required level of acceptance under the circumstances of the tissues in this case. . . . Since there have never been any attempts to demonstrate the presence of *d*-tubocurarine in embalmed, buried tissue . . . the State cannot even assert that the techniques it wishes to utilize to demonstrate this have been generally accepted.

The defense presented affidavits from a variety of forensic scientists, from which we present one example:

It should be noted that even though the newer analytical methods and some of the sophisticated equipment are extremely sensitive for drug detection, the sensitivity of some method is not a criterion of its specificity. Sensitivity is the minimum amount of an unknown substance below which a test gives a negative result. Specificity is the ability of a test to establish the individual characteristics and/or configuration of a particular substance by differentiating it from all other substances, especially in a biologic mixture.

Currently, the reported analytical methods, which include ultraviolet absorption spectrophotometry, thin layer chromatography and radioimmunoassay, alone or in conjunction, lack such a degree of specificity with any degree of scientific certainty required to support the opinion that they identified the isolated material as *d*-tubocurarine in embalmed, decomposed and skeletonizing tissues that have been in the ground for ten years under varying climatic conditions [Abraham Stolman, Chief Toxicologist, State of Connecticut Department of Health].

On June 20 the judge ruled that the analytical evidence was admissible. He stated,

> All I'm saying is under the law the evidence is admissible. I'm not going to comment on the value or trustworthiness of the witnesses [who testified]. The ultimate decision must be made by the jury.

Following this decision, the jury began listening to the scientific evidence, with the State's and the defense's witnesses in the process explaining such points as: What is curare, and specifically *d*-tubocurarine? What is radioimmunoassay? What is an antibody, and how is the antibody for *d*-tubocurarine created? What is high-pressure liquid chromatography?

Dr. Richard Coumbis testified about his finding tubocurarine in tissues from four of the five patients: ". . . can only state there is presumptive evidence" that curare was discovered in the fifth patient. Under cross-examination by defense attorney Raymond Brown, Coumbis maintained that the RIA and HPLC procedures were valid methods of detecting curare because "on the basis of my personal experience, I did not find any other substance interfering with curare."

The toxicologist admitted that the counting efficiencies of the instruments he used to get the RIA displacement values varied from day to day and were subject to error. Brown disagreed with the displacement figures Coumbis arrived at, and wanted to know whether there was a "cut-off point" whereby he arrived at the conclusion that curare was or was not present in tissues. The RIA results ranged from as low as 77 counts all the way up to 700. Somewhere within that range, Brown argued, was a point at which Coumbis arrived at the decision that the drug was detected or not. Where, he asked, was that point? The toxicologist responded by saying that the higher the figure, the more likely curare was present. He said in many instances, however, he had to use his discretion to determine the cut-off point.

Dr. David Beggs of Hewlett-Packard then testified that he found curare in the Savino lung and liver samples using mass spectrometry. He said the Biggs and Arzt samples contained possible traces of curare; however, he could not be scientifically certain of this. He stated that mass spectrometry "is not an absolute test" for curare, but "just indicated that it is probably there." He did carry out a solvent blank as a means of eliminating false positives. He held under cross-examination that the electron impact technique used by him resulted in a spectrum with 12 major peaks and that 10 were sufficient for "fingerprint" identification of curare.

Dr. Sidney Spector of the Roche Institute testified about how he had developed the antibody for *d*-tubocurarine and applied it in RIA analysis of body fluids such as urine and blood. He had not himself run any tests for curare in human tissue samples and stated, "If there were curare in tissues, there is the possibility it could be detected." He said that the State's RIA experiments were "inadequate" in relying on aqueous solutions of curare to develop a standard curve. He held that the RIA procedure could give an indication that curare was present, but that the finding would only be presumptive evidence and not sufficient to say that the muscle-relaxant drug was positively present. He made the same point about HPLC and said that even if the two techniques were used together, there still would only be presumptive proof that the drug was present.

Dr. Leo Dal Cortivo then took the witness stand and testified that he had found curare in tissue remains of three of the patients using HPLC. He also had measured curare in vials found in the defendant's locker at Riverdell Hospital in 1966, which the defense contended had been used in animal experiments conducted by Jascalevich at the College of Medicine in Jersey City. It was necessary to use RIA for the detection of curare in the HPLC eluates. The samples were prepared for LC analysis by an extraction procedure which Dal Cortivo stated gave a 75% recovery. He rejected the contention that the extraction and LC method might have allowed positive results because of an interfering substance.

The prosecution then completed its case. At this point Judge Arnold dismissed two counts of murder and stated that the prosecution had not presented scientific evidence for the presence of curare in the bodies of Emma Arzt and Margaret Henderson. The defense then began presentation of its case with testimony about the medical aspects.

In September, attention returned to the analytical data. Drs. Frederick Rieders and Bo Holmstedt testified about the experiments they carried out on the samples provided by the prosecution. The major question they addressed was that of the long-term stability of curare under the conditions to which the bodies were subjected between 1966 and 1976.

Dr. Rieders maintained that, in his opinion, the RIA was not specific enough and "could only raise suspicions that something is there but it might not be there." The only procedure he found specific enough to be confident of identification of curare is mass spectrometry, using the entire spectrum, not just selected ion monitoring. In critical analyses, a four-step extraction procedure was used to isolate *d*-tubocurarine from the samples. . . .

Rieders tested for the stability of curare and found that both embalming fluids and tissue juices (from the patients) had destructive effects on this compound. He added curare to these liquids and could detect it by TLC initially, but after a few days could find no trace of it or other nitrogenous bases. These liquids altered curare chemically to the point where it was no longer recognizable as such. He concluded that the rapid rate of decomposition meant that to detect curare in the specimens in 1976 would have required huge, medically impossible amounts to have been present in 1966.

Rieders tested the samples for curare and found it only in the liver specimen of Nancy Savino. He stated that mass spectrometry indicated that the curare in this sample was highly pure and could not have been present in the ground for 10 years. Furthermore, if curare was present in the liver, it should also have been found in the child's muscle tissue. That it was not detected in the latter specimen was a "tremendous inconsistency."

Dr. Bo Holmstedt then stated that curare could not survive in embalmed bodies for 10 years, especially because of the effects of bacteria and repeated fluctuations in temperature of the bodies. He reviewed experiments which showed that curare, upon injection, shows levels of the same order of magnitude in liver and muscle tissues. After 10 min., "40% of the drug is to be found in the muscle and 3% in the liver."

On October 14 the defense rested its case. On October 23, after both sides had presented summations of their cases, Judge Arnold gave his charge to the jury. The next day, October 24, 1978—seven and a half months after the trial had begun—the jury received the case. After just over 2 h of deliberations, the jury returned a unanimous verdict of not guilty on all three remaining counts of murder. Two years and five months after the indictments against him had been returned, Dr. Mario Jascalevich was free.

2

The Crime Scene

As automobiles run on gasoline, crime laboratories "run" on **physical evidence**. Physical evidence encompasses any and all objects that can establish that a crime has been committed or can provide a link between a crime and its victim or a crime and its perpetrator. But if physical evidence is to be effectively used for aiding the investigator, its presence first must be recognized at the crime scene. If *all* the natural and commercial objects within a reasonable distance of a crime were gathered so that the scientist could uncover significant clues from them, the deluge of material would quickly immobilize the laboratory facility. Physical evidence can only achieve its optimum value in criminal investigations when its collection is performed with a selectivity governed by the collector's thorough knowledge of the crime laboratory's techniques, capabilities, and limitations.

Forthcoming chapters will be devoted to discussions of methods and techniques available to forensic scientists for the evaluation of physical evidence. Although it is true that present-day technology has given the crime laboratory capabilities far exceeding those of past decades, these advances are no excuse for complacency on the part of criminal investigators. Crime laboratories do not solve crimes; only a thorough and competent investigation conducted by professional police officers will enhance the chances for the successful outcome of a criminal investigation. To be sure, forensic science is, and will continue to be, an important element of the total investigative process; but it is only one aspect of an endeavor that must be a team effort. The investigator who believes the crime laboratory to be a panacea for laxity or ineptness is in for a rude awakening.

Forensic science begins at the crime scene. If the investigator cannot recognize physical evidence or cannot properly preserve it for laboratory examination, no amount of sophisticated laboratory instrumentation or technical expertise can salvage the situation. The know-how for conducting a proper crime-scene search for physical evidence is not beyond the grasp of any police department, regardless of its size. With proper training, police agencies can assure themselves of competent performance at crime scenes. In many jurisdictions, police agencies have delegated this task to a specialized team of technicians. However, whether this task is carried out by a specialist or by a patrolman, it must be emphasized that the techniques of crime-scene investigation are not difficult to master and certainly lie within the bounds of comprehension of the average police officer.

Not all crime scenes require retrieval of physical evidence, and in reality, limited resources and manpower have forced many police agencies to restrict their efforts in this area to crimes of a more serious nature. However, once the commitment is made to completely process a crime site for physical evidence it is imperative that certain fundamental practices be adhered to.

SECURE AND ISOLATE THE CRIME SCENE

It is the responsibility of the first officer arriving on the scene of a crime to take steps to preserve and protect the area to the greatest extent possible. Of course, first priority should be given to obtaining medical assistance for individuals in need of it, and to arresting the perpetrator. However, as soon as it is possible, extensive efforts must be taken to exclude all unauthorized personnel from the scene. As additional officers arrive, measures are immediately initiated to isolate the area. Ropes or barricades along with the strategic positioning of guards will prevent unauthorized access to the area.

Sometimes the exclusion of unauthorized personnel proves to be a more difficult task than expected. Crimes of violence are especially susceptible to attention by higher level police officials and members of the press, as well as by emotionally charged neighbors and curiosity seekers. Every individual who enters the scene is a potential destroyer of physical evidence, even if it is by unintentional carelessness. If proper control is to be exercised over the crime scene, the officer charged with the responsibility for protecting it must have the authority to exclude everyone, including fellow police officers not directly involved in processing the site or in conducting the investigation. Seasoned criminal investigators are always prepared to relate horror stories about crime scenes made totally valueless for physical evidence by hordes of people who, for one reason or another, trampled through them.

Securing and isolating the crime scene are critical steps in an investigation, the accomplishment of which is the mark of a trained and professional crime-scene investigative team.

RECORD THE SCENE

Investigators will only have a limited amount of time to work a crime site in its untouched state. The opportunity to permanently record the scene in its original state must not be lost. Such records will not only prove useful during the subsequent investigation, but they are also required for presentation at a trial in order to document the condition of the crime site and to delineate the location of physical evidence. Photography, sketches, and notes are the three methods for crime-scene recording (Figure 2-1). Ideally all three should be employed; however, as is often the case, manpower and monetary limitations may prohibit the utilization of photography at every crime site. Under these circumstances departmental guidelines will establish priorities for deploying photographic resources. However, no reason exists for a failure to utilize sketches and notes at the crime scene.

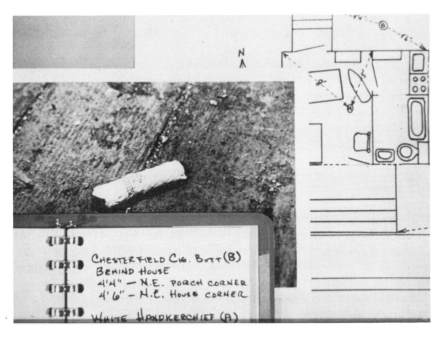

Figure 2-1. The finding of an evidential cigarette butt at the crime scene requires photographing it, making a sketch showing its relation to the crime scene, and recording the find in field notes. *Courtesy* Police Science Services, Niles, Illinois.

Photography. The most important prerequisite for photographing a crime scene is to have it in an unaltered condition. Unless there are injured parties involved, objects must not be moved until they have been photographed from all necessary angles. If objects are removed, positions changed, or items added, the photographs may not be admissible as evidence at a trial, and their intended value will be lost.

Each crime scene should be photographed as completely as possible. This means that the crime scene should include the area in which the crime actually took place and all adjacent areas where important acts occurred immediately before or after the commission of the crime. Overview photographs of the entire scene and surrounding area, including points of exit and entry, must be taken from various angles. If the crime has taken place indoors, the entire room should be photographed to show each wall area. Rooms adjacent to the actual crime site must be similarly photographed. If the crime scene includes a body, photographs must be taken to show the body's position and location relative to the entire scene. Close-up photos depicting injuries and weapons lying near the body are also necessary.

As items of physical evidence are discovered, they are photographed to show their position and location relative to the entire scene. After these overviews are taken, there should be close-ups to record the details of the object itself. When the size of an item is of significance, a ruler or other measuring scale may be inserted near the object and included in the photograph as a point of reference.

The use of videotape at crime scenes is becoming increasingly popular as the cost of this equipment is decreasing. The same principles used in crime-scene photographs apply to videotaping. As with conventional photography, videotaping should include the entire scene and the immediate surrounding area. Long shots as well as close-ups should be taken in a slow and systematic manner. Furthermore, it is desirable to have one crime-scene investigator narrate the events and scenes being taped while another does the actual shooting.

Sketching. Once photographs are taken, the crime-scene investigator will sketch the scene. The investigator may have neither the skill nor the time to make a polished sketch of the scene. However, this is not required during the early phase of the investigation. What is necessary is a "rough" sketch containing an accurate depiction of the dimensions of the scene and showing the location of all objects having a bearing on the case.

A rough sketch is illustrated in Figure 2-2. It shows all recovered items of physical evidence, as well as other important features of the crime scene. Objects are located in the sketch by distance measurements from two fixed points, such as the walls of a room. It is important that distances shown on the sketch be accurate and not the result of a guess or estimate. For this reason, all measurements are made with a tape measure. The simplest way to

2741 ARAGON ST.
6/7/81
9:30 PM
DEATH (SHOOTING)

SKETCH by OFFICER
JOHN SMITH

DINING ROOM

A — DINING ROOM TABLE
B — CHAIR
C — OVERTURNED CHAIR
D — 0.38 REVOLVER
E — MALE BODY
F — TABLE
G — CHAIR

Figure 2-2. Diagram of a crime scene.

designate an item in a sketch is to assign it a number or letter. A legend or list placed below the sketch will then correlate the letter to the item's description. The sketch should also show a compass heading designating *north*.

Unlike the rough sketch, the finished sketch is drawn with care and concern for aesthetic appearance. It is usually prepared with the aid of templates and drafting tools by a skilled individual and is frequently drawn to scale. When the finished sketch is completed, it must reflect information contained within the rough sketch in order to be admissible evidence in a courtroom.

Notes. Note taking must be a constant activity throughout the processing of the crime scene. These notes must include a detailed written description of the scene with the location of items of physical evidence recovered. They must also identify the time an item of physical evidence was discovered, by whom, how and by whom it was packaged and marked, and the disposition of the item after it was collected. The note taker has to keep in mind that this written record may be the only source of information for refreshing one's memory months, perhaps years, after a crime scene has been processed. The notes must be sufficiently detailed to anticipate this need.

CONDUCT A SYSTEMATIC SEARCH
FOR EVIDENCE

The search for physical evidence at a crime scene must be thorough and systematic. For a factual, unbiased reconstruction of the crime, the investigator, through his training and experience, must not overlook any pertinent evidence. Even in those cases in which suspects are immediately seized and the motives and circumstances of the crime are readily apparent, it is imperative that a thorough search for physical evidence be conducted at once. Failure in this, even though it may seem at the time to be unnecessary, can lead to accusations of negligence or charges that the investigative agency knowingly "covered up" evidence that would be detrimental to its case.

Assigning those responsible for searching a crime scene is a function of the investigator in charge. Except in major crimes, or where the evidence is very complex, it is usually not necessary to have the assistance of a forensic scientist at the crime scene; his or her role appropriately begins with the submission of evidence to the crime laboratory. As has already been observed, some police agencies do have trained field evidence technicians to conduct the search for physical evidence at the crime scene. They have the equipment and skill to photograph the scene and examine it for the presence of fingerprints, footprints, tool marks, or any other type of evidence that may be relevant to the crime.

How one proceeds to carry out a crime-scene search will depend on the locale and size of the area, as well as on the actions of the suspect(s) and victim(s) at the scene. When possible, it is advisable to have one person supervising and coordinating the collection of evidence. Without proper control the search may be conducted in an atmosphere of confusion with needless duplication of effort. Evidence collectors may choose to subdivide the scene into segments and search each segment individually, or the search may start at some outer point and gradually move toward the center of the scene in a circular fashion (see Figure 2-3). The areas searched must include all probable points of entry and exit used by the criminals.

What to search for will be determined by the particular circumstances of the crime. Obviously, the skill of crime-scene investigators at recognizing

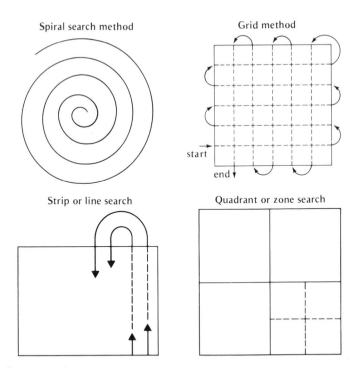

Spiral search method
Grid method
Strip or line search
Quadrant or zone search

Figure 2-3. Several typical examples of crime-scene search patterns are illustrated. The pattern selected will normally depend on the size and locale of the scene and the number of collectors participating in the search.

evidence and searching relevant locations is paramount to the successful processing of the crime scene. While training will impart general knowledge for conducting a proper crime-scene investigation, ultimately the investigator must rely on the experience gained from numerous investigations to formulate a successful strategy for recovering relevant physical evidence at crime scenes. For example, in the case of homicide, the search will be centered on the weapon and for any type of evidence left as a result of contact between the victim and assailant. The cross-transfer of evidence, such as hairs, fibers, and blood, between individuals involved in the crime is particularly useful for linking suspects to the crime site and for corroborating events transpiring during the commission of the crime. During the investigation of a burglary, efforts will be made to locate tool marks at the point of entry. In most crimes a thorough and systematic search for latent fingerprints is required.

Vehicle searches must be carefully planned and systematically carried out. The nature of the case determines how detailed the search must be. In hit-and-run cases, the outside and undercarriage of the car must be examined with care. Particular attention is paid to looking for any evidence resulting from a cross-transfer of evidence between the car and the victim—this includes blood, tissue, hair, fibers, and fabric impressions. Traces of paint or broken glass may be located on the victim. In cases of homicide, burglary, kidnapping, etc., all areas of the vehicle, inside and outside, are searched with equal care for physical evidence.

Physical evidence can be anything from massive objects to microscopic traces. Often, many items of evidence are obvious in their presence, but others may only be detected through examination in the crime laboratory. For example, minute traces of blood may be discovered on garments only after a thorough search in the laboratory; or the presence of hairs and fibers may be revealed in vacuum sweepings or on garments only after close laboratory scrutiny. For this reason, it is important to collect *possible* carriers of trace evidence in addition to more discernible items. Hence, it may be necessary to take custody of all clothing worn by the participants in a crime. Each clothing item should be handled carefully and wrapped separately to avoid loss of trace materials. Critical areas of the crime scene should be vacuumed and the sweepings submitted to the laboratory for analysis. The sweepings from different areas must be collected and packaged separately. A portable vacuum cleaner equipped with a special filter attachment is suitable for this purpose (see Figure 2-4). Additionally, fingernail scrapings from individuals who were in contact may contain minute fragments of evidence capable of providing a link between assailant and victim. The undersurface of each nail is best scraped with a dull object such as a toothpick to avoid cutting the skin. These scrapings will be subjected to microscopic examination in the laboratory.

The search for physical evidence must extend beyond the crime scene to the autopsy room of a deceased victim. Here, the medical examiner or

Figure 2-4. Vacuum sweeper attachment, constructed of clear plastic in two pieces that are joined by a threaded joint. A metal screen is mounted in one-half to support a filter paper to collect debris. The unit attaches to the hose of the vacuum sweeper. After a designated area of the crime scene is vacuumed, the filter paper is removed and retained for laboratory examination. *Courtesy* Sirchie Laboratories, Inc., Raleigh, N. Carolina.

coroner will carefully examine the victim to establish a cause and manner of death. As a matter of routine, tissues and organs will be retained for pathological and toxicological examination. At the same time, arrangements must be made between the examiner and investigator to secure a variety of items that may be obtainable from the body for laboratory examination. As a matter of routine the following are to be collected and sent to the forensic laboratory:

1. Victim's clothing.
2. Fingernail scrapings.
3. Head and pubic hairs.
4. Blood (for typing purposes).
5. Vaginal, anal, and oral swabs (in sex-related crimes).
6. Recovered bullets from the body.
7. Hand swabs or washings from shooting victims (for gunshot residue analysis).

Once the body is buried, efforts at obtaining these items may prove difficult or futile. Furthermore, a lengthy time delay in obtaining many of the above items will diminish or destroy their forensic value.

In recent years many police departments have gone to the expense of purchasing and equipping "mobile crime laboratories" (see Figure 2-5) for their evidence technicians. However, the term *mobile crime laboratory* is a misnomer. These vehicles carry the necessary supplies to protect the crime

Figure 2-5. Evidence collection vehicle. *Courtesy* Sirchie Laboratories, Inc., Raleigh, N. Carolina.

scene, photograph, collect and package physical evidence, and perform latent print development. They are not designed to carry out the functions of a chemical laboratory. *Crime-scene search vehicle* would be a more appropriate but perhaps less dramatic name for such a vehicle.

COLLECT AND PACKAGE PHYSICAL EVIDENCE

Physical evidence must be handled and processed in a way that prevents any change from taking place between the time it is removed from the crime scene and the time it is received by the crime laboratory. Changes can arise through such ways as contamination, breakage, evaporation, accidental scratching or bending, or loss through improper or careless packaging.

The integrity of evidence is best maintained when the item is kept in its original condition as found at the crime site. Whenever possible, evidence should be submitted to the laboratory intact. Blood, hairs, fibers, soil particles, and other types of trace evidence should not normally be removed from garments, weapons, or other articles that bear them. Instead, the entire object is to be sent to the laboratory for processing. Of course, if evidence is adhering to an object in a precarious manner, good judgment is best exercised by removing and packaging the item. If evidence is found adhering to large structures, such as a door, wall, or floor, common sense must be used; remove the specimen with a forceps or other appropriate tool. In the case of a bloodstain, one has the option of either scraping the stain off the surface, transferring the stain to a moistened swab, or cutting out the area of the object bearing the stain.

Each different item or similar items collected at different locations must be placed in separate containers. Packaging evidence separately prevents damage through contact and prevents cross-contamination.

The well-prepared evidence collector will arrive at a crime scene with a large assortment of packaging materials and tools ready to encounter any type of situation. Forceps and similar tools may have to be used to pick up small items. Unbreakable plastic pill bottles with pressure lids are excellent containers for hairs, glass, fibers, and various other kinds of small or trace evidence. Alternately, manila envelopes, screw-cap glass vials, or cardboard pillboxes are adequate containers for most trace evidence encountered at crime sites. Ordinary mailing envelopes should not be used as evidence containers because powders and fine particles will leak out of their corners. Small amounts of trace evidence can also be conveniently packaged in a carefully folded paper, using what is known as a "druggist fold." This consists of folding one end of the paper over one-third, then folding the other end (one-third) over that, and repeating the process from the other two sides. After being folded in this manner, the outside two edges are tucked into each other to produce a closed container that keeps the specimen from falling out.

Although pill bottles, vials, pillboxes, or manila envelopes are good universal containers for most trace evidence, two frequent finds at crime scenes warrant special attention. If bloodstained materials are stored in airtight containers, the accumulation of moisture may encourage the growth of mold, which can destroy the evidential value of blood. In these instances, wrapping paper, manila envelopes, or paper bags are recommended packaging materials. As a matter of routine, all items of clothing are to be air-dried and placed individually in separate paper bags to ensure a constant circulation of air through them. This will prevent the formation of mold and mildew. On the other hand, charred debris recovered from the scene of a suspicious fire must be sealed in an airtight container to prevent the evaporation of volatile petroleum residues. New paint cans or tightly sealed jars are recommended in such situations.

A detailed description of the proper collection and packaging of various types of physical evidence will be discussed in forthcoming chapters; additionally, most of this information is summarized in the evidence guide found in Appendix I.

MAINTAIN CHAIN OF CUSTODY

Continuity of possession, or the chain of custody, must be established whenever evidence is presented in court as an exhibit. Adherence to standard procedures in recording the location of evidence, marking it for identification, and properly completing evidence submission forms for laboratory analysis is the best guarantee that the evidence will withstand inquiries of what happened to it from the time of its findings to its presentation in court. This means that every person who handled or examined the evidence must be accounted for. Failure to substantiate the evidence's chain of custody may lead to serious questions regarding the authenticity and integrity of the evidence and the examinations rendered upon it.

All items of physical evidence should be carefully packaged and marked upon their retrieval at crime sites. This should be done with the utmost care to avoid destroying their evidential value or restricting the number and kind of examinations to which they may be subjected by the criminalist. If at all possible, the evidence itself should be marked for identification. Normally, the collector's initials and the date of collection are inscribed directly on the article. However, if the evidence collector is unsure of the necessity of marking the item itself, or has doubts as to where to mark it, it is best to omit this step. Where appropriate, the evidence is to be tagged for identification. Once an evidence container is selected for the evidence, whether it be box, bag, vial, or can, it also must be marked for identification. A minimum record would show the collector's initials, location of the evidence, and date of collection. If the evidence is turned over to another individual for care or delivery to the laboratory, this transfer must be recorded in notes and other appropriate forms. In fact, every individual who has occasion to possess the evidence must maintain a written record of its acquisition and disposition. Frequently, all of the individuals involved in the collection and transportation of the evidence may be requested to testify in court. Thus, to avoid confusion and to retain complete control of the evidence at all times, the chain of custody should be kept to a minimum.

OBTAIN CONTROLS

The examination of evidence, whether it is soil, blood, glass, hair, fibers, etc., often requires comparison with a known standard or control. Although most investigators have little difficulty in recognizing and collecting relevant crime-scene evidence, few seem aware of the like necessity and importance of providing the crime lab with a thorough sampling of control materials. Such materials may be obtained from the victim, a suspect, or other sources. For instance, investigation of a hit-and-run incident might require the removal of control paint from a suspect vehicle. This will permit its comparison to paint recovered at the scene. Similarly, hair found at a crime scene will only be of optimum value when compared to control hairs removed from the suspect and victim. Likewise, bloodstained evidence must be accompanied by whole blood controls obtained from all relevant crime-scene participants. The quality and quantity of control specimens often determine the evidential value of crime-scene evidence, and these control specimens must be treated with equal care. The thorough collection and proper packaging of control specimens are the mark of a skilled investigator.

SUBMISSION OF EVIDENCE
TO THE LABORATORY

Evidence is usually submitted to the laboratory either by personal delivery or by mail shipment. The method of transmittal will usually be determined by the distance the submitting agency must travel to the laboratory and the urgency of the case. If personal delivery of the evidence is undertaken, the deliverer should be someone who is familiar with the case. This arrangement will facilitate any discussions that may ensue between laboratory personnel and the deliverer concerning specific aspects of the case.

If desired, most evidence can be conveniently shipped through the mails. However, postal regulations do restrict the shipment of certain chemicals and live ammunition and prohibit the mailing of explosives. In such situations the laboratory must be consulted to determine the disposition of these substances. Care must also be exercised in the packaging of evidence in order to prevent breakage or other accidental destruction while it is in transit to the laboratory.

Most laboratories require that an evidence submission form accompany all evidence submitted. One such form is shown in Figure 2-6. It is essential

DEPARTMENT OF LAW AND PUBLIC SAFETY
DIVISION OF STATE POLICE

REQUEST FOR EXAMINATION OF EVIDENCE

Crime Rape & Murder _____ In County of Burlington _____ Lab. No. _____

Victim Mary F. Jones, w-f, age 34 _____ Suspect _____ George White, w-m, age 22

Submitting Agency N. J. State Police, Troop C, Bordentown, N. J. _____

Forward Replies to _____ Capt. F. J. Smith, Commanding, Troop C, Princeton, N. J. 08540

Invest. by ____ DSG. J. F. Brown _____ Delivered by _____
                                                            SIGNATURE OF PERSON DELIVERING EVIDENCE

Brief History of Case: Victim found dead in bed, Apt. 9-A, Bordentown Arms Apts. Face of the victim bruised around cheekbones. Pink bedspread crumpled on floor next to bed. On night table one (1) prescription bottle containing two (2) blue pills (pharmacy check, prescription Amo-barbital). Bits of pink thread discovered in victim's mouth. Apt. door forced. Suspect was seen in the general area of Apt. 9-A. Pink threads on suspect's sweater. Screwdriver found in his pocket.

Examination Requested:

1. Nos. 1 & 2 - general toxicology for narcotics, poisons, alcohol.
2. No. 3 for pill content.
3. Compare threads, #4, removed from victim's mouth with fibers of bedspread #5.
4. Compare specimen #5 with #6 - threads adhering to sweater with fiber of bedspread.
5. Comparison, blade of #7 with mark on #8.
6. Nos. 9 through 19 for the presence of semen or stains.

List of Specimens:

1. Blood - 25 cc (Oxalated) from victim.
2. Urine - 20 cc from bladder of victim.
3. Prescription bottle containing two (2) blue pills, labeled "Bardly Pharmacy - Prescription #56789 - Dr. S. Johnson - Patient Mary F. Jones".
4. Four (4) strands of pink thread.
5. One (1) pink bedspread.
6. One (1) blue "Darwin" sweater with pink threads adhering to same - suspects.
7. One (1) five inch (5") "Handyman" screwdriver - suspects.
8. One (1) door latch from front door of apartment with possible toolmarks on same.
9. One (1) white bra - victims.
10. One (1) pair of white panties - victims.
11. One (1) housecoat, light blue - victims.
12. One (1) bed sheet, 72" x 108", white.
13. One (1) pillow case, white with blue design.
14. Rectal swab from victim.
15. Vaginal swab from victim.
16. Mouth swab from victim.
17. One (1) white "T" shirt - suspects.
18. One (1) pair of white "Jockey" shorts - suspects.
19. One (1) pair of light brown trousers - suspects.

NOTE: Photos of above scene and autopsy to be forwarded to Laboratory by Troop C Identification Bureau.

Figure 2-6. An example of a properly completed evidence submission form. *Courtesy* New Jersey State Police.

that this form be properly completed. Its information will enable the laboratory analyst to make an intelligent and complete examination of the evidence. Particular attention should be paid to providing the laboratory with a brief description of the case history. This information will allow the examiner to analyze the specimens in a logical sequence and make the proper comparisons, and it will also facilitate the search for trace quantities of evidence.

The particular kind of examination requested for each type of evidence is to be delineated. However, it must be made clear that the analyst will not be bound to adhere strictly to the specific tests requested by the investigator. As the examination proceeds, new evidence may be uncovered, and as a result the complexity of the case may change. Furthermore, the analyst may find the initial requests to be incomplete or not totally relevant to the case. Finally, a list of items submitted for examination must be included in the evidence submission form. Each item is to be packaged separately and assigned a number or letter, which should be listed in an orderly and logical sequence on the form.

LEGAL CONSIDERATIONS AT THE CRIME SCENE

In police work, there is perhaps no experience more exasperating or demoralizing than to watch valuable evidence excluded from use against the accused because of legal considerations. This situation most often arises from what is deemed to be an "unreasonable" search and seizure of evidence. Therefore, the removal of any evidence from a person or from the scene of a crime must be done in conformity with Fourth Amendment privileges:

> The right of the people to be secure in their persons, houses, papers, and effects, against unreasonable searches and seizure, shall not be violated, and no warrants shall issue, but upon probable cause, supported by oath or affirmation, and particularly describing the place to be searched, and the persons or things to be seized.

Since the 1960s, the Supreme Court has been particularly concerned with defining the circumstances under which the police can search for evidence in the absence of a court-approved search warrant. A number of allowances have been made to justify a warrantless search: (1) the existence of emergency circumstances, (2) the need to prevent the immediate loss or destruction of evidence, (3) a search of a person and property within the immediate control of the person provided it is made incident to a lawful arrest, and (4) a search made by consent of the parties involved. In cases other than the above, police must be particularly cautious about processing a crime scene without a search warrant. In 1978, the Supreme Court addressed this very issue and in so doing set forth guidelines for investigators to follow in determining the propriety of conducting a warrantless search at a crime scene. Significantly, the two cases decided on this issue related to homicide and arson crime scenes, both of which are normally subjected to the most intensive forms of physical evidence searches by police.

In the case of *Mincey* v. *Arizona*,[1] the Court dealt with the legality of a four-day search at a homicide scene. The case involved a police raid on the home of Rufus Mincey, who had been suspected of dealing in drugs. Under the pretext of buying drugs, an undercover police officer forced entry into Mincey's apartment and was killed in a scuffle that ensued. Without a search warrant, the police spent four days searching the apartment, recovering among other things, bullets, drugs, and drug paraphernalia. These items were subsequently introduced as evidence at the trial. Mincey was convicted and on appeal contended that the evidence gathered from his apartment, without a warrant and without his consent, was illegally seized. The Court unanimously upheld Mincey's position, stating:

> We do not question the right of the police to respond to emergency situations. Numerous state and federal cases have recognized that the Fourth Amendment does not bar police officers from making warrantless entries and searches when they reasonably believe that a person within is in need of immediate aid. Similarly, when the police come upon the scene of a homicide they may make a prompt warrantless search of the area to see if there are other victims or if a killer is still on the premises. . . . Except for the fact that the offense under investigation was a homicide, there were no exigent circumstances in this case. . . . There was no indication that evidence would be lost, destroyed or removed during the time required to obtain a search warrant. Indeed, the police guard at the apartment minimized that possibility. And there is no suggestion that a search warrant could not easily and conveniently have been obtained. We decline to hold that the seriousness of the offense under investigation itself creates exigent circumstances of the kind that under the Fourth Amendment justify a warrantless search.

In *Michigan* v. *Tyler*,[2] a business establishment leased by Loren Tyler and a business partner was destroyed by fire. The fire was finally extinguished in the early hours of the morning; however, hampered by smoke, steam, and darkness, fire officials and police were prevented from thoroughly examining the scene for evidence of arson. The building was then left unattended until 8 A.M. of that day when officials returned and began an inspection of the burned premise. During the morning search assorted items of evidence were recovered and removed from the building. On three other occasions, 4 days, 7 days, and 25 days after the fire, investigators re-entered the premise and removed additional items of evidence. Each of these searches was made with-

---

[1] 57 L.Ed.2d 290 (1978).
[2] 56 L.Ed.2d 486 (1978).

out a warrant or without consent, and the evidence seized was used to convict Tyler and his partner of conspiracy to burn real property and related offenses. The Supreme Court upheld the reversal of the conviction, holding the initial morning search to be proper but contending that evidence obtained from subsequent reentries to the scene was inadmissible.

> We hold that an entry to fight a fire requires no warrant, and that once in the building, officials may remain there for a reasonable time to investigate the cause of a blaze. Thereafter, additional entries to investigate the cause of the fire must be made pursuant to the warrant procedures. . . .

The message from the Supreme Court is clear: When time and circumstances permit, obtain a search warrant before investigating and retrieving physical evidence at the crime scene.

REVIEW QUESTIONS

1. The term _____ encompasses all objects that can establish whether a crime has been committed or can provide a link between a crime and its victim or perpetrator.
2. Scientific evaluation of crime-scene evidence can usually overcome the results of a poorly conducted criminal investigation. (True, False)
3. The techniques of physical evidence collection require a highly skilled individual who must specialize in this area of investigation. (True, False)
4. All unauthorized personnel must be _____ from crime scenes.
5. Three methods for recording the crime scene are _____, _____, and _____.
6. The most important prerequisite for photographing a crime scene is to have it in an _____ condition.
7. Photographs of physical evidence must include overviews as well as _____ to record the details of objects.
8. An investigator need only draw a _____ sketch at the crime scene to show its dimensions and pertinent objects.
9. A detailed search of the crime scene for physical evidence must be conducted in a _____ manner.
10. Besides the more obvious items of physical evidence, possible _____ of trace evidence must be collected for detailed examination in the laboratory.
11. In cooperation with the medical examiner or coroner, what type of evidence retrieved from a deceased victim is to be submitted to the crime laboratory?

12. Whenever possible, trace evidence (is, is not) to be removed from the object that bears it.
13. Each item collected at the crime scene must be placed in _____ containers.
14. An ordinary mailing envelope is considered to be a good general-purpose evidence container. (True, False)
15. An airtight container (is, is not) recommended packaging material for bloodstained garments.
16. As a matter of routine, all items of clothing are to be _____ before packaging.
17. Charred debris recovered from the scene of an arson is best placed in a porous container. (True, False)
18. The possibility of future legal proceedings requires that a _____ be established with respect to the possession and location of physical evidence.
19. Most physical evidence collected at the crime site will require the accompanying submission of _____ material for comparison purposes.
20. In the case of *Mincey* v. *Arizona* the Supreme Court restricted the practice of conducting a _____ search at a homicide scene.
21. In the case of *Michigan* v. *Tyler* the Supreme Court dealt with search and seizure procedures at an _____ scene.

FURTHER REFERENCES

Fox, Richard H., and Carl L. Cunningham, *Crime Scene Search and Physical Evidence Handbook.* Washington, D.C.: U.S. Government Printing Office, 1973.

Geberth, Vernon J., *Practical Homicide Investigation.* New York: Elsevier Science Publishing Co., 1983.

Goddard, Kenneth W., *Crime Scene Investigation.* Reston, Va.: Reston Publishing Company, 1977.

Handbook of Forensic Science. Washington, D.C.: U.S. Government Printing Office, 1984.

Peterson, Joseph L., *The Utilization of Criminalistic Services by the Police.* Washington, D.C.: U.S. Government Printing Office, 1974.

Peterson, Joseph L., Steven Mihajlovic, and Michael Gilliand, *Forensic Evidence and the Police: The Effects of Scientific Evidence on Criminal Investigations.* Washington, D.C.: U.S. Government Printing Office, 1984.

Svenson, A., Otto Wendel, and Barry J. Fisher, *Techniques of Crime Scene Investigation*, 3rd ed. New York: Elsevier North-Holland, Inc., 1981.

Swanson, Charles R., Jr., Ned C. Chamelin, and Leonard Territo, *Criminal Investigation*. Santa Monica, Calif.: Goodyear Publishing Co., 1977.

Weston, Paul B., and Kenneth M. Wells, *Criminal Investigation*, 3rd ed. Englewood Cliffs, N.J.: Prentice-Hall, Inc., 1980.

AUDIOVISUAL PRESENTATIONS

Care, Custody and Control (filmstrip and audio tape). Robert J. Brady Co., Bowie, Md.

The Crime Scene (filmstrip and audio tape). Robert J. Brady Co., Bowie, Md.

Physical Evidence (80 35-mm slides and audio tape). Police Science Services, Niles, Ill.

Physical Evidence (114 35-mm slides and accompanying script). Motorola Teleprograms Inc., Shiller Park, Ill.

3

Physical Evidence

It would be impossible to list all the objects that could conceivably be of importance to a crime; every crime scene obviously has to be treated on an individual basis, having its own peculiar history, circumstances, and problems. It is practical, however, to list those items whose scientific examination are likely to yield significant results in ascertaining the nature and circumstances of a crime. The investigator who is thoroughly familiar with the recognition, collection, and analysis of these items, as well as with laboratory procedures and capabilities, can make logical decisions when the uncommon and unexpected are encountered at the crime scene. Just as important, a qualified evidence collector cannot rely on collection procedures memorized from a pamphlet but must be able to make innovative, on-the-spot decisions at the crime scene.

COMMON TYPES OF PHYSICAL EVIDENCE

1. Blood, Semen, and Saliva. All suspected blood, semen, or saliva—liquid or dried, animal or human—present in a form to suggest a relation to the offense or persons involved in a crime. This category includes blood or semen dried onto fabrics or other objects, as well as cigarette butts that may contain saliva residues. These substances are subjected to serological and biochemical analysis for determination of identity and possible origin.

2. Documents. Any handwriting and typewriting submitted so that authenticity or source can be determined. Related items include paper, ink, indented writings, obliterations, and burned or charred documents.

3. Drugs. Any substance seized in violation of laws regulating the sale, manufacture, distribution, and use of drugs.

4. Explosives. Any device containing an explosive charge, as well as all objects removed from the scene of an explosion that are suspected to contain the residues of an explosive.

5. Fibers. Any natural or synthetic fiber whose transfer may be useful in establishing a relationship between objects and/or persons.

6. Fingerprints. All prints of this nature, latent and visible, are included.

7. Firearms and Ammunition. Any firearm, as well as discharged or intact ammunition, suspected of being involved in a criminal offense.

8. Glass. Any glass particle or fragment that may have been transferred to a person or object involved in a crime. Windowpanes containing holes made by a bullet or other projectile are included in this category.

9. Hair. Any animal or human hair present that could link a person with a crime.

10. Impressions. This category includes tire markings, shoe prints, depressions in soft soils, and all other forms of tracks. Glove and other fabric impressions, as well as bite marks in skin or foodstuffs, are also included.

11. Organs and Physiological Fluids. Body organs and fluids are submitted for toxicology to detect possible existence of drugs and poisons. This category includes blood to be analyzed for the presence of alcohol and other drugs.

12. Paint. Any paint, liquid or dried, that may have been transferred from the surface of one object to another during the commission of a crime. A common example is the transfer of paint from one vehicle to another during an automobile collision.

13. Petroleum Products. Any petroleum product removed from a suspect or recovered from a crime scene. The most common examples are gasoline residues removed from the scene of an arson, or grease and oil stains whose presence may suggest involvement in a crime.

14. Powder Residues. Any item suspected of containing firearm discharge residues.

15. Serial Numbers. This category includes all stolen property submitted to the laboratory for the restoration of erased identification numbers.

16. Soils and Minerals. All items containing soil or minerals that could link a person or object to a particular location. Common examples are soil imbedded in shoes and safe insulation found on garments.

17. Tool Marks. This category includes any object suspected of containing the impression of another object that served as a tool in a crime. For example, a screwdriver or crowbar could produce tool marks by being impressed into or scraped along a surface of a wall.

18. Wood and Other Vegetative Matter. Any fragments of wood, sawdust, shavings, or vegetative matter discovered on clothing, shoes, or tools that could link a person or object to a crime location.

THE SIGNIFICANCE OF PHYSICAL EVIDENCE

The examination of physical evidence by a forensic scientist is usually undertaken for identification or comparison.

IDENTIFICATION

Identification has as its purpose the determination of the physical or chemical identity of a substance with as near absolute certainty as existing analytical techniques will permit. For example, the crime laboratory is frequently requested to identify the chemical composition of an illicit drug preparation that may contain heroin, cocaine, barbiturates, etc. It may be asked to identify gasoline in residues recovered from the debris of a fire, or it may have to identify the nature of explosive residues—e.g., dynamite or TNT. Also, the identification of blood, semen, hair, or wood would, as a matter of routine, include a determination for species origin. For example, did an evidential bloodstain originate from a human as opposed to a dog or cat? Each of these requests requires the analysis and ultimate identification of a specific physical or chemical substance to the exclusion of all other possible substances.

The process of identification first requires the adoption of testing procedures that give characteristic results for specific standard materials. Once these test results have been established, they may be permanently recorded and used repeatedly to prove the identity of suspect materials. For example, if one wants to ascertain that a particular suspect powder is heroin, the test results on the powder must be identical to those that have been previously obtained from a known heroin sample. Second, identification requires that the number and type of tests needed to identify a substance be sufficient to exclude all other substances. This means that the examiner must devise a specific analytical scheme that will eliminate all but one substance from consideration. Hence, if a conclusion is reached that a white powder contains heroin, the examiner's test results must have been comprehensive enough to have excluded all other drugs, or for that matter, all other substances, from consideration.

Simple rules cannot be devised for defining what constitutes a thorough and foolproof analytical scheme. Each type of evidence obviously requires different tests, and each test has a different degree of specificity. Thus, one substance could conceivably be identified by one test, whereas another may require the combination of five or six different tests to arrive at an identification. In a science in which the practitioner has little or no control over the quality and quantity of the specimens received, a standard series of tests cannot encompass all possible problems and pitfalls. So, it is left to the forensic scientist to determine at what point the analysis can be concluded and the criteria for positive identification satisfied; for this, he/she must rely on knowledge gained through education and experience. Ultimately, the conclusion will have to be substantiated beyond any reasonable doubt in a court of law.

COMPARISON

A comparison analysis subjects a suspect specimen and a control specimen to the same tests and examinations for the ultimate purpose of determining whether or not they have a common origin. For example, the forensic scientist may assist in placing a suspect at a particular location by noting the similarities of a hair found at the crime scene to hairs removed from a suspect's head. Or a paint chip found on a hit-and-run victim's garment may have to be compared with paint removed from a vehicle suspected of being involved in the incident. The forensic comparison is actually a two-step procedure. First, a combination of select properties are chosen from the suspect and the control specimen for comparison. The question of which and how many properties are to be selected will obviously depend on the type of materials being examined. (This is a subject that will receive a good deal of discussion in forthcoming chapters.) The overriding consideration must be the ultimate evidential value of the conclusion. This brings us to the second objective. Once the examination has been completed, the forensic scientist must be prepared to render a conclusion with respect to the origin of the specimens. Do they or do they not come from the same source? Certainly if one or more of the properties selected for comparison do not agree, the analyst will not hesitate in concluding that the specimens are not the same, and hence could not have originated from the same source. Suppose, on the other hand, that all the properties do compare and the specimens, as far as the examiner can determine, are indistinguishable. Does it logically follow that they come from the same source? Not necessarily so.

In order to comprehend the evidential value of a comparison, one must appreciate the role that probability has in ascertaining the origin of two or more specimens. Simply defined, probability is the frequency of occurrence of an event. If a coin is flipped 100 times, in theory we can expect heads to come up 50 times. Hence, the probability of the event (heads) occurring is 50 in a hundred. In other words, probability defines the odds at which a certain event will occur.

Individual Characteristics. Evidence that can be associated with a common source with an extremely high degree of probability is said to possess **individual characteristics.** Examples of this are the matching ridge characteristics of two fingerprints, the comparison of random striation markings on bullets or tool marks, the comparison of irregular and random wear patterns in tire or footwear impressions, the comparison of handwriting characteristics, the fitting together of the irregular edges of broken objects in the manner of a jigsaw puzzle (Figure 3-1), or matching sequentially made plastic bags by

Figure 3-1. The body of a woman was found with evidence of beating about the head and a stablike wound in the neck. Her husband was charged with the murder. The pathologist found a knife blade tip in the wound in the neck. The knife blade tip was compared with the broken blade of a penknife found in the trousers pocket of the accused. Note that in addition to the fit of the indentations on the edges, there are scratch marks running across the blade tip corresponding in detail to those on the broken blade. *Courtesy* Centre of Forensic Sciences, Toronto, Canada.

striation marks running across the bags (see Figure 3-2). In all of these cases it is not possible to state with mathematical exactness the probability that the specimens are of common origin; it can only be concluded that this probability is so high as to defy mathematical calculations or human comprehension. Furthermore, the conclusion of common origin must be substantiated by the practical experience of the examiner. For example, the French scientist Victor Balthazard has mathematically determined that the probability of two individuals having the same fingerprints is one out of 1×10^{60}, or 1 followed by 60 zeros. This probability value is so small as to exclude the possibility of any two individuals having the same fingerprints. This contention is also supported by the experience of fingerprint examiners who, after classifying millions of prints over the past 80 years, have never found any two to be exactly alike.

Class Characteristics. One of the disappointments awaiting the investigator unfamiliar with the limitations of forensic science is the frequent inability of the laboratory to relate physical evidence to a common origin with a high degree of certainty. Evidence is said to possess **class characteristics** when it can only be associated with a group and never with a single source.

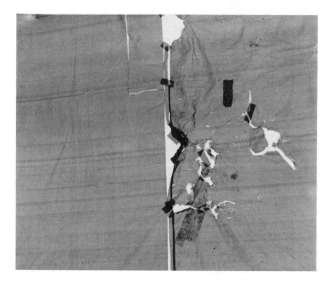

Figure 3-2. The bound body of a young woman was recovered from a river. Her head was covered with a black polyethylene trash bag (shown on the right). Among the items recovered from one of several suspects was a black polyethylene trash bag (shown on the left). A side-by-side comparison of the two bags' extrusion marks and pigment bands showed them to be consecutively manufactured. This information allowed investigators to focus their attention on one suspect who ultimately was convicted of the homicide. *Courtesy* New Jersey State Police.

Here again probability is a determining factor. For example, if we were to compare two one-layer automobile paint chips of a similar color, the chances of their having originated from the same car is not nearly as great as when we compare two paint chips each having *seven* similar layers of paint, not all of which were part of the car's original color. The former will have class characteristics and could only be associated at best to one car model (which may number in the thousands), whereas the latter may be judged to have individual characteristics and to have a high probability of originating from one specific car.

Blood offers another good example of evidence that has class characteristics. For example, two blood specimens are compared: both are found to be of human origin, and both are typed as O. The frequency of occurrence in the population of type O blood is 43 percent—hardly offering a basis for establishing the common origin of the stains. However, if other blood factors are also determined in each stain and are found to compare, the probability that the two stains originated from a common source increases. The following blood factors may be used as an illustration:

Blood Factors	Frequency
O	43%
D	85%
PGM 2	5.5%
AK 2-1	9%
EsD 2-1	19%
EAP A	13%

The product of all the frequencies shown above will determine the probability that any one individual will possess such a combination of blood factors. In this instance, 0.004 percent or 4 in 100,000 would be expected to have this particular combination of blood factors. Although the forensic scientist has still not individualized the bloodstains to one person, data has been provided that will permit the investigator and the court to better assess the evidential value of the two stains.

One of the present weaknesses of forensic science is the inability of the examiner to assign exact or even approximate probability values to the comparison of most class physical evidence. For example, what is the probability that a nylon fiber originated from a particular sweater, or that a hair came from a particular person's head, or that a paint chip came from a suspect car involved in a hit-and-run accident? There is very little statistical data available from which to derive this information, and in a society that is increasingly dependent on mass-produced products, the gathering of such data is becoming an increasingly elusive goal. One of the primary endeavors of forensic scientists must be to create and update statistical data bases for evaluating the significance of class physical evidence. Of course, when such information—e.g., the population frequency of blood factors—is available, it is utilized; but for the most part the forensic scientist must rely on personal experience when he is called upon to interpret the significance of class physical evidence.

Disappointment is often expressed when someone unfamiliar with the realities of modern criminalistics learns that most items of physical evidence retrieved at crime scenes cannot be linked definitively to a single person or object. Although efforts are always made to uncover physical evidence possessing individual characteristics—i.e., fingerprints, tool marks, and bullets—the chances of finding class physical evidence are far greater. To deny or belittle the value of such evidence is to reject the potential role that criminalistics can play in a criminal investigation. In practice, criminal cases are fashioned for the courtroom around a collection of diverse elements, each pointing to the guilt or involvement of a party in a criminal act. Often, the majority of the evidence gathered is subjective in nature, prone to human error and bias. The believability of eyewitness accounts, confessions, and informant testimony can all be disputed, maligned, and subjected to severe attack and skepticism in the courtroom. Under these circumstances, errors in human judgment are often magnified to detract from the credibility of the witness.

The value of class physical evidence lies in its ability to provide corroboration of events with data that is, as nearly as possible, free of human error and bias. It is the thread that binds together other investigative findings that are more dependent on human judgments and, therefore, more prone to human failings. The fact that scientists have not yet learned to individualize many kinds of physical evidence only means that the criminal investigator should not abdicate or falter in his pursuit of all investigative leads. However, the ability of scientists to achieve a high degree of success in evaluating class physical evidence does mean that the criminal investigator can pursue his work with a much greater chance of success.

Admittedly, in most situations, the problem of trying to define the significance of an item of class evidence in exact mathematical terms is difficult if not impossible to solve. While class evidence is by its very nature not unique, our common experience tells us that meaningful items of physical evidence, such as those listed on pages 47–49 are extremely diverse in our environment. Select, for example, a colored fiber from an article of clothing and try to locate the exact same color on the clothing of individuals you randomly come in contact with, or select a car color and try to match it to other automobiles you see on local streets or roads. Furthermore, keep in mind that a forensic comparison actually goes beyond a mere color comparison and involves examining and comparing a variety of chemical and/or physical properties. The point to be made is that the chances of encountering two indistinguishable items of physical evidence at a crime scene which actually originated from different sources are at best slight. Obviously, given these circumstances, only those objects which exhibit a significant amount of diversity in our environment are deemed appropriate for classification as physical evidence.

In the same way, when one is dealing with more than one type of class evidence, their collective presence may lead to an extremely high certainty that they originated from the same source. As the number of different objects linking an individual to a crime increases, the probability of involvement increases dramatically. A classic example of this situation can be found with evidence presented at the trial of Wayne Williams (see the case reading at the end of this chapter). Wayne Williams was charged with the murders of two individuals in the Atlanta, Georgia, metropolitan area; he was also linked to the murders of ten other boys or young men. An essential element of the State's case involved the association of Williams with the victims through a variety of fiber evidence. Actually, 28 different types of fibers linked Williams to the murder victims, evidence that the forensic examiner characterized as "overwhelming."

In further evaluating the contribution of physical evidence, one cannot overlook one important reality in the courtroom: The weight or significance accorded physical evidence is a determination left entirely to the trier of fact, usually a jury of laypersons. Given the high esteem in which scientists are generally held by society and the infallible image created by books and television for forensic science, it is not hard to understand why scientifically evaluated evidence often takes on an aura of special reliability and trustworthiness in the courtroom. Often physical evidence, whether it be individual or class, is accorded great weight during jury deliberations and becomes a primary factor in reinforcing or overcoming lingering doubts about guilt or innocence. In fact, a number of jurists have already cautioned against giving carte blanche approval to admitting scientific testimony without first giving due consideration to its relevancy in a case. Given the potential weight of scientific evidence, failure to take proper safeguards may unfairly prejudice a case against the accused.

Physical evidence may also serve to exclude or exonerate a person from suspicion. For instance, if type A blood is linked to the suspect, all individuals that have types B, AB, and O blood can be eliminated from consideration. Because it is not possible to assess at the crime scene what value, if any, the scientist will find in the evidence collected, or what significance such findings will ultimately have to a jury, it is imperative that a thorough collection and scientific evaluation of physical evidence become a routine part of all criminal investigations.

Just when an item of physical evidence crosses the line that distinguishes class from individual is a most difficult question to answer and is often the source of heated debate and honest disagreement among forensic scientists.

How many striations are necessary to individualize a mark to a single tool and no other? How many color layers will individualize a paint chip to a single car? How many ridge characteristics individualize a fingerprint, and how many handwriting characteristics will tie a person to a signature? These are all questions that defy simple solutions. It is the task of the forensic scientist to find as many characteristics as possible to compare one substance with another. The significance that is attached to the findings is a matter that is decided by the quality and composition of the evidence, the case history, and the examiner's experience. Ultimately, the conclusion can range from mere speculation to near certainty.

There are practical limits to the properties and characteristics the forensic scientist can select for comparison. Carried to the extreme, no two things in this world are alike in every detail. Modern analytical techniques have become so sophisticated and sensitive that the criminalist must be careful to define the limits of natural variation that exist among materials when interpreting the data gathered from a comparative analysis. For example, we will learn in the next chapter that two properties, density and refractive index, are best suited for comparing two pieces of glass. But the latest techniques that have been developed to measure these properties are so sensitive that they can even distinguish glass originating from a single pane of glass. Certainly, this goes beyond the desires of the criminalist who is just trying to determine if two glass particles originated from the same window. Similarly, if the surface of a paint chip is magnified 1600 times with a powerful scanning electron microscope, it is apparent that the fine details that are revealed could not be duplicated in any other paint chip. Under these circumstances, no two paint chips, even those coming from the same surface, could ever compare in the true sense of the word. Therefore, practicality dictates that such examinations be conducted at a less revealing, but more meaningful, magnification [see Figure 3-3 (a) and (b)].

Distinguishing evidential variations from natural variations is not always an easy task. Learning how to use the microscope and all the other modern instruments in a crime laboratory properly is one thing; gaining the proficiency needed to interpret the observations and data is another. As new crime laboratories are created and others expand to meet the requirements of the law enforcement community, many individuals are starting new careers in forensic science. They must be cautioned that merely reading relevant textbooks and journals is not and cannot be a substitute for experience in this most practical of sciences.

REVIEW QUESTIONS

1. The process of _____ determines a substance's physical or chemical identity with as near absolute certainty as existing analytical techniques will permit.

(a)

(b)

Figure 3-3. (a) Two-layer paint chip magnified 244 times with a scanning electron microscope. (b) The same paint chip as viewed at a magnification of 1600 times. Both photos *courtesy* Jeff Albright.

57

2. The number and type of tests needed to identify a substance must be sufficient to _____ all other substances from consideration.
3. A _____ analysis subjects a suspect and a control specimen to the same tests and examination for the ultimate purpose of determining whether they have a common origin.
4. _____ is the frequency of occurrence of an event.
5. Evidence that can be traced to a common source with an extremely high degree of probability is said to possess _____ characteristics.
6. Evidence associated with a group and not to a single source is said to possess _____ characteristics.
7. One of the major deficiencies of forensic science is the inability of the examiner to assign exact or approximate probability values to the comparison of most class physical evidence. (True, False)
8. The value of class physical evidence lies in its ability to provide _____ of events that is as nearly as possible free of human error and bias.
9. The _____ accorded physical evidence during a trial is left entirely to the trier of fact.
10. Physical evidence cannot be used to exclude or exonerate a person from suspicion of committing a crime. (True, False)
11. The distinction between individual and class evidence is always easy to make. (True, False)
12. Modern analytical techniques have become so sensitive that the forensic examiner must be aware of the _____ that exists among materials when interpreting the significance of comparative data.

FURTHER REFERENCES

Kirk, Paul L., *Crime Investigation*, 2nd ed., John I. Thornton, ed. New York: Wiley & Sons, 1974.

Osterburg, James W., "The Evaluation of Physical Evidence in Criminalistics: Subjective or Objective Process?" *Journal of Criminal Law, Criminology and Police Science*, 60 (1969), 97.

Walls, H. J., "What Is Reasonable Doubt? A Forensic Scientist Looks at the Law," in *Forensic Science*, Joseph L. Peterson, ed. New York: AMS Press, Inc., 1975.

CASE READING

FIBER EVIDENCE
AND THE
WAYNE WILLIAMS TRIAL

Harold A. Deadman

Special Agent
Microscopic Analysis Unit
Laboratory Division
Federal Bureau of Investigation
Washington, D.C.

On February 26, 1982, a Fulton County, Ga., Superior Court jury returned a verdict of "guilty as charged" on two counts of murder brought against Wayne Bertram Williams by a Fulton County grand jury in July 1981. Williams had been on trial since December 28, 1981, for the asphyxial murders of Nathaniel Cater and Jimmy Payne in April and May of 1981. During the 8-week trial, evidence linking Williams to those murders and to the murders of 10 other boys or young men was introduced.

An essential part of this case, presented by the Fulton County District Attorney's Office, involved the association of fibrous debris removed from the bodies of 12 murder victims with objects from the everyday environment of Williams.

Fiber evidence has often been an important part of criminal cases, but the Williams trial differed from other cases in several respects. Fiber evidence has not played a significant role in any case involving a large number of murder victims. The victims whose deaths were charged to Williams were 2 of 30 black children and black young men who were reported missing or who had died under suspicious circumstances in the Atlanta area over a 22-month period beginning in July 1979. During the trial, fiber evidence was used to associate Williams with 12 of those victims.

Fiber evidence is often used to corroborate other evidence in a case—it is used to support other testimony and validate other evidence presented at a trial. This was not the situation in the Williams trial. Other evidence and other aspects of the trial were important but were used to support and complement the fiber evidence, not the usual order of things. The "hair and fiber matches" between Williams' environment and 11 of the 12 murder victims discussed at the trial were so significant that in the author's opinion,

Reprinted in part from *FBI Law Enforcement Bulletin*, March and May, 1984.

these victims were positively linked to both the residence and automobiles that were a major part of the world of Wayne Williams.

Another difference between this case and most other cases was the extremely large amount of publicity surrounding both the investigation of the missing and murdered children and the arrest and subsequent trial of Williams. Few other murder trials have received the attention that the Williams case received. . . .

It is often difficult to get an accurate picture from press reports of the physical evidence introduced at a trial and the significance of that evidence. This article will also set forth in some detail the fiber evidence that linked Williams to the murder victims.

By discussing only the fiber evidence introduced at the trial, many other other aspects of the case against Williams are being neglected. Additional evidence dealing with Williams' motivations—his character and behavior, his association with several of the victims by eyewitness accounts, and his link to a victim recovered from a river in Atlanta—was also essential to the case. . . .

Development of Williams as a
Murder Suspect

Before Wayne Williams became a suspect in the Nathaniel Cater murder case, the Georgia State Crime Laboratory located a number of yellowish-green nylon fibers and some violet acetate fibers on the bodies and clothing of the murder victims whose bodies had been recovered during the period of July 1979 to May 1981. The names of those victims were included on the list of missing and murdered children that was compiled by the Atlanta Task Force (a large group of investigators from law enforcement agencies in the Atlanta area). The yellowish-green nylon fibers were generally similar to each other in appearance and properties and were considered to have originated from a single source. This was also true of the violet acetate fibers. Although there were many other similarities that would link these murders together, the fiber linkage was notable since the possibility existed that a source of these fibers might be located in the future.

Initially, the major concern with these yellowish-green nylon fibers was determining what type of object could have been their source. This information could provide avenues of investigative activity. The fibers were very coarse and had a lobed cross-sectional appearance, tending to indicate that they originated from a carpet or a rug. The lobed cross-sectional shape of these fibers, however, was unique, and initially, the manufacturer of these fibers could not be determined. Photomicrographs of the fibers were prepared for display to contacts within the textile industry. On one occasion, these photomicrographs were distributed among several chemists attending a meeting at the research facilities of a large fiber producer. The chemists concurred that the yellowish-green nylon fiber was very unusual in cross-sectional shape and was consistent with being a carpet fiber, but again, the manufacturer of this fiber could not be determined. Contacts with other textile producers and textile chemists likewise did not result in an identification of the manufacturer.

In February 1981, an Atlanta newspaper article publicized that several different fiber types had been found on two murder victims. Following the publication of this article, bodies recovered from rivers in the Atlanta metropolitan area were either nude or clothed only in undershorts. It appeared possible that the victims were being disposed of in this undressed state and in rivers in order to eliminate fibers from being found on their bodies.*

On May 22, 1981, a four-man surveillance team of personnel from the Atlanta Police Department and the Atlanta Office of the FBI was situated under and at both ends of the James Jackson Parkway Bridge over the Chattahoochee River in northwest Atlanta. Around 2:00 A.M., a loud splash alerted the surveillance team to the presence of an automobile being driven slowly off the bridge. The driver was stopped and identified as Wayne Bertram Williams.

Two days after Williams' presence on the bridge, the nude body of Nathaniel Cater was pulled from the Chattahoochee River, approximately 1 mile downstream from the James Jackson Parkway Bridge. A yellowish-green nylon carpet-type fiber, similar to the nylon fibers discussed above, was recovered from the head hair of Nathaniel Cater. When details of Williams' reason for being on the bridge at 2:00 A.M. could not be confirmed, search warrants for Williams' home and automobile were obtained and were served on the afternoon of June 3, 1981. During the late evening hours of the same day, the initial associations of fibers from Cater and other murder victims were made with a green carpet in the home of Williams. Associations with a bedspread from Williams' bed and with the Williams' family dog were also made at that time.

An apparent source of the yellowish-green nylon fibers had been found. It now became important to completely characterize these fibers in order to verify the associations and determine the strength of the associations resulting from the fiber matches. Because of the unusual cross-sectional appearance of the nylon fiber and the difficulty in determining the maufacturer, it was

---

*Prior to the publication of the February 11, 1981, newspaper article, one victim from the task force list, who was fully clothed, had been recovered from a river in the Atlanta area. In the 2½-month period after publication, the nude or nearly nude bodies of seven of the nine victims added to the task force list were recovered from rivers in the Atlanta area.

believed that this was a relatively rare fiber type, and therefore, would not be present in large amounts (or in a large number of carpets).

The Williams Carpet

Shortly after Williams was developed as a suspect, it was determined the yellowish-green nylon fibers were manufactured by the Wellman Corporation. The next step was to ascertain, if possible, how much carpet like Williams' bedroom carpet had been sold in the Atlanta area—carpet composed of the Wellman fiber and dyed with the same dye formulation as the Williams' carpet. Names of Wellman Corporation customers who had purchased this fiber type, technical information about the fiber, and data concerning when and how much of this fiber type had been manufactured were obtained.

It was confirmed that the Wellman Corporation had, in fact, manufactured the fiber in Williams' carpet and that no other fiber manufacturer was known to have made a fiber with a similar cross section. It was also determined that fibers having this cross-sectional shape were manufactured and sold during the years 1967 through 1974. Prior to 1967, this company manufactured only a round cross section; after 1974, the unusual trilobal cross section seen in Williams' carpet was modified to a more regular trilobal cross-sectional shape. A list of sales of that fiber type during the period 1967 through 1974 was compiled. . . .

Through numerous contacts with yarn spinners and carpet manufacturers, it was determined that the West Point Pepperell Corporation of Dalton, Ga., had manufactured a line of carpet called "Luxaire," which was constructed in the same manner as the Williams' carpet. One of the colors offered in the "Luxaire" line was called "English Olive," and this color was the same as that of the Williams' carpet (both visually and by the use of discriminating chemical and instrumental tests).

It was learned that the West Point Pepperell Corporation had manufactured the "Luxaire" line for a 5-year period from December 1970 through 1975; however, it had only purchased Wellman 181B fiber for this line during 1970 and 1971. In December 1971, the West Point Pepperell Corporation changed the fiber composition of the "Luxaire" line to a different nylon fiber, one that was dissimilar to the Wellman 181B fiber in appearance. Accordingly, "Luxaire" carpet, like the Williams' carpet, was only manufactured for a 1-year period. This change of carpet fiber after only 1 year in production was yet another factor that made the Williams' carpet unusual.

It is interesting to speculate on the course the investigation would have taken if the James Jackson Parkway Bridge had not been covered by the surveillance team. The identification of the manufacturer of the nylon fibers showing up on the bodies could still have occurred and the same list of purchasers of the Wellman fiber could have been obtained. The same contacts with the yarn and carpet manufacturers could have been made; however, there would not have been an actual carpet sample to display. It is believed that eventually the carpet manufacturer could have been determined. With a sample of carpet supplied by West Point Pepperell—which they had retained in their files for over 10 years—it would have been possible to conduct a house-by-house search of the Atlanta area in an attempt to find a similar carpet. Whether this very difficult task would have been attempted, of course, will never be known. A search of that type, however, would have accurately answered an important question that was discussed at the trial—the question of how many other homes in the Atlanta area had a carpet like the Williams' carpet. An estimation, to be discussed later, based on sales records provided by the West Point Pepperell Corporation indicated that there was a very low chance (1/7792) of finding a carpet like Williams' carpet by randomly selecting occupied residences in the Atlanta area.

Only the West Point Pepperell Corporation was found to have manufactured a carpet exactly like the Williams' carpet. Even though several manufacturers had gone out of business and could not be located, it was believed that considering the many variables that exist in the manufacture of carpet and the probable uniqueness of each carpet manufacturer's dye formulations, it would be extremely unlikely for two unrelated companies to construct a carpet or dye the carpet fibers in exactly the same way. A large number of other green fibers, visually similar in color to Williams' carpet, were examined. None was found to be consistent with fibers from the Williams carpet.

Probability Determinations

To convey the unusual nature of the Williams residential carpet, an attempt was made to develop a numerical probability—something never before done in connection with textile materials used as evidence in a criminal trial.* The following information was gathered from the West Point Pepperell Corporation:

1. West Point Pepperell reported purchases of Wellman 181B fiber for the "Luxaire" line during a 1-year period. The Wellman 181B fiber was used to manufacture "Luxaire" carpet from December 1970 until December 1971, at which time a new fiber type replaced that Wellman fiber.
2. In 1971, West Point Pepperell sold 5,710 square yards of English Olive

---

*E. J. Mitchell and Holland, "An Unusual Case of Identification of Transferred Fibers," *Journal of the Forensic Science Society*, vol. 19, 1979, p. 23. This article describes a case in which carpet fibers transferred to a murder victim's body in England were traced back to the carpet manufacturer and finally to an automobile owned by the person who eventually confessed to the murder.

"Luxaire" and "Dreamer" carpet to Region C (10 southeastern States which include Georgia). "Dreamer" was a line of carpet similar to "Luxaire" but contained a less dense pile. In order to account for the carpet manufactured during 1971, but sold after that time, all of the "Luxaire" English Olive carpet sold during 1972 to Region C (10,687 square yards) was added to the 1971 sales. Therefore, it was estimated that a total of 16,397 square yards of carpet containing the Wellman 181B fiber and dyed English Olive in color was sold by the West Point Pepperell Corporation to retailers in 10 southeastern States during 1971 and 1972. (In 1979, existing residential carpeted floor space in the United States was estimated at 6.7 billion square yards.)*

3. By assuming that this carpet was installed in one room, averaging 12 feet by 15 feet in size, per house, and also assuming that the total sales of carpet were divided equally among the 10 southeastern States, then approximately 82 rooms with this carpet could be found in the State of Georgia.

4. Information from the Atlanta Regional Commission showed that there were 638,995 occupied housing units in the Atlanta metropolitan area in November 1981. † Using this figure, the chance of randomly selecting an occupied housing unit in metropolitan Atlanta and finding a house with a room having carpet like Williams' carpet was determined to be 1 chance in 7,792—a very low chance.

To the degree that the assumptions used in calculating the above probability number are reasonable, we can be confident in arriving at a valid probability number. . . .

The probability figures illustrate clearly that the Williams' carpet is, in fact, very uncommon. To enhance the figures even further, it is important to emphasize that these figures are based on the assumption that none of the carpet of concern had been discarded during the past 11 years. In fact, carpet of this type, often used in commercial settings, such as apartment houses, would probably have had a normal life span of only 4 or 5 years. . . .††

---

*This information was taken from a study by E.I. du Pont de Nemours & Co. concerned with the existing residential floor space with carpet in the United States. This study was reported in the marketing survey conducted by the Marketing Corporation of America, Westport, Conn.

†Information regarding the number of housing units in the Atlanta metropolitan area was obtained from a report provided by the Atlanta Regional Commission. The report, dated November 11, 1981, contained population and housing counts for counties, super districts, and census tracts in the Atlanta metropolitan area.

††Information about carpet similar to Williams' carpet was developed through contacts with carpet manufacturers and carpet salesmen in Georgia. It was determined that this type carpet was often installed in commercial settings, such as apartments, and in those settings, had an average life span of 4 to 5 years.

The Williams Trial

To any experienced forensic fiber examiner, the fiber evidence linking Williams to the murder victims was overwhelming. But regardless of the apparent validity of the fiber findings, it was during the trial that its true weight would be determined. Unless it could be conveyed meaningfully to a jury, its effect would be lost. Because of this, considerable time was spent determining what should be done to convey the full significance of the fiber evidence. Juries are not usually composed of individuals with a scientific background, and therefore, it was necessary to "educate" the jury in what procedures were followed and the significance of the fiber results. In the Williams case, over 40 charts with over 350 photographs were prepared to illustrate exactly what the crime laboratory examiners had observed. . . .

Representatives of the textile fiber industry, including technical representatives from the Wellman and West Point Pepperell Corporations, were involved in educating the jury regarding textile fibers in general and helped lay the foundation for the conclusions of the forensic fiber examiners. The jury also was told about fiber analysis in the crime laboratory.

The trial, as it developed, can be divided into two parts. Initially, testimony was given concerning the murders of Nathaniel Cater and Jimmy Ray Payne, the two victims included in the indictment drawn against Williams in July 1981. Testimony was then given concerning Williams' association with 10 other murder victims.

The fiber matches made between fibers in Williams' environment and fibers from victims Payne and Cater were discussed. The items from Williams' environment that were linked to either or both of the victims are shown in the center of the chart. (See Fig. 1.) Not only is Payne linked to the Williams' environment by seven items and Cater linked by six items, but both of the victims are linked strongly to each other based on the fiber matches and circumstances surrounding their deaths.

In discussing the significance or strength of an association based on textile fibers, it was emphasized that the more uncommon the fibers, the stronger the association. None of the fiber types from the items in Williams' environment shown in the center of Figure 1 is by definition a "common" fiber type. Several of the fiber types would be termed "uncommon."

One of the fibers linking the body of Jimmy Ray Payne to the carpet in the 1970 station wagon driven by Williams was a small rayon fiber fragment recovered from Payne's shorts. Data were obtained from the station wagon's manufacturer concerning which automobile models produced prior to 1973 contained carpet made of this fiber type. These data were coupled with additional information from Georgia concerning the number of these models registered in the Atlanta metropolitan area during 1981. This allowed a calculation to be made relating to the probability of randomly selecting an automobile having carpet like that in the 1970 Chevrolet station wagon

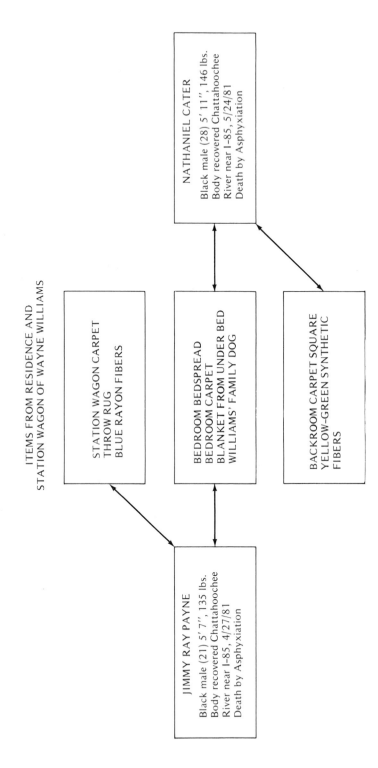

ITEMS FROM RESIDENCE AND
STATION WAGON OF WAYNE WILLIAMS

NATHANIEL CATER
Black male (28) 5′ 11′′, 146 lbs.
Body recovered Chattahoochee
River near I-85, 5/24/81
Death by Asphyxiation

STATION WAGON CARPET
THROW RUG
BLUE RAYON FIBERS

BEDROOM BEDSPREAD
BEDROOM CARPET
BLANKET FROM UNDER BED
WILLIAMS' FAMILY DOG

BACKROOM CARPET SQUARE
YELLOW-GREEN SYNTHETIC
FIBERS

JIMMY RAY PAYNE
Black male (21) 5′ 7′′, 135 lbs.
Body recovered Chattahoochee
River near I-85, 4/27/81
Death by Asphyxiation

Figure 1. Items from residence and station wagon of Wayne Williams.

from the 2,373,512 cars registered in the Atlanta metropolitan area. This probability is 1 chance in 3,828, a very low probability representing a significant association.

Another factor to consider when assessing the significance of fiber evidence is the increased strength of the association when multiple fiber matches become the basis of the association. This is true if different fiber types from more than one object are found and each fiber type either links two people together or links an individual with a particular environment. As the number of different objects increases, the strength of an association increases dramatically. That is, the chance of randomly finding several particular fiber types in a certain location is much smaller than the chance of finding one particular fiber type.

The following example can be used to illustrate the significance of multiple fiber matches linking two items together. If one were to throw a single die one time, the chance or probability of throwing a particular number would be one chance in six. The probability of throwing a second die and getting that same number also would be one chance in six. However, the probability of getting 2 of the same numbers on 2 dice thrown simultaneously is only 1 in every 36 double throws—a much smaller chance than with either of the single throws. This number is a result of the product rule of probability theory. That is, the probability of the joint occurrence of a number of mutually independent events equals the product of the individual probabilities of each of the events (in this example—$\frac{1}{6} \times \frac{1}{6} = \frac{1}{36}$). Since numerous fiber types are in existence, the chance of finding one particular fiber type, other than a common type, in a specific randomly selected location is small. The chance then of finding several fiber types together in a specific location is the product of several small probabilities, resulting in an extremely small chance. . . .

However, no attempt was made to use the product rule and multiply the individual probability numbers together to get an approximation of the probability of finding carpets like Williams' residential carpet and Williams' automobile carpet in the same household. The probability numbers were used only to show that the individual fiber types involved in these associations were very uncommon. . . .*

In addition to the two probability numbers already discussed (bedroom and station wagon carpets), each of the other fiber types linking Williams to both Cater and Payne has a probability of being found in a particular location. The chance of finding all of the fiber types indicated on the chart

---

*Joseph L. Peterson, ed. *Forensic Science* (New York: AMS Press, Inc., 1975), pp. 181-225. This collection of articles, dealing with various aspects of forensic science, contains five papers concerned with using statistics to interpret the meaning of physical evidence. It is a good discussion of probability theory and reviews cases where probability theory has been used in trial situations.

[Fig. 1] in one location (seven types on Payne's body and six types on Cater's body) would be extremely small. Although an actual probability number for those findings could not be determined, it is believed that the multiple fiber associations shown on this chart are proof that Williams is linked to the bodies of these two victims, even though each fiber match by itself does not show a positive association with Williams' environment.

Studies have been conducted in England that show that transferred fibers are usually lost rapidly as people go about their daily routine.* Therefore, the foreign fibers present on a person are most often from recent surroundings. The fibrous debris found on a murder victim reflects the body's more recent surroundings, especially important if the body was moved after the killing. Accordingly, the victims' bodies in this particular case are not only associated with Williams but are apparently associated with Williams shortly before or after their deaths.

It was also pointed out during the trial that the locations of the fibers—on Payne's shorts and in Cater's head hairs and pubic hairs—were not those where one would expect to find fibrous debris transferred from an automobile or a house to victims who had been fully clothed.

Although from these findings it would appear that the victims were in the residence of Williams, there was one other location that contained many of the same fibers as those in the composition of various objects in his residence—Williams' station wagon. The environment of a family automobile might be expected to reflect, to some extent, fibers from objects located within the residence. This was true of the 1970 station wagon. With one exception, all of the fiber types removed from Payne and Cater, consistent with originating from items shown in the center of Figure 1, were present in debris removed by vacuuming the station wagon. The automobile would be the most logical source of the foreign fibers found on both Payne and Cater if they were associated with Williams shortly before or after their deaths. It should also be pointed out that two objects, the bedspread and the blanket, were portable and could have at one time been present inside the station wagon.

Both Payne and Cater were recovered from the Chattahoochee River. Their bodies had been in the water for several days. Some of the fibers found on these victims were like fibers in the compositions of the bedroom carpet and bedspread except for color intensity. They appeared to have been bleached. By subjecting various known fibers to small amounts of Chattahoochee River water for different periods of time, it was found that bleaching did occur. This was especially true with the carpet and bedspread fibers from Williams' bedroom.

---

*C. A. Pounds and K. W. Smalldon, "The Transfer of Fibers between Clothing Materials During Simulated Contacts and Their Persistence During Wear," *Journal of the Forensic Science Society*, vol. 15, 1975, pp. 29-37.

Two crime laboratory examiners testified during the closing stages of the first part of the trial about Williams' association with Payne and Cater. They concluded that it was highly unlikely that any environment other than that present in Wayne Williams' house and car could have resulted in the combination of fibers and hairs found on the victims and that it would be virtually impossible to have matched so many fibers found on Cater and Payne to items in Williams' house and car unless the victims were in contact with or in some way associated with the environment of Wayne Williams.

After testimony was presented concerning the Payne and Cater cases, the Fulton County District Attorney's Office asked the court to be allowed to introduce evidence in the cases of 10 other victims whose murders were similar in many respects. Georgia law allows evidence of another crime to be introduced ". . . if some logical connection can be shown between the two from which it can be said that proof of the one tends to establish the other as relevant to some fact other than general bad character."* There need be no conviction for the other crime in order for details about that crime to be admissible.

It was ruled that evidence concerning other murders could be introduced in an attempt to prove a "pattern or scheme" of killing that included the two murders with which Williams was charged. The additional evidence in these cases was to be used to help the jury ". . . decide whether Williams had committed the two murders with which he is charged."†

There were similarities between these additional victims and Payne and Cater. (See Fig. 2.) Although some differences can also be seen on this chart, the prosecution considered these differences to fit within the "pattern of killing" of which Payne and Cater were a part. The most important similarities between these additional victims were the fiber matches that linked 9 of the 10 victims to Williams' environment. The fiber findings discussed during the trial and used to associate Williams to the 12 victims were illustrated during the trial. (See Fig. 3.)

The 12 victims were listed in chronological order based on the dates their bodies were recovered. The time period covered by this chart, approximately 22 months, is from July 1979, until May 1981. During that time period, the Williams family had access to a large number of automobiles, including a number of rental cars. Three of these automobiles are listed at the top of Figure 3. If one or more of the cars was in the possession of the Williams family at the time a victim was found to be missing, the space under that car(s) and after the particular victim's name is shaded.

Four objects (including the dog) from Williams' residence are listed horizontally across the top of Figure 3, along with objects from three of his

---

Encyclopedia of Georgia Law, vol. 11A (The Harrison Company, 1979), p. 70.

†*The Atlanta Constitution*, "Williams Jury Told of Other Slayings," Sec. 1-A, 1/26/82, p. 25.

VICTIM'S NAME	DATE VICTIM MISSING	DAYS MISSING	BODY RECOVERY AREA	CAUSE OF DEATH	AGE	WEIGHT	HEIGHT
EVANS	7/25/79	3	WOODED AREA S.W. ATLANTA	PROBABLE ASPHYXIATION/ STRANGULATION	13	87 LBS.	5'4"
MIDDLEBROOKS	5/18/80	1	NEAR STREET S.E. ATLANTA	BLUNT TRAUMA TO HEAD	14	88 LBS.	4'10"
STEPHENS	10/9/80	1	NEAR STREET S.E. ATLANTA	ASPHYXIATION	10	120 LBS.	5'0"
GETER	1/3/81	33	WOODED AREA FULTON COUNTY	MANUAL STRANGULATION	14	130 LBS.	5'4"
PUE	1/22/81	1	NEAR HIGHWAY ROCKDALE CO.	LIGATURE STRANGULATION	15	105 LBS.	5'5"
BALTAZAR	2/6/81	7	NEAR HIGHWAY DEKALB CO.	LIGATURE STRANGULATION	12	125 LBS.	5'4"
BELL	3/2/81	31	SOUTH RIVER DEKALB CO.	ASPHYXIATION	16	100 LBS.	5'2"
ROGERS	3/30/81	10	NEAR STREET N.W. ATLANTA	ASPHYXIATION/ STRANGULATION	20	110 LBS.	5'3"
PORTER	4/10/81	1	NEAR STREET IN S.W. ATLANTA	ASPHYXIATION	28	123 LBS.	5'7"
PAYNE	4/22/81	5	CHATTAHOOCHEE RIVER FULTON COUNTY	ASPHYXIATION	21	135 LBS.	5'7"
BARRETT	5/11/81	1	NEAR STREET DEKALB CO.	LIGATURE STRANGULATION (3 PUNCTURE WOUNDS)	17	125 LBS.	5'4"
CATER	5/21/81	3	CHATTAHOOCHEE RIVER FULTON COUNTY	ASPHYXIATION/ STRANGULATION	28	146 LBS.	5'11"

Figure 2. Chart used during the trial to show similarities between Payne and Cater and ten other murder victims.

NAME OF VICTIM	VIOLET-GREEN BEDSPREAD WILLIAMS' BEDROOM	GREEN CARPET WILLIAMS' BEDROOM	YELLOW BLANKET WILLIAMS' BEDROOM	DOG HAIRS WILLIAMS' DOG	BLUE RAYON FIBERS DEBRIS FROM WILLIAMS' HOME	TRUNK LINER 1978 PLYMOUTH	CARPET 1979 FORD	CARPET 1970 CHEVROLET	ADDITIONAL ITEMS FROM WILLIAMS' HOME, AUTOMOBILES OR PERSON
Alfred Evans	X	X				X			
Eric Middlebrooks	X	X					X		YELLOW NYLON FORD TRUNK LINER
Charles Stephens	X	X	X		X				YELLOW NYLON WHITE POLYESTER BACKROOM CARPET FORD TRUNK LINER
Lubie Geter	X	X						X	KITCHEN CARPET
Terry Pue	X	X							WHITE POLYESTER BACKROOM CARPET
Patrick Balazar	X	X		X				X	YELLOW NYLON WHITE POLYESTER HEAD HAIR GLOVE JACKET PIGMENTED POLYPROPYLENE BACKROOM CARPET
Joseph Bell	X	X			X				
Larry Rogers	X	X		X				X	YELLOW NYLON PORCH BEDSPREAD
John Porter	X	X		X	X			X	PORCH BEDSPREAD
Jimmy Payne	X	X		X	X			X	BLUE THROW RUG
William Barrett	X	X		X	X			X	GLOVE
Nathaniel Cater	X	X		X					BACKROOM CARPET YELLOW-GREEN SYNTHETIC

Figure 3. Fiber findings discussed during the trial and used to associate Williams to the twelve victims.

automobiles. An "X" on the chart indicates an apparent transfer of textile fibers from the listed object to a victim. Other objects from Williams' environment which were linked to various victims by an apparent fiber transfer are listed on the right side of the chart. Fiber types from objects (never actually located) that were matched to fiber types from one or more victims are also listed either at the top or on the right side of the chart. Fourteen specific objects and five fiber types (probably from five other objects) listed on this chart are linked to one or more of the victims. More than 28 different fiber types, along with the dog hairs, were used to link up to 19 objects from Williams' environment to 1 or more of the victims. Of the more than 28 fiber types from Williams' environment, 14 of these originated from a rug or carpet.

The combination of more than 28 different fiber types would not be considered so significant if they were primarily common fiber types. In fact, there is only 1 light green cotton fiber of the 28 that might be considered common. This cotton fiber was blended with acetate fibers in Williams' bedspread. Light green cotton fibers removed from many victims were not considered or compared unless they were physically intermingled with violet acetate fibers which were consistent with originating from the bedspread. It should be noted that a combination of cotton and acetate fibers blended together in a single textile material, as in the bedspread, is in itself uncommon. . . .

The previous discussion concerning the significance of multiple fiber matches can be applied to the associations made in the cases of all the victims except Bell, but especially to the association of Patrick Baltazar to William's environment. Fibers and animal hairs consistent with having originated from 10 sources were removed from Baltazar's body. These 10 sources include the uncommon bedroom carpet and station wagon carpet. In addition to the fiber (and animal hair) linkage, two head hairs of Negroid origin were removed from Baltazar's body that were consistent with originating from the scalp area of Williams. Head hair matches were also very significant in linking Williams to Baltazar's body. In the opinion of author, the association based upon the hair and fiber analyses is a positive association.

Another important aspect of the fiber linkage between Williams and these victims is the correspondence between the fiber findings and the time periods during which Williams had access to the three automobiles listed on the chart. Nine victims are linked to automobiles used by the Williams family. When Williams did not have access to a particular car, no fibers were recovered that were consistent with having originated from that automobile. Trunk liner fibers of the type used in the trunks of many late model Ford Motor Company automobiles were also recovered from the bodies of two victims.

One final point should be made concerning Williams' bedroom and station wagon carpets where probability numbers had been determined. Fibers consistent with having originated from both of these "unusual" carpets were recovered from Payne's body. Of the nine victims who were killed during the time period when Williams had access to the 1970 station wagon, fibers consistent with having originated from both the station wagon carpet and the bedroom carpet were recovered from six of these victims.

The apparent bleaching of several fibers removed from the bodies of Payne and Cater was consistent with having been caused by river water. Several fibers similar to those from Payne and Cater were removed from many of the victims whose bodies were recovered on land. Consistent with the bleaching argument, none of the fibers from the victims found on land showed any apparent bleaching. The finding of many of the same fiber types on the remaining victims, who were recovered from many different locations, refutes the possibility that Payne's and Cater's bodies picked up foreign fibers from the river.

The fact that many of the victims were involved with so many of the same fiber types, all of which linked the victims to Williams' environment, is the basis for arguing conclusively against these fibers originating from a source other than Williams' environment.

It is hoped that this article has provided valuable insight concerning the use of fiber evidence in a criminal trial, has provided answers to questions from those in the law enforcement community about textile fiber evidence in general, and has presented convincing arguments to establish Wayne Williams' association with the bodies of the murder victims.

4

Physical Properties: Glass and Soil

The forensic scientist must constantly determine those properties that impart distinguishing characteristics to matter, giving it a unique identity. The search for distinctive properties is a continuing one and ends only when the scientist has completely individualized a substance to one correct source. Properties are the identifying characteristics of substances. In this and succeeding chapters we will examine properties that are most useful for characterizing soil, glass, and other physical evidence. However, before we begin this task, our understanding of the nature of properties can be made easier by classifying them into two broad categories: physical and chemical.

Physical properties describe a substance without reference to any other substance. For example, weight, volume, color, boiling point, and melting point are typical physical properties that can be measured for a particular substance without reference to other materials; they are associated only with the physical existence of that substance. **A chemical property describes the behavior of a substance when it reacts or combines with another substance.** For example, when wood burns, it chemically combines with oxygen in the air to form new substances; this transformation describes a chemical property of wood. In the crime laboratory a routine procedure for determining the presence of heroin in a suspect specimen is to react it with a chemical reagent known as the Marquis reagent. In the presence of heroin, the Marquis reagent turns purple. This color transformation thus becomes a chemical property of heroin and provides a convenient test for its identification.

Which physical and chemical properties the forensic scientist ultimately chooses to observe and measure will depend on the type of material that is being examined. Logic requires, however, that if the property can be assigned a numerical value, it must be one that relates to a standard system of measurement accepted throughout the scientific community.

THE METRIC SYSTEM

Although scientists throughout the world have been using the metric system of measurement for more than a century, the United States still uses the cumbersome "English System" to express length in inches, or feet, or yards; weight in ounces or pounds; and volume in pints or quarts. The inherent difficulty of this system is that no simple numerical relationship exists between the various units of measurement. For example, to convert inches to feet one must know that 1 foot is equal to 12 inches; the conversion of ounces to pounds requires the knowledge that 16 ounces is equivalent to 1 pound. In 1791, the French Academy of Science devised the simple system of measurement known as the metric system. This system uses a simple decimal relationship so that a unit of length, volume, or mass can be converted into a subunit by simply multiplying or dividing by a multiple of ten—e.g., 10, 100, or 1000.

Even though the United States has not yet adopted the metric system, its system of currency is decimal and hence analogous to the metric system. The basic unit of currency is the dollar, a dollar is divided into ten equal units called dimes, and each dime is further divided into ten equal units of cents.

The metric system has basic units of measurement for length, mass, and volume; they are the meter, gram, and liter, respectively. These three basic units can be converted into subunits that are decimal multiples of the basic unit by simply attaching a prefix to the unit name. The following are common prefixes and their equivalent decimal value:

Prefix	Equivalent Value
deci	1/10 or 0.1
centi	1/100 or 0.01
milli	1/1000 or 0.001
micro	1/1,000,000 or 0.000001
nano	1/1,000,000,000 or 0.000000001
kilo	1000
mega	1,000,000

Hence, 1/10 or 0.1 of a gram is the same as a decigram (dg), 1/100 or 0.01 of a meter is equal to a centimeter (cm), and 1/1000 of a liter is a milliliter (ml). A metric conversion is simply carried out by moving the decimal point to the right or left and inserting the proper prefix to show the direction and number of places that the decimal point has been moved. For example, if the weight of a powder is 0.0165 gram, it may be more convenient to multiply this value by 100 and express it as 1.65 centigrams or by 1000 to show it as its equivalent value of 16.5 milligrams. Similarly, an object that weighs 264,450 grams may be expressed as 264.450 kilograms simply by dividing it by 1000. It is important to remember that in any of these conversions, the value of the measurement has not changed; 0.0165 gram is still equivalent to 1.65 centigrams, just as one dollar is still equal to 100 cents. We have simply adjusted the position of the decimal and shown the extent of the adjustment with a prefix.

One interesting aspect of the metric system is that volume can be defined in terms of length. A liter by definition is the volume of a cube, each side having a length of 10 centimeters. One liter is therefore equivalent to a volume of 10 cm × 10 cm × 10 cm, or 1000 cubic centimeters (cc). Thus, one-thousandth of a liter or one milliliter (ml) is equal to one cubic centimeter (cc). It is common for scientists to use the subunits ml and cc interchangeably to express volume.

At times, it may be necessary to convert units from the metric system into the English system, or vice versa (see Figure 4-1). In order to accomplish this, we must consult references that list English units and their metric equivalents. Some of the more useful equivalents are shown below:

1 inch   = 2.54 centimeters
1 meter   = 39.37 inches
1 pound   = 453.6 grams
1 liter   = 1.06 quarts
1 kilogram = 2.2 pounds

The general mathematical procedures for converting from one system to another can be illustrated by the conversion of 12 inches into centimeters. To change inches into centimeters we need to know that there are 2.54 centimeters per inch. Hence, if we multiply 12 inches by 2.54 centimeter/inch (12 in. × 2.54 cm/in.), the unit of inches will cancel out, leaving the product 30.48 cm. Similarly, applying the conversion of grams to pounds, 227 grams is equivalent to 227 gm × 1 lb/453.6 gm or 0.5 lb.

Figure 4-1. Comparison of the metric and English systems of length measurement; 2.54 centimeters = 1 inch.

PHYSICAL PROPERTIES

TEMPERATURE

The determination of the physical properties of any material will often require the measurement of temperature. For instance, the temperatures at which a substance melts or boils are readily determinable characteristics that will help identify a substance. Temperature is a measure of heat intensity, or the hotness or coldness of a substance. Temperature is usually measured by causing a thermometer to come into contact with a substance. The familiar mercury-in-glass thermometer functions because mercury expands more than glass when heated and contracts more than glass when cooled. Thus, the length of the mercury column in the glass tube provides a measure of the surrounding environment's temperature. The construction of a temperature scale requires two reference points and a choice of units. The reference points most conveniently chosen are the freezing point and boiling point of water. The two most common temperature scales used are the Fahrenheit and Celsius (formerly called centigrade) scales.

The Fahrenheit scale is based on the assignment of the value 32°F to the freezing point of water and 212°F to its boiling point. The difference between the two points is evenly divided into 180 units. Thus, a degree Fahrenheit is 1/180th of the temperature change between the freezing point and boiling point of water. The Celsius scale is derived by assigning the freezing point of water a value of 0°C and its boiling point a value of 100°C. A degree Celsius is thus 1/100th of the temperature change between the two reference points. Scientists in most countries use the Celsius scale to measure temperature. A comparison of the two scales is shown in Figure 4-2.

WEIGHT AND MASS

The force with which gravity attracts a body is called *weight*. If your weight is 180 lb, this means that earth's gravity is pulling you down with a force of 180 lb; on the moon, where the force of gravity is one-sixth that of earth, your weight would be 30 lb.

Mass differs from weight because it refers to the amount of matter an object contains, and is independent of its location on earth or any other place in the universe. The mathematical relationship between weight (w), and mass (m) is shown in Equation (4-1), where g is the acceleration imparted to a body by the force of gravity.

$$W = mg \qquad (4\text{-}1)$$

The weight of a body is seen to be directly proportional to its mass; hence, a large mass weighs more than a small mass.

In the metric system it is always the mass of an object rather than its weight that is specified. The basic unit of mass is the gram. An object that has a mass of 40 grams on earth will have a mass of 40 grams anywhere else in this universe. Normally however, the terms *mass* and *weight* are used inter-

Figure 4-2. Comparison of Celsius and Fahrenheit temperature scales.

changeably, and we often speak of the weight of an object when we really mean its mass.

The mass of an object is determined by comparing it against the known mass of standard objects. This comparison is confusingly called *weighing*, and the standard objects are called *weights* (*masses* would be a more correct term). The comparison is performed on a balance. The simplest type of balance for weighing is the equal-arm balance shown in Figure 4-3. The object to be weighed is placed on the left pan and the standard weights are placed on the right pan; when the pointer between the two pans is at the center mark, the total mass on the right pan is equal to the mass of the object on the left pan.

The modern laboratory has progressed beyond the simple equal-arm balance, and either the top-loading balance or the single-pan analytical balance [Figure 4-4 (a) and (b)] is now likely to be used. The choice depends

Figure 4-3. The measurement of mass.

(a)

(b)

Figure 4-4. (a) Top-loading balance. (b) Single-pan analytical balance. Both *courtesy* Mettler Instrument Corp., New Jersey.

on the accuracy required and the amount of material being weighed. Each works on the same counterbalancing principle as the simple equal-arm balance, but the second pan, the one on which the standard weights are placed, is hidden from view within the balance's housing. Once the object whose weight is to be determined is placed on the visible pan, the operator selects the proper standard weights (also contained with the housing) by manually turning a set of knobs located on the front side of the balance. At the point of balance, the weights selected are automatically recorded on digital and optical readout scales. The top-loading balance can accurately weigh an object to the nearest one milligram or 0.001 gram; the analytical balance is even more accurate, weighing to the nearest tenth of a milligram or 0.0001 gram.

DENSITY

A most important physical property of matter with respect to the analysis of certain kinds of physical evidence is density. Density is defined as mass per unit volume, Equation (4-2).

$$\text{Density} = \frac{\text{mass}}{\text{volume}} \qquad (4\text{-}2)$$

Density is an intensive property of matter—that is, it is the same regardless of the size of a substance; thus, it is a characteristic property of a substance and can be used as an aid in identification. Solids tend to be more dense than liquids, and liquids more dense than gases. The densities of some common substances are shown in Table 4-1.

A simple procedure for determining the density of a solid is illustrated in Figure 4-5. First, the solid is weighed on a balance against known standard gram weights, and its mass is determined. The solid's volume is then determined from the volume of water it displaces. This is easily measured by filling a cylinder with a known volume of water (V_1), adding the object, and measuring the new water level (V_2). The difference $V_2 - V_1$ in ml is equal to the volume of the solid. Density can now be calculated from Equation (4-2) in grams per milliliter.

The volumes of gases and liquids vary considerably with temperature; hence, when determining density, it is important to control and record the temperature at which the measurements are made. For example, one gram of water occupies a volume of one milliliter at $4°C$ and thus has a density of 1.0 g/ml. However, as the temperature of water increases, its volume will expand. Therefore, at $20°C$ (room temperature) one gram of water will occupy a volume of 1.002 ml and will have a density of 0.998 g/ml.

The observation that a solid object will either sink, float, or remain suspended when immersed in a liquid is one that can be accounted for by the

Table 4-1.

DENSITIES OF SELECTED MATERIALS
(AT 20°C UNLESS OTHERWISE STATED)

Substance	Density (g/ml)
Solids	
Silver	10.5
Lead	11.5
Iron	7.8
Aluminum	2.7
Window Glass	2.47–2.54
Ice (0°C)	0.92
Liquids	
Mercury	13.6
Benzene	0.88
Ethyl Alcohol	0.79
Gasoline	0.69
Water at 4°C	1.00
Water at 20°C	0.998
Gases	
Air (0°C)	0.0013
Chlorine (0°C)	0.0032
Oxygen (0°C)	0.0014
Carbon Dioxide (0°C)	0.0020

Mass

Volume

Figure 4-5. A simple procedure for determining the density of a solid is to first weigh it and then measure its volume by noting the volume of water it displaces.

property of density. For instance, if the density of a solid is greater than the liquid medium in which it is immersed, the object will sink; if the solid has a density that is less than the liquid, it will float; and when the solid and liquid both have equal densities, the solid will remain suspended in the liquid medium. As we will shortly see, these observations provide the criminalist with a convenient technique for comparing the densities of solid objects.

REFRACTIVE INDEX

Light, as we will learn in the next chapter, can have the property of a wave. Lightwaves travel in air at a constant velocity of nearly 300,000,000 meters per second until they penetrate another medium, such as glass or water, at which point they are suddenly slowed, causing the rays to bend. The bending of a lightwave because of a change in velocity is called **refraction**.

The phenomenon of refraction is apparent when we view an object that is immersed in a transparent medium; because we are accustomed to thinking that light travels in a straight line, we often forget to take refraction into account. For instance, suppose a ball is observed at the bottom of a pool of water, the light rays reflected from the ball will travel through the water and into the air to reach the eye. As the rays leave the water and enter the air, their velocity suddenly increases, causing them to be refracted. However, because of our assumption that light travels in a straight line, our eyes deceive us and make us think we see an object lying at a higher point than is actually the case. This phenomenon is illustrated in Figure 4-6.

The ratio of the velocity of light in a vacuum to that in any medium determines the refractive index of that medium and is expressed as:

$$\text{Refractive index} = \frac{\text{velocity of light in vacuum}}{\text{velocity of light in medium}} \qquad (4\text{-}3)$$

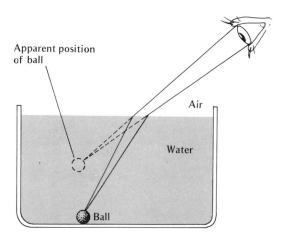

Apparent position of ball

Air

Water

Ball

Figure 4-6. Light is refracted when it travels obliquely from one medium to another.

For example, at 25°C the refractive index of water is 1.333. This means that light travels 1.333 times faster in a vacuum than it does in water at this temperature.

Like density, refractive index is an intensive physical property of matter and will serve to characterize a substance. However, any procedure used to determine a substance's refractive index must be performed under carefully controlled temperature and lighting conditions because the refractive index of a substance varies with its temperature and the frequency wavelength of light passing through it. Nearly all tabulated refractive indices are determined at a standard wavelength, usually 589.3 nonometers; this is the predominant wavelength emitted by sodium light and is commonly known as the sodium D light.

When a transparent solid is immersed in a liquid having a similar refractive index, light will not be refracted as it passes from the liquid into the solid. For this reason, the eye will not be able to distinguish the liquid-solid boundary, and the solid seems to disappear from view. This observation, as we will see, offers the forensic scientist a rather simple method for comparing the refractive indices of transparent solids.

Normally, a solid or a liquid would be expected to exhibit only one refractive index value for each frequency of light; however, many solids that are crystalline in nature will have two refractive indices whose values in part depend on the direction in which the light enters the crystal with respect to the crystal axis. Solids that are crystalline have definite geometric forms because of the orderly arrangement of the fundamental particle of a solid, the atom. In any type of crystal the relative location and distance between its atoms are repetitive throughout the solid. Figure 4-7 shows the crystalline structure of sodium chloride, or ordinary table salt. Sodium chloride is an example of a cubic crystal in which each sodium atom is surrounded by six chloride atoms and each chloride atom by six sodium atoms, except at the

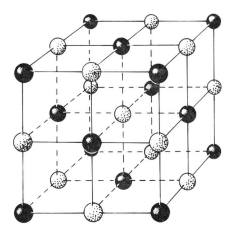

Figure 4-7. Diagram of sodium chloride crystal. Sodium is represented by the black spheres, chlorine by the white spheres.

crystal surface. Not all solids are crystalline in nature; some such as glass have their atoms arranged randomly throughout the solid; these materials are known as **amorphous solids**.

Most crystals, excluding those that have cubic configurations, will refract a beam of light into two different light-ray components. This phenomenon is known as **double refraction** and can be illustrated by studying the behavior of the crystal calcite. When the calcite is laid on a printed page, the observer sees not one but two images of each word covered. The two light rays that give rise to the double image are refracted at different angles, and each has a different refractive index value. The indices of refraction for calcite are 1.486 and 1.658, and subtracting the two values yields a difference of 0.172; this difference is known as **birefringence**. Thus, the optical properties of crystals provide points of identification that will help characterize a crystal.

Many of us have at one time or another had the experience of holding a glass prism up toward the sunlight and watching it transform light into the colors of the rainbow. This observation serves to demonstrate that visible "white light" is not homogeneous but is actually composed of many different component colors. The process of separating light into component colors is called **dispersion**. The ability of a prism to disperse light into its component colors is explained by the property of refraction. Each color component of light, on passing through the glass, will be slowed to a speed slightly different from the others, thus causing each component to bend at a different angle as it emerges from the prism. As shown in Figure 4-8, the component colors of visible light extend from red to violet. We will learn in Chapter 5 that each color actually corresponds to a different range of frequencies or wavelengths of light. Dispersion thus separates light into its component frequencies and demonstrates that glass has a slightly different index of refraction for each frequency of light passing through it.

Now that we have investigated various physical properties of objects, we are ready to apply such properties to the characterization of two substances—glass and soil—that commonly must be examined by the criminalist.

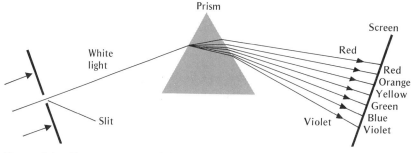

Figure 4-8.   Representation of the dispersion of light by a glass prism.

COMPARING GLASS FRAGMENTS

Glass that is broken and shattered into fragments and minute particles during the commission of a crime can be used to place a suspect at the crime scene. For example, chips of broken glass from a window may be lodged in a suspect's shoes or garments during the act of a burglary, or particles of headlight glass found at the scene of a hit-and-run accident may offer clues that can confirm the identity of a suspect vehicle. All of these possibilities require the comparison of glass fragments found on the suspect, whether a person or vehicle, with the shattered glass remaining at the crime scene.

Glass is a hard, brittle amorphous substance that is composed of silicon oxides mixed with various metal oxides. When sand is mixed with other metal oxides, melted at high temperatures, and then cooled to a rigid condition without crystallization, the product is glass. The main ingredient in ordinary glass is sand. By adding soda (Na_2CO_3) to the sand, its melting point and viscosity are both lowered, making it much easier to work. Lime (CaO) is added to the sand and soda mixture so that the "soda-lime" glass will not dissolve in water. The forensic scientist is often requested to analyze soda-lime glass, which is used for manufacturing most window and bottle glass. The common metal oxides found in this type of glass are sodium, calcium, magnesium, and aluminum. In addition, a wide variety of special glasses can be made by substituting in whole or in part other metal oxides for the silica, sodium, and calcium oxides. For example, automobile headlights and heat-resistant glass, such as Pyrex, are manufactured by adding boron oxide to the oxide mix. These glasses are therefore known as **borosilicates**.

Another type of glass that the reader may be familiar with is tempered glass. This glass is made stronger than ordinary window glass by introducing stress through rapid heating and cooling of the glass surfaces. When tempered glass breaks, it does not shatter but rather fragments or "dices" into small squares with little splintering. Because of this safety feature, tempered glass is used in the side and rear windows of automobiles made in the United States, as well as in the windshields of some foreign-made cars. The windshields of all cars manufactured in the United States are constructed from laminated glass. This glass derives its strength by sandwiching one layer of plastic between two pieces of ordinary window glass.

For the forensic scientist the problem of glass comparison is one that depends on the need to find and measure those properties that will associate one glass fragment to another while minimizing or eliminating the possible existence of other sources. Needless to say, considering the prevalency of glass in our society, it is easy to develop an appreciation for the magnitude of this analytical problem. Obviously, glass will possess its greatest evidential value when it can be individualized to one source. Such a determination, however, can only be made when the suspect and crime-scene fragments are assembled and physically fitted together. Comparisons of this type will require piecing together irregular edges of broken glass as well as the matching of all irregularities and striations on the broken surfaces (see Figure 4-9). The possibility that two pieces of glass originating from different sources will fit exactly together is so unlikely as to exclude all other sources from practical consideration.

Unfortunately, the majority of glass evidence presented to the criminalist is either too fragmentary or too minute to permit a comparison of this type. In such instances, the search for individual properties has proven to be a fruitless one. For example, the general chemical composition of various window glasses within the capability of current analytical methods has so far been found to be relatively uniform among various manufacturers and thus offers no basis for individualization. However, as more sensitive analytical techniques are developed, trace elements present in glass may eventually prove to be distinctive and measurable characteristics.

At this time, the physical properties of density and refractive index are used most successfully for characterizing glass particles. However, these properties are class characteristics and as such will not provide the sole criteria for individualizing glass to a common source. They do, however, give the analyst sufficient data to evaluate the significance of a glass comparison, and the absence of comparable density and refractive index values will certainly serve to exclude glass fragments that originate from different sources.

It was previously indicated that a solid particle will either float, sink, or

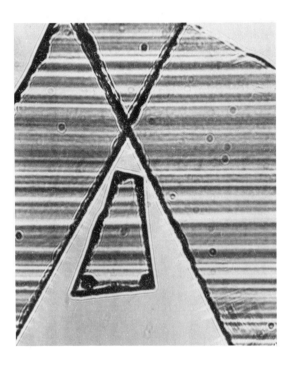

Figure 4-9. Match of broken glass. Note that in addition to the physical fit of the edges, glass ream patterns are used to establish a relationship between the fragments. The normally invisible reams are visualized by focusing a point of light source on the glass so that it casts a shadow of the sample on photographic film. *Courtesy* Centre of Forensic Sciences, Toronto, Canada.

remain suspended in a liquid depending on its density relative to the liquid medium. This knowledge gives the criminalist a rather precise and rapid method for comparing densities of glass. In a method known as flotation, a control glass particle is immersed in a liquid; a mixture of bromoform and bromobenzene may be used. The composition of the liquid is carefully adjusted by the addition of small amounts of bromoform or bromobenzene until the glass chip remains suspended in the liquid medium. At this point, the control glass and liquid each have the same density. Glass chips of approximately the same size and shape as the control are now added to the liquid for comparison. If both the unknown and the control particles remain suspended in the liquid, their densities are equal to each other and to that of the liquid.[1] Particles of different densities will either sink or float, depending on whether they are more or less dense than the liquid.

It is interesting to note that the density of a single sheet of window glass is not completely homogeneous throughout. It has a range of values that can differ by as much as 0.0003 g/ml. Therefore, in order to distinguish between the normal internal density variations of a single sheet of glass and those of glasses of different origins, it is advisable to let the comparative density approach but not exceed a sensitivity value of 0.0003 g/ml. The flotation method meets this requirement and can adequately distinguish glass particles that differ in density by 0.001 g/ml.

Once glass has been distinguished by a density determination, different origins are immediately concluded. Comparable density results, however, require the added comparison of refractive indices. This determination is best accomplished by an immersion method. For this, glass particles are immersed in a liquid medium whose refractive index is varied until it is equal to that of the glass particles. At this point, known as the match point, the observer will note the disappearance of the Becke line and minimum contrast between the glass and liquid medium. The Becke line is a bright halo that is observed near the border of a particle that is immersed in a liquid of a different refractive index. This halo disappears when the medium and fragment have similar refractive indices.

The refractive index of an immersion fluid is best varied by adjusting the temperature of the liquid. Temperature control is of course critical to the success of the procedure and is accomplished by heating the liquid in a special apparatus known as a hot stage. The glass is immersed in a high boiling liquid, usually a silicone oil, and heated at the rate of 0.2°C per minute until the match point is reached. Increasing the temperature of the liquid

---

[1] As an added step, the analyst can determine the exact numerical density value of the particles of glass by transferring the liquid to a density meter. This instrument will electrically measure and calculate the liquid's density. See A. P. Beveridge and C. Semen, "Glass Density Measurement Using a Calculating Digital Density Meter," *The Canadian Society of Forensic Science Journal*, 12 (1979), 113.

has a negligible effect on the refractive index of glass, while the liquid's index decreases at the rate of approximately 0.0004 per degree Celsius. The hot stage, as shown in Figure 4-10, is designed to be used in conjunction with a microscope, through which the examiner can observe the disappearance of the Becke line on minute glass particles that are illuminated with sodium D light or at other wavelengths of light. If all the glass fragments examined have similar match points, it can be concluded that they have comparable refractive indices (see Figure 4-11). Furthermore, the examiner can determine the refractive index value of the immersion fluid as it changes with temperature. With this information the exact numerical value of the glass refractive index can be calculated at the match point temperature.

As with density, glass fragments removed from a single sheet of plate glass may not have a uniform refractive index value; instead, their values may vary by as much as 0.0002. Hence, for comparison purposes, the difference in refractive index between a control and questioned glass must exceed this value. This allows the examiner to differentiate between the normal internal variations present in a sheet of glass and those present in glasses that originate from completely different sources.

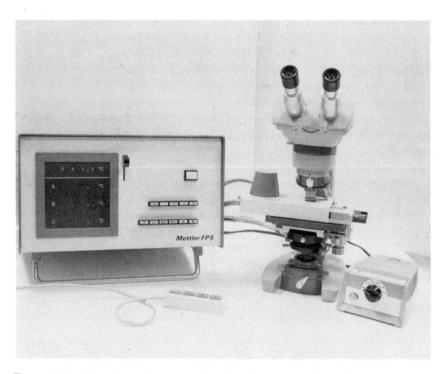

Figure 4-10.   Hot-stage microscope. *Courtesy* New Jersey State Police.

(c)   (d)

Figure 4-11. Determination of the refractive index of glass. **(a)** Glass particles are immersed in a liquid of a much higher refractive index at a temperature of 77°C. **(b)** At 87°C the liquid still has a higher refractive index than the glass. **(c)** The refractive index of the liquid is closest to that of the glass at 97°C as shown by the disappearance of the glass and the Becke lines. **(d)** At the higher temperature of 117°C, the liquid has a much lower index than the glass, and the glass is plainly visible. *Courtesy* Walter C. McCrone.

A significant difference in either density or refractive index proves that the glasses examined do not have a common origin. But what if two pieces of glass exhibit comparable densities and comparable refractive indices? How certain can one be that they did indeed come from the same source? After all, there are untold millions of windows and other glass objects in this world. In order to provide a reasonable answer to this question, the FBI Laboratory has set about to collect density and refractive indices values from glass submitted to it for examination. What has emerged is a data bank correlating these values to their frequency of occurrence in the glass population of the United States. This collection is available to all forensic laboratories in the United States. Likewise, in England, the Central Research Establishment is continually updating a refractive index data bank for glass specimens received by that country's forensic laboratories.

What this means is that once a criminalist has completed a comparison of glass fragments, he or she can correlate their density and refractive index values to their frequency of occurrence and can make a meaningful assessment as to the probability the fragments were at one time from the same source. Figure 4-12 shows the distribution of refractive index values (measured with sodium D light) for nearly 1200 glasses analyzed by the FBI. The wide distribution of values clearly demonstrates that the refractive index is a highly distinctive property of glass and is thus useful for defining its frequency of occurrence and hence its evidential value. For example, a glass fragment having a refractive index value of 1.5290 is found in only 1 out of 1200 specimens, while glass with a value of 1.5180 occurs in 22 glasses out of 1200.

GLASS FRACTURES

Glass bends in response to any force that is exerted on any one of its surfaces; when the limit of its elasticity is reached, the glass fractures. Frequently, fractured window glass will reveal information that can be related to the force and direction of an impact; such knowledge may be useful for reconstructing events at a crime-scene investigation.

The penetration of ordinary window glass by a projectile, whether it is a bullet or stone, produces a familiar fracture pattern in which cracks both radiate outward and encircle the hole, as shown in Figure 4-13. The radiating lines are appropriately known as **radial fractures**, and the circular lines are termed **concentric fractures**.

Often it is difficult to determine just from the size and shape of a hole in glass whether it was made by a bullet or by some other projectile. For instance, a small stone thrown at a comparatively high speed against a pane of glass will often produce a hole very similar to that of a bullet. On the other hand, a large stone can completely shatter a pane of glass in a manner

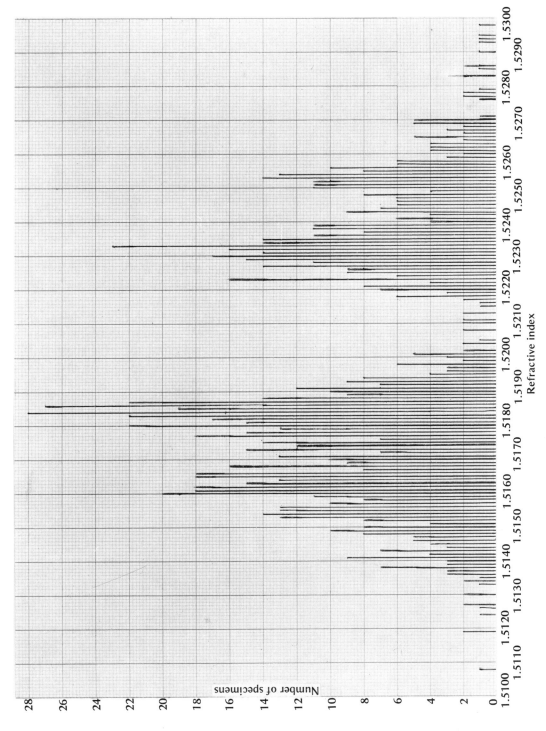

Figure 4-12. Frequency of occurrence of refractive index values (measured with sodium D light) for approximately 1200 flat glass specimens received by the F.B.I. Laboratory. *Courtesy* F.B.I. Laboratory, Washington, D.C.

Figure 4-13. Radial and concentric fracture lines in a sheet of glass. *Courtesy* New Jersey State Police.

closely resembling the result of a close-range shot. However, in the latter instance, the presence of gunpowder deposits on the shattered glass fragments does point to damage caused by a firearm.

When it penetrates glass, a high-velocity projectile such as a bullet often leaves a round crater-shaped hole that is surrounded by a nearly symmetrical pattern of radial and concentric cracks. The hole is inevitably wider at the exit side (Figure 4-14), and hence its examination is an important factor in determining the direction of impact. However, as the velocity of the penetrating projectile decreases, the irregularity of the shape of the hole and of its surrounding cracks increases, so that at some point the hole shape will provide no assistance for determining the direction of impact. At this time information derived from an examination of the radial and concentric fracture lines may prove a useful alternative for determining the direction of impact.

Figure 4-14. Crater-shaped hole made by a pellet passing through glass. The upper surface is the exit side of the projectile. *Courtesy* New Jersey State Police.

When a force pushes on one side of a pane of glass, the elasticity of the glass permits it to bend in the direction of the force applied. Once the elastic limit is exceeded, the glass begins to crack. As shown in Figure 4-15, the first fractures form on the surface opposite that of the penetrating force, and these fractures develop into radial lines. The continued motion of the force places tension on the front surface of the glass, resulting in the formation of concentric cracks. An examination of the edges of the radial and concentric cracks frequently reveals stress markings whose shape can be related to the side on which the window first cracked.

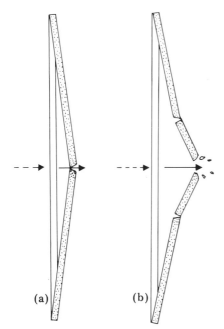

(a)   (b)

Figure 4-15. Diagram showing the production of radial and concentric fractures in glass. (a) Radial cracks are formed first, commencing on the side of the glass opposite to the destructive force. (b) Concentric cracks occur afterwards, starting on the same side as the force.

Stress marks, shown in Figure 4-16, are shaped like arches that are perpendicular to one glass surface and curved nearly parallel to the opposite surface. The importance of stress marks stems from the observation that the perpendicular edge always faces the surface on which the crack originated. Thus, in examining the stress marks on the edge of a radial crack near the point of impact, the perpendicular end is always found to be located opposite the side from which the force of impact was applied. For a concentric fracture the perpendicular end always faces the surface on which the force originated. A convenient way for remembering these observations is the 3R rule—*R*adial cracks form *R*ight angle on the *R*everse side of the force. These facts will enable the examiner to determine readily the side on which a window was broken. Unfortunately, the absence of radial or concentric fracture

Figure 4-16. Stress marks on the edge of a radial glass fracture. Arrow indicates direction of force. *Courtesy* New Jersey State Police.

lines prevents the above observations from being applied to broken tempered glass.

When there have been successive penetrations of glass, it is frequently possible to determine the sequence of impact by observing the existing fracture lines and their points of termination. **A fracture always terminates at an existing line of fracture.** In Figure 4-17, the fracture on the left preceded that on the right; we know this because the latter's radial fracture lines terminate at the cracks of the former.

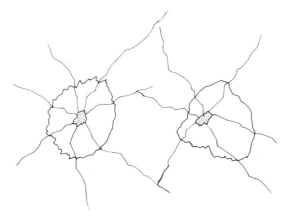

Figure 4-17. Two bullet holes in a piece of glass. The left hole preceded the right hole.

COLLECTION AND PRESERVATION OF GLASS EVIDENCE

The gathering of glass evidence at the crime scene and from the suspect must be thorough if the examiner is to have any chance to individualize the fragments to a common source. If even the remotest possibility exists that fragments may be pieced together, every effort must be made to collect all the glass found. For example, collection of evidence at hit-and-run scenes must include all the broken parts of the headlight and reflector lenses. This evidence may ultimately prove to be an invaluable means of placing a suspect vehicle at the accident scene by actually matching the fragments with glass remaining in the headlight or reflector shell of the suspect vehicle. In addition, an examination of the headlight's filaments may resolve any questions regarding whether or not an automobile's headlights were on or off before the impact (see Figure 4-18).

When an individual fit is thought improbable, the evidence collector must submit all glass evidence found in the possession of the suspect along with a representative sample of broken glass remaining at the crime scene. This control glass should always be taken from any remaining glass in the window or door frames, as close as possible to the point of breakage. About

Figure 4-18. Presence of oxides on the lower filament indicates the filament was hot when it was exposed to air. Thus, the filament must have been on prior to impact. *Courtesy* New Jersey State Police.

one square inch of sample is usually adequate for this purpose. The glass fragments should be packaged in solid containers to avoid further breakage. If the suspect's shoes or clothing are to be examined for the presence of glass fragments, they should be individually wrapped in paper and transmitted to the laboratory. It is best that the field investigator avoid removing such evidence from garments unless it is thought absolutely necessary for its preservation.

When a determination of the direction of impact is desired, all broken glass must be recovered and submitted for analysis. Wherever possible, the exterior and interior surfaces of the glass must be indicated. In cases in which this is not immediately apparent, the presence of dirt, paint, grease, or putty may provide an indication as to the exterior surface of the glass.

FORENSIC CHARACTERISTICS OF SOIL

There are many definitions for the term *soil*; however, for forensic purposes, soil may be thought of as including any disintegrated surface material, both natural and artificial, that lies on or near the earth's surface. Therefore, the forensic examination of soil is not only concerned with the analysis of naturally occurring rocks, minerals, vegetation, and animal matter—it also encompasses the detection of such manufactured objects as glass, paint chips, asphalt, brick fragments, and cinders, whose presence may impart soil with characteristics that will make it unique to a particular location. When this material is collected accidentally or deliberately in a manner that will associate it with a crime under investigation, it becomes valuable physical evidence.

The value of soil as evidence rests with its prevalence at crime scenes and its transferability between the scene and the criminal. Thus, soil or dried mud found adhering to a suspect's clothing, shoes, or to an automobile, when compared to soil samples collected at the crime site, may provide associative evidence that can link a suspect or object to the crime scene. As with most types of physical evidence, forensic soil analysis is comparative in nature; soil found in the possession of the suspect must be carefully collected to be compared to soil samplings from the crime scene and the surrounding vicinity. However, one should not rule out the value of soil even if the site of the crime has not been ascertained. For instance, a person or object containing small amounts of soil may be found far from the actual site of a crime. A geologist having knowledge of local geology, and with the aid of geological maps, may be able to direct police to the general vicinity where the soil was originally picked up and the crime committed.

Most soils can be differentiated and distinguished by their gross appearance. A side-by-side visual comparison of the color and texture of soil specimens is easy to perform and provides a sensitive property for distinguishing soils that originate from different locations. It is important to remember that the color of soil is darker when it is wet; therefore, color comparisons must always be made when all the samples are dried under identical laboratory conditions. It is estimated that there are nearly 1100 distinguishable soil colors; hence the comparison of color offers a logical first step in a forensic soil comparison.

Low-power microscopic examination of soil will reveal the presence of plant and animal materials as well as of man-made debris. Further high-power microscopic examination will aid in the characterization of minerals and rocks present in earth materials. Although this approach to the forensic identification of soil requires the expertise of an investigator trained in geology, it can provide the most varied and significant points of comparison between soil samples. Only through a careful examination and comparison of the minerals and rocks naturally present in soil can one take advantage of the large number of variations that exist between soils and thus add to the evidential value of a positive comparison.[2] A mineral is a naturally occurring crystal, and like any other crystal its physical properties—e.g., color, geometric shape, density, and refractive index or birefringence—are most useful for identification. More than 2200 minerals are known to exist; however, most of these are so rare that the forensic geologist will usually encounter only about 40 of the more common ones. Rocks are composed of a combination of minerals and therefore exist in thousands of varieties on the earth's surface. Their identification is usually made by characterizing their mineral content and grain size.

Considering the vast variety of minerals, rocks, and the possible occurrence of man-made debris that may be present in soil, the forensic geologist is presented with many points of comparison between two or more specimens. The number of comparative points and their frequency of occurrence must all be taken into consideration before similarity between specimens is concluded and the probability of common origin judged.

Rocks and minerals are not only present in earth materials, they are also used by man to manufacture a wide variety of industrial and commercial products. For example, it is not uncommon to find that the tools and garments of an individual suspected of breaking into a safe will contain traces of safe insulation. Safe insulation may be made from a wide combination of mineral mixtures that can provide significant points of identification. Similarly, building materials, such as brick, plaster, and concrete blocks, are combinations of minerals and rocks that can easily be recognized and compared microscopically to similar minerals found on the breaking and entering suspect.

Many forensic laboratories presently rely on the **density-gradient tube**

---

[2] W. J. Graves, "A Mineralogical Soil Classification Technique for the Forensic Scientist," *Journal of Forensic Sciences*, 24 (1979), 323.

technique to compare soil specimens. Typically, glass tubes 6 to 10 mm in diameter and from 25 to 40 cm in length are filled with layers of two liquids mixed in varying proportions so that each layer has a different density value. For example, tetrabromoethane (density 2.96 g/ml) and ethanol (density 0.789 g/ml) may be mixed so that the ratios of the two liquids in each layer are such that each successive layer has a lower density than the preceding one, from the bottom to the top of the tube. The simplest gradient tube may have from six to ten layers in which the bottom layer is pure tetrabromoethane and the top layer is pure ethanol, with corresponding variations of concentration in the layers between these two extremes. When soil is added to the density-gradient tube, its particles will sink to the portion of the tube that has a density of equal value; the particle will remain suspended in the liquid at this point. In this way, a density distribution pattern of soil particles can be obtained and compared to other specimens treated in a similar manner (Figure 4-19). This procedure is used by many crime laboratories to compare soil evidence. However, there is evidence that this test is far from definitive in that many soils collected from different locations yield similar density distribution patterns.[3] At best, the density-gradient test has been shown to be useful for comparing soils when it's used in combination with other tests.

Figure 4-19. A soil comparison by density-gradient tubes. *Courtesy* Philadelphia Police Dept. Laboratory.

---

[3]K. Chaperlin and P. S. Howarth, "Soil Comparison by the Density Gradient Method—A Review and Evaluation," *Forensic Science International*, 23 (1983), 161-77.

The ultimate forensic value of soil evidence depends on its variation at the crime scene. If, for example, soil is indistinguishable for miles surrounding the location of a crime, with the methods used in the examination, it will have limited value in associating soil found on the suspect to that particular site. Significant conclusions relating the suspect to a particular crime-scene location through a soil comparison may be made when variations in soil composition occur every 10 to 100 yards from the crime site. However, even when such variations do exist, it is usually not possible for the forensic geologist to individualize soil to any one location unless an unusual combination of rare minerals, rocks, or man-made debris can be located.

Up to this time, there have been no statistically valid forensic studies on the variability of soil evidence. A pilot study recently conducted in southern Ontario, Canada, seems to indicate that this part of Canada has soil showing extensive diversity. It was found that the probability is smaller than 1 in 50 of finding two soils that are indistinguishable in both color and mineral properties but that originate in two different locations separated by a distance in the order of 1000 feet. Based on these preliminary results, similar diversity may be expected in the northern United States, Canada, northern Europe, and much of the U.S.S.R. However, such probability values can only serve as a general indication of the variation of soil within these geographical areas. It must be emphasized that each crime scene must be evaluated separately to establish its own soil variation probabilities.

COLLECTION AND PRESERVATION OF SOIL EVIDENCE

The importance of establishing the variation of soil at the crime-scene area must be given primary consideration when the evidence collector gathers soil specimens. For this reason, control soils are to be collected at various intervals within a 100-yard radius of the crime scene, as well as at the site of the crime, for comparison to the questioned soil. Additionally, soil specimens should also be collected at all possible alibi locations that the suspect may claim. It is important that the specimens gathered be representative of the soil that was removed by the suspect. In most cases this means that only the top-surface layer of soil will be picked up during the commission of a crime. Thus, control specimens must be removed from the surface without digging too deeply into the unrepresentative subsurface layers. A quantity of soil equal to approximately a tablespoon or two is all that is required by the laboratory for a thorough comparative analysis. All specimens collected should be packaged in individual containers, such as plastic vials. Each vial is marked to indicate the location at which the sampling was made.

Soil found on a suspect must be carefully preserved for analysis. If it is found adhering to an object, as in the case of soil on a shoe, the investigator must not remove it. Instead, each object is individually wrapped in paper with the soil intact, and transmitted to the laboratory. Similarly, no effort should be made to remove loose soil adhering to garments; these items should be carefully wrapped individually in paper bags and sent to the laboratory for analysis. Care must be taken that all particles that may accidentally fall off the garment during transportation will remain within the paper bag.

When a lump of soil is found, it should be collected and preserved intact. For example, an automobile tends to collect and build up layers of soil under fenders, body, etc. In some situations the impact of an automobile with another object may jar some of this soil loose. Once the suspect car has been apprehended, a comparison of the soil left at the scene with soil remaining on the automobile may help establish that the car was present at the accident scene. In these situations, separate samples are collected from under all the fender and frame area of the vehicle; care is taken to remove the soil in lump form in order to preserve the order in which the soil was deposited onto the car. Undoubtedly, during the normal use of an automobile, soil will be picked up from numerous locations over a period of months and years. This layering effect may serve to impart soil with greater variation, and hence greater evidential value, than that which is normally associated with loose soil.

The prevalence of glass and soil in our environment makes them common types of physical evidence at crime scenes. Their proper collection and preservation by the criminal investigator will help ensure that a proper scientific examination can support investigative conclusions placing a suspect or object at the crime scene. Equally important is that glass and soil, like other types of physical evidence, when properly collected and examined may serve to exonerate the innocent from involvement in a crime.

REVIEW QUESTIONS

1. A _____ property describes the behavior or a substance without reference to any other substance.
2. A _____ property is one that describes the behavior of a substance when it reacts or combines with another substance.
3. The _____ system of measurement was devised by the French Academy of Science in 1791.
4. The basic units of measurement for length, mass, and volume in the metric system are the _____, _____, and _____, respectively.
5. A centigram is equivalent to _____ of a gram.
6. A milliliter is equivalent to _____ liter.
7. 0.2 grams is equivalent to _____ milligrams.

8. One cubic centimeter (cc) is equivalent to one _____.
9. One meter is slightly longer than a yard. (True, False)
10. The equivalent of one pound in grams is _____.
11. A liter is slightly larger than a quart. (True, False)
12. _____ is a measure of a substance's heat intensity.
13. There are _____ degrees Fahrenheit between the freezing and boiling points of water.
14. There are _____ degrees of Celsius between the freezing and boiling points of water.
15. The amount of matter an object contains determines its _____.
16. The simplest type of balance for weighing is the _____.
17. Mass per unit volume defines the property of _____.
18. If an object is immersed in a liquid of greater density, it will (sink, float).
19. The bending of a light wave because of a change in velocity is called _____.
20. The physical property of _____ is determined by the ratio of the velocity of light in a vacuum to light's velocity in a substance.
21. Solids having an orderly arrangement of their constituent atoms are crystalline. (True, False)
22. Solids that have their atoms randomly arranged are said to be _____.
23. The crystal calcite has two indices of refraction. The difference between these two values is known as _____.
24. The process of separating light into its component colors or frequencies is known as _____.
25. A hard, brittle amorphous substance composed mainly of silicon oxides is _____.
26. Glass that can be physically pieced together has _____ characteristics.
27. The two most useful physical properties of glass for forensic comparisons are _____ and _____.
28. Comparing the relative densities of glass fragments is readily accomplished by a method known as _____.
29. When glass is immersed in a liquid of similar refractive index, its _____ will disappear, and minimum contrast between the glass and liquid will be observed.
30. The exact numerical density and refractive indices of glass can be correlated to _____ in order to assess the evidential value of the comparison.
31. The fracture lines radiating outward from a crack in glass are known as _____ fractures.

32. A crater-shaped hole in glass is (narrower, wider) on the side where the projectile entered the glass.

33. It is easy to determine from the size and shape of a hole in glass whether it was made by a bullet or some other projectile. (True, False)

34. Stress marks on the edge of a radial crack are always perpendicular to the edge of the surface on which the impact force originated. (True, False)

35. A fracture line (will, will not) terminate at an existing line fracture.

36. The vast majority of soils have indistinguishable color and texture. (True, False)

37. Naturally occurring crystals commonly found in soils are _____.

38. A comparison of the density of soil particles is readily accomplished through the use of _____ tubes.

39. The ultimate value of soil as evidence is dependent on its variation at the crime scene. (True, False)

FURTHER REFERENCES

Dolan, D. N., "Vehicle Lights and Their Use as Evidence," *Journal of the Forensic Science Society*, 11 (1971), 69-82.

Dudley, R. J., and K. Smalldon, "The Evaluation of Methods for Soil Analysis under Simulated Scenes of Crime Conditions," *Forensic Science International*, 12 (1978), 49-60.

Hickman, D. A., "Linking Criminals to the Scene of the Crime with Glass Analysis," *Analytical Chemistry*, 56 (1984) 844A-52A.

McJunkins, Steven P., and John I. Thornton, "Glass Fracture Analysis— A Review," *Forensic Science*, 2 (1973), 1-27.

Miller, Elmer T., "Forensic Glass Comparisons," in *Forensic Science Handbook*, R. Saferstein, ed. Englewood Cliffs, N.J.: Prentice-Hall, Inc., 1982.

Murray, Raymond C., "Forensic Examination of Soil," in *Forensic Science Handbook*, R. Saferstein, ed. Englewood Cliffs, N.J.: Prentice-Hall, Inc., 1982.

Murray, Raymond C., and John C. F. Tedrow, *Forensic Geology*. New Brunswick, N.J.: Rutgers University Press, 1975.

Ojena, S. M., and P. R. De Forest, "Precise Refractive Index Determination by the Immersion Method, Using Phase Contract Microscopy and the Mettler Hot Stage," *Journal of the Forensic Science Society*, 12 (1973), 315-29.

Svensson, A., O. Wendel, and B. A. J. Fisher, *Techniques of Crime Scene Investigations*, 3rd ed. New York: Elsevier North-Holland, Inc., 1981.

AUDIOVISUAL PRESENTATION

Basic Principles in Chemistry Measurement, Series 820 (35-mm slides and audio tapes). Prentice-Hall Media, Tarrytown, N.Y.

5

Organic Analysis

In the previous chapter some physical properties were described and used to characterize glass and soil evidence. Before we can apply other physical properties, as well as chemical properties, to the identification and comparison of evidence, we need to gain an insight into the composition of matter. Beginning with knowledge of the fundamental building block of all substances—the element—it will be convenient for us to classify all evidence as either organic or inorganic. The procedures used to measure the properties associated with each class are distinctly different and merit separate chapters for their description. In later chapters we will continually return to these procedures as we discuss the examination of the various kinds of physical evidence. This chapter will be devoted, in large part, to reviewing a variety of techniques and instruments that have become the indispensable tools of the forensic scientist for examining organic evidence.

ELEMENTS AND COMPOUNDS

Matter is anything that has a mass and occupies space. As we examine the world that surrounds us and consider the countless variety of materials that we encounter, we must consider it one of man's most remarkable accomplishments to have discovered the concept of the atom to explain the composition of all matter. This search had its earliest contribution from the ancient Greek philosophers, who suggested air, water, fire, and earth as

104

matter's fundamental building blocks. It culminated with the development of the atomic theory and the discovery of matter's simplest identity, the element.

An element is the simplest substance known· to man and provides the building block from which all matter is composed. At present, 107 elements have been identified (see Table 5-1); of these, 89 occur naturally on earth, and the remainder have been created in the laboratory. In Figure 5-1, all the elements are listed by name and symbol in a form that has become known as the **periodic table**. This table is most useful to chemists because it systematically arranges elements with similar chemical properties in the same vertical row or group.

For convenience, chemists have chosen letter symbols to represent the elements. Many of these symbols come from the first letter of the element's English name—for example, carbon (C), hydrogen (H), and oxygen (O). Others are two-letter abbreviations of the English name—calcium (Ca), zinc (Zn). Some of the symbols are derived from the first letters of Latin or

Table 5-1.
LIST OF ELEMENTS WITH THEIR SYMBOLS AND ATOMIC MASSES

Element	Symbol	Atomic Mass[a] (amu)	Element	Symbol	Atomic Mass[a] (amu)
Actinum	Ac	(227)	Erbium	Er	167.26
Aluminum	Al	26.9815	Europium	Eu	151.96
Americium	Am	(243)	Fermium	Fm	(153)
Antimony	Sb	121.75	Fluorine	F	18.9984
Argon	Ar	39.948	Francium	Fr	(223)
Arsenic	As	74.9216	Gadolinium	GD	157.25
Astatine	At	(210)	Gallium	Ga	69.72
Barium	Ba	137.34	Germanium	Ge	72.59
Berkelium	Bk	(247)	Gold	Au	196.9665
Beryllium	Be	9.01218	Hafnium	Hf	178.49
Bismuth	Bi	208.9806	[Hahnium][b]	[Ha]	(260)
Boron	B	10.81	Helium	He	4.00260
Bromine	Br	79.904	Holmium	Ho	164.9303
Cadmium	Cd	112.40	Hydrogen	H	1.0080
Calcium	Ca	40.08	Indium	In	114.82
Californium	Cf	(251)	Iodine	I	126.9045
Carbon	C	12.011	Iridium	Ir	192.22
Cerium	Ce	140.12	Iron	Fe	55.847
Cesium	Cs	132.9055	Krypton	Kr	83.80
Chlorine	Cl	35.453	Lanthanum	La	138.9055
Chromium	Cr	51.996	Lawrencium	Lr	(257)
Cobalt	Co	58.9332	Lead	Pb	207.2
Copper	Cu	63.546	Lithium	Li	6.941
Curium	Cm	(247)	Lutetium	Lu	174.97
Dysprosium	Dy	162.50	Magnesium	Mg	24.305
Einsteinium	Ds	(254)	Manganese	Mn	54.9380

(continued on next page)

Table 5-1. (continued)
LIST OF ELEMENTS WITH THEIR SYMBOLS AND ATOMIC MASSES

Element	Symbol	Atomic Mass[a] (amu)	Element	Symbol	Atomic Mass[a] (amu)
Mendelevium	Md	(256)	[Rutherfordium][b]	[Rf]	(261)
Mercury	Hg	200.59	Samarium	Sm	105.4
Molybdenum	Mo	95.94	Scandium	Sc	44.9559
Neodymium	Nd	144.24	Selenium	Se	78.96
Neon	Ne	20.179	Silicon	Si	28.086
Neptunium	Np	237.0482	Silver	Ag	107.868
Nickel	Ni	58.71	Sodium	Na	22.9898
Niobium	Nb	92.9064	Strontium	Sr	87.62
Nitrogen	N	14.0067	Sulfur	S	32.06
Nobelium	No	(253)	Tantalum	Ta	180.9479
Osmium	Os	190.2	Technetium	Tc	98.9062
Oxygen	O	15.9994	Tellurium	Te	127.60
Palladium	Pd	106.4	Terbium	Tb	158.9254
Phosphorus	P	30.9738	Thallium	Tl	204.37
Platinum	Pt	195.09	Thorium	Th	232.0381
Plutonium	Pu	(244)	Thulium	Tm	168.9342
Polonium	Po	(209)	Tin	Sn	118.69
Potassium	K	39.102	Titanium	Ti	47.90
Praseodymium	Pr	140.9077	Tungsten	W	183.85
Promethium	Pm	(145)	Uranium	U	238.029
Protactinium	Pa	231.0359	Vanadium	V	50.9414
Radium	Ra	226.0254	Xenon	Xe	131.30
Radon	Rn	(222)	Ytterbium	Yb	173.04
Rhenium	Re	186.2	Yttrium	Y	88.9059
Rhodium	Rh	102.9055	Zinc	Zn	65.57
Rubidium	Rb	85.4678	Zirconium	Zr	91.22
Ruthenium	Ru	101.07			

[a] *Based on the assigned relative atomic mass of C = exactly 12; parentheses denote the mass number of the isotope with the longest half-life.*
[b] *Name and symbol not officially approved.*

Greek names. Thus, the symbol for silver, Ag, comes from the Latin name *argentum*, copper, Cu, from the Latin *cuprium*, and helium, He, from the Greek name *helios*.

The smallest particle of an element that can exist and still retain its identity as that element is the atom. When we write the symbol C we mean one atom of carbon; the chemical symbol for carbon dioxide, CO_2, signifies one atom of carbon combined with two atoms of oxygen. When two or more elements are combined to form a substance, as with carbon dioxide, there is created a new substance, different in its physical and chemical properties from its elemental components. This new material is called a **compound**. Compounds contain at least 2 elements. Considering that there are 89 natural elements, it is not difficult to imagine the large number of possible elemental

PERIODIC CHART OF THE ELEMENTS

Period	IA	IIA	IIIB	IVB	VB	VIB	VIIB	VIII	VIII	VIII	IB	IIB	IIIA	IVA	VA	VIA	VIIA	O
1	1 H																	2 He
2	3 Li	4 Be											5 B	6 C	7 N	8 O	9 F	10 Ne
3	11 Na	12 Mg											13 Al	14 Si	15 P	16 S	17 Cl	18 Ar
4	19 K	20 Ca	21 Sc	22 Ti	23 V	24 Cr	25 Mn	26 Fe	27 Co	28 Ni	29 Cu	30 Zn	31 Ga	32 Ge	33 As	34 Se	35 Br	36 Kr
5	37 Rb	38 Sr	39 Y	40 Zr	41 Nb	42 Mo	43 Tc	44 Ru	45 Rh	46 Pd	47 Ag	48 Cd	49 In	50 Sn	51 Sb	52 Te	53 I	54 Xe
6	55 Cs	56 Ba	57 La a	72 Hf	73 Ta	74 W	75 Re	76 Os	77 Ir	78 Pt	79 Au	80 Hg	81 Tl	82 Pb	83 Bi	84 Po	85 At	86 Rn
7	87 Fr	88 Ra	89 Ac b	104 Rf	105 Ha	106	107											

a Lanthanide series

58 Ce	59 Pr	60 Nd	61 Pm	62 Sm	63 Eu	64 Gd	65 Tb	66 Dy	67 Ho	68 Er	69 Tm	70 Yb	71 Lu

b Actinide series

90 Th	91 Pa	92 U	93 Np	94 Pu	95 Am	96 Cm	97 Bk	98 Cf	99 Es	100 Fm	101 Md	102 No	103 Lw

Figure 5-1. The Periodic Table.

combinations that may exist to form compounds. Not surprisingly, over five million known compounds have already been identified.

Just as the atom is the basic particle of an element, the molecule is the smallest unit of a compound. Thus, a molecule of carbon dioxide is represented by the symbol CO_2, and a molecule of table salt is symbolized by NaCl, representing the combination of one atom of the element sodium (Na) with one atom of the element chlorine (Cl).

As we look around us and view the materials that comprise our home planet, Earth, it becomes an awesome task even to attempt to estimate the number of different kinds of matter that exists. A much more logical approach is to classify matter according to the physical form it takes. These forms are called **physical states**. There are three such states: **solid, liquid, and gas (vapor)**. A solid is rigid and therefore has a definite shape and volume. A liquid also occupies a specific volume, but its fluidity causes it to take the shape of the container in which it is residing. A gas has neither a definite shape nor volume, and it will completely fill any container into which it is placed.

Substances can change from one state to another. For example, as water is heated, it is converted from a liquid form into a vapor. At a high enough temperature (100°C), water boils and is rapidly changed into steam. Similarly, at 0°C, water solidifies or freezes into ice. Under certain conditions some solids can be converted directly into a gaseous state. For instance, a piece of dry ice (solid carbon dioxide) left standing at room temperature will quickly form carbon dioxide vapor and disappear. This change of state from a solid to a gas is called sublimation.

In each of these examples it is important to recognize that no new chemical species are formed; matter is simply being changed from one physical state to another. Water, whether it is in the form of liquid, ice, or steam, remains chemically H_2O. Simply, what has been altered are the attractive forces that exist between the water molecules. In a solid these forces are very strong, and the molecules are held closely together in a rigid state. In a liquid the attractive forces are not as strong, and the molecules have more mobility. Finally, in the vapor state, there are no longer appreciable attractive forces between the molecules; thus they are permitted to move in any and all directions at will.

Chemists are forever combining different substances, no matter whether they are in the solid, liquid, or gaseous states, hoping to create new and useful products. Our everyday observations should make it apparent that not all attempts at mixing matter can be productive. For instance, oil spills testify to the fact that oil and water do not mix. **Whenever a situation exists in which substances can be distinguished by a visible boundary, different phases are said to exist.** Thus, oil floating on water is an example of a two-phase system. The oil and water each constitute a separate liquid phase, clearly distinct from each other. Similarly, when sugar is first added to water, it will not dissolve, and there exist two distinctly different phases, the solid sugar and the liquid water. However, after stirring, all the sugar will dissolve leaving just one liquid phase.

SELECTING AN ANALYTICAL TECHNIQUE

Now that the basic components of matter have been defined, the proper selection of analytical techniques that will allow the forensic scientist to identify or compare matter can best be understood by categorizing all substances into one of two broad groups: **organics** and **inorganics.**

Organic substances contain the element carbon, commonly in combination with one or more of the following elements: hydrogen, oxygen, nitrogen, sulfur, phosphorus, chlorine, and bromine. Inorganic substances encompass all other chemical substances known to man. Each of these two broad groups has properties that are quite distinctive and characteristic. Thus, once the analyst has determined whether a material is organic or inorganic, the properties to be measured and the choice of analytical techniques to be used will generally be the same for all materials falling into each group.

Another consideration in selecting an analytical technique is the need for either a **qualitative** or a **quantitative** determination. The former relates just to the identity of the material, whereas the latter requires the determination of the percent combination of the components of a mixture. Hence, a qualitative identification of a powder may reveal the presence of heroin and quinine, whereas a quantitative analysis may conclude the presence of 10 percent heroin and 90 percent quinine. Obviously, a qualitative identification must precede any attempt at quantitation, for little value is served by attempting to quantitate a material without first determining its identity. Essentially, a qualitative analysis of a material will require the determination of numerous properties using a variety of analytical techniques. On the other hand, a quantitative measurement is usually accomplished by the precise measurement of a single property of the material.

Most of the evidence currently received by crime laboratories requires the identification of organic compounds. These compounds may include substances such as commonly abused drugs (e.g., alcohol, marijuana, heroin, amphetamines, and barbiturates), synthetic fibers, petroleum products, paint binders, and high-order explosives. As we have already observed, organic compounds are composed of a combination of a relatively small number of elements that must include carbon; fortunately, the nature of the forces or bonds that exist between these elements is such that the resultant compounds can readily be characterized by their absorption of light. The study of the absorption of light by chemical substances is known as spectrophotometry and serves as a basic tool for the characterization and identification of organic materials. Although spectrophometry is most applicable to organic analysis, its optimum utilization requires that a material be in a relatively pure state. Because the purity of physical evidence is almost always beyond the control of the criminalist, this criterion often is not met. For this reason, the analytical technique of chromatography is widely applied for the analysis of physical evidence. **Chromatography is a means of separating and tentatively identifying the components of a mixture.** We will discuss both of these techniques in this chapter.

CHROMATOGRAPHY

THEORY OF CHROMATOGRAPHY

Chromatography as a technique for purifying substances is particularly useful for analyzing the multicomponent specimens that are frequently received in the crime laboratory. For example, illicit drugs sold on the street are not manufactured to meet government labeling standards; instead, they may be diluted with practically any material that is at the disposal of the drug dealer in order to increase the quantity of the product that is made available to prospective customers. Hence, the task of identifying an illicit drug preparation would be an arduous one without the aid of chromatographic methods to first separate the mixture into its components.

The theory of chromatography has as its basis the observation that chemical substances have a tendency to partially escape into the surrounding environment when dissolved in a liquid or when absorbed on a solid surface. This is best illustrated by a gas dissolved in a beaker of water kept at a constant temperature. It will be convenient for us to characterize the water in the beaker as the liquid phase and the air above it as the gas phase. If the beaker is covered with a bell jar, as shown in Figure 5-2, some of the gas molecules (represented by the dark balls) will escape from the water into the

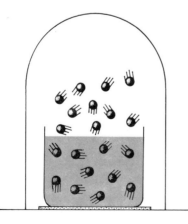

Figure 5-2.   Evaporation of a liquid.

surrounding enclosed air. The molecules remaining behind are said to be in the liquid phase; those molecules that have found their way into the air are said to be in the gas phase. As the gas molecules continue their escape into the surrounding air, they will begin to accumulate above the water; here, random motion will carry some of them back into the water. Eventually, a point will be reached at which the number of molecules leaving the water will be equal to the number returning. At this time the liquid and gas phases are said to be in **equilibrium**. If the temperature of the water is increased, the equilibrium state will readjust itself to a point where more gas molecules will move into the gas phase.

This behavior was first observed in 1803 by a British chemist, William Henry. His explanation of this phenomenon is known appropriately as Henry's Law and may be stated as follows: *When a volatile chemical compound is dissolved in a liquid and is brought to equilibrium with air, there is a fixed ratio between the concentration of the volatile compound in air and its concentration in the liquid, and this ratio remains constant for a given temperature.*

The distribution or partitioning of a gas between the liquid and gas phase is determined by the solubility of the gas in the liquid. The higher its solubility, the greater the tendency of the gas molecules to remain in the liquid phase. If two different gases are simultaneously dissolved in the same liquid, each will reach a state of equilibrium with the surrounding air independently of the other. For example, as shown in Figure 5-3, gas A (black balls) and gas B (white balls) are both dissolved in water. At equilibrium, gas A has a greater number of its molecules dissolved in the water as compared to B. This is so because A is more soluble in water than B.

Now return to the concept of chromatography. In Figures 5-2 and 5-3, both phases—the liquid and gas—were kept stationary; that is, they were not moving. During a chromatographic process this is not the case; instead, one phase is always made to move continuously in one direction over a station-

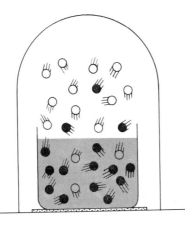

Figure 5-3. At equilibrium there are a greater number of gas A molecules (black balls) in the liquid phase than there are gas B molecules (white balls).

ary or fixed phase. For example, in Figure 5-3 showing the two gases A and B dissolved in water, chromatography will occur only when the air is forced to move continuously in one direction over the water. Because B has a greater percentage of its molecules in the moving gas phase as compared to A, its molecules will travel over the liquid at a faster pace than those of A. Eventually, when the moving phase has advanced a reasonable distance, B will become entirely separated from A and the chromatographic process will be complete. This process is illustrated in Figure 5-4.

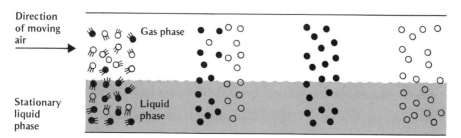

Figure 5-4. In this illustration of chromatography, the molecules represented by the white balls have a greater affinity for the upper phase and hence will be pushed along at a faster rate by the moving air. Eventually, the two sets of molecules will separate from each other, completing the chromatographic process.

Simply, we can think of chromatography as being analogous to a race between chemical compounds. At the starting line all the participating substances are mixed together; however, as the race progresses, those materials that have a preference for the moving phase will slowly pull ahead of those substances that prefer to remain in the stationary phase. Finally, at the completion of the race, all the participants will be separated, each crossing the finish line at different times.

The different types of chromatographic systems that can exist are as varied as the possible number of stationary and moving-phase combinations that can be devised. However, three chromatographic processes—gas chromatography (GC), high-performance liquid chromatography (HPLC), and thin-layer chromatography (TLC)—are found to be most applicable for solving many of the analytical problems encountered in the crime laboratory.

GAS CHROMATOGRAPHY (GC)

Gas chromatography (GC) separates mixtures on the basis of their distribution between a stationary liquid phase and a moving-gas phase. This technique is widely utilized because of its ability to resolve a highly complex mixture into its components within a time period that is usually measured in minutes.

In gas chromatography the moving phase is actually a gas called the *carrier gas* which flows through a column constructed of stainless steel or glass. The stationary phase is a thin film of liquid contained within the column. Two types of columns are in current use: the **packed column** and the **capillary column**. With the packed column the stationary phase is a thin film of liquid which is fixed onto small granular particles packed into the column. This column is usually constructed of stainless steel or glass and is 2 to 6 meters in length and about 3 millimeters in diameter. Capillary columns are composed of glass and are much longer than packed columns—15 to 60 meters in length. These types of columns are very narrow, ranging from .25 to .75 millimeter in diameter. Capillary columns can be made narrower than packed columns since their stationary liquid phase is actually coated as a very thin film directly onto the column's inner wall. In any case, as the carrier gas flows through the packed or capillary column, it carries along with it the components of a mixture that has been injected into the column. Those components having a greater affinity for the moving-gas phase will travel through the column at a faster rate as compared to those having a greater affinity for the stationary liquid phase. Eventually, after the mixture has traversed the length of the column, it will emerge separated into its components.

A simplified scheme of the gas chromatograph is shown in Figure 5-5. The operation of the instrument can be summed up briefly as follows: A gas stream, the so-called carrier gas, is fed into the column at a constant rate. The carrier gas is chemically inert and is generally nitrogen or helium. The

1 SAMPLE

2 INJECTOR

3 CARRIER GAS

4 COLUMN

5 DETECTOR

6 POWER SUPPLY

7 RECORDER

8 CHROMATOGRAM

Figure 5-5. Basic gas chromatography. Gas chromatography permits the rapid separation of complex mixtures into individual compounds and allows identification and quantitative determination of each compound. As shown, a sample is introduced by a syringe (1) into a heated injection chamber (2). A constant stream of nitrogen gas (3) flows through the injector carrying the sample into the column (4) which contains a thin film of liquid. The sample is separated in the column, and the carrier gas and separated components emerge from the column and enter the detector (5). Signals developed by the detector activate the recorder (7), which makes a permanent record of the separation by tracing a series of peaks on the chromatograph (8). The time of elution identifies the component present, and the peak area identifies the concentration. *Courtesy* Varian Instruments, California.

sample under investigation is injected as a liquid into a heated injection port with a syringe, where it is immediately vaporized and swept into the column by the carrier gas. The column itself is heated in an oven in order to keep the sample in a vapor state as it travels through the column. In the column, the components of the sample travel in the direction of the carrier gas flow at speeds that are determined by their distribution between the stationary and moving phases. Assuming that the analyst has selected the proper liquid phase and has made the column long enough, the components of the sample will be completely separated as they emerge from the column.

As each component emerges from the column, it enters a detector. One type of detector uses a flame to ionize the emerging chemical substance, thus generating an electrical signal. The signal is recorded onto a strip-chart recorder as a function of time. This written record of the separation is called a **chromatogram**. A gas chromatogram is a plot of the recorder response (vertical axis) versus time (horizontal axis). A typical chromatogram will show a series of peaks, each peak corresponding to one component of the mixture. The time required for a component to emerge from the column from the time of its injection onto the column is known as the **retention time**. This serves as a useful identifying characteristic of a material. Figure 5-6 (a) shows the chromatogram of two barbiturates; each barbiturate has tentatively been identified by comparing its retention time to those of known barbiturates, shown in Figure 5-6 (b). (See Appendix III for chromatographic conditions.) However, because it is always possible that other substances may have comparable retention times under similar chromatographic conditions, gas chromatography cannot be considered an absolute means of identification. Conclusions derived from this technique must be confirmed by other testing procedures.

Gas chromatography has an added advantage in that it is extremely sensitive and can yield quantitative results. The amount of substance passing through the GC detector is proportional to the peak area recorded; therefore, by chromatographing a known concentration of a material and comparing it to the unknown, the amount of the sample may be determined by proportion. Gas chromatography has sufficient sensitivity to detect and quantitate materials at the nanogram (0.000000001 gram or 1×10^{-9} gram) level.[1]

An important extension of the application of gas chromatography to forensic science is the technique of **pyrolysis gas chromatography**. Many solid materials commonly encountered as physical evidence—e.g., paint chips, fibers, and plastics—cannot be readily dissolved in a solvent for injec-

---

[1] For ease of handling large or small numbers, the power of ten notion is quite useful and simple. The power of ten expresses the number of places that the decimal point must be moved. If it is positive, the decimal point is moved to the right; if it is negative, the decimal point is moved to the left. Thus, to express 1×10^{-9} as a number, the decimal point is simply moved nine places to the left of 1.

Figure 5-6. (a) An unknown mixture of barbiturates is identified by comparing its retention times to (b). (b) A known mixture of barbiturates. *Courtesy* Varian Instruments, California.

tion into the gas chromatograph. Thus, under normal conditions these substances cannot be subjected to gas chromatographic analysis. However, materials such as these can be heated or pyrolyzed to high temperatures (500–1000°C) so that they will decompose into numerous gaseous products. Pyrolyzers have been designed to permit these gaseous products to enter the carrier gas stream where they flow into and through the GC column. The pyrolyzed material can then be characterized by the pattern produced by its chromatogram or **pyrogram**. As an example, Figure 5-7 illustrates the pyrogram of a paint chip. The complexity of the paint pyrogram in essence serves as a "fingerprint" of the material and gives the examiner many points to compare with other paints that are analyzed in a similar fashion.

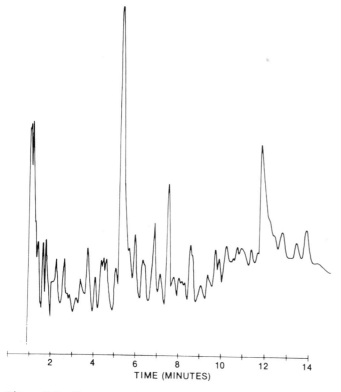

TIME (MINUTES)

Figure 5-7. Pyrogram of a GM automobile paint. *Courtesy* Varian Instruments, California.

HIGH-PERFORMANCE LIQUID
CHROMATOGRAPHY (HPLC)

As was previously mentioned, a chromatographic system requires having a moving phase and a stationary phase in contact with each other. In the previous section, gas chromatography was described. Here, the stationary phase is a thin film and the moving phase a gas. However, by changing the nature of these phases, one can create different forms of chromatography. One form finding increasing utility in crime laboratories is high-performance liquid chromatography (HPLC). Its moving phase is a liquid which is pumped under pressure through a column filled with fine solid particles. In one form of HPLC the surfaces of these solid particles are chemically treated and act as the stationary phase. As the liquid moving phase is being pumped through the column, a sample is injected onto the column. As the liquid carries the sample through the column, different components are retarded to different degrees depending on their interaction with the stationary phase. This leads to a separation of the different components making up the sample mixture.

The major advantage of HPLC is that the entire process takes place at room temperature. With GC the sample must be first vaporized and made to travel through a heated column. Hence, any materials sensitive to high temperatures may fail to survive their passage through the column. In such situations the analyst may turn to HPLC as the method of choice. Organic explosives are generally heat-sensitive and are therefore more readily separated by HPLC. Likewise heat-sensitive drugs, such as LSD, lend themselves to analysis by HPLC.

THIN-LAYER CHROMATOGRAPHY (TLC)

The technique of thin-layer chromatography incorporates a solid stationary phase and a moving liquid phase to effect the separation of the constituents of a mixture. A thin-layer plate is prepared by coating a glass plate with a thin film of a granular material. Commonly, silica gel or aluminum oxide is used. This granular material serves as the solid stationary phase, and is usually held in place on the plate with a binding agent such as plaster of Paris. If the sample to be analyzed is a solid, it first must be dissolved in a suitable solvent and a few microliters of the solution spotted with a capillary tube onto the granular surface near the lower edge of the plate. A liquid sample may be applied directly to the plate in the same manner. The plate is then placed upright into a closed chamber that contains a selected liquid, with care that the liquid does not touch the sample spot.

The liquid will slowly begin to rise up the plate by capillary action. It is the rising liquid that serves as the moving phase in thin-layer chromatography. As it moves past the sample spot, the components of the sample will become distributed between the stationary solid phase and the moving liquid phase. Those components with the greatest affinity for the moving phase will travel up the plate at a faster speed as compared to those that have greater affinity for the stationary phase. When the liquid front has moved a sufficient distance (usually 10 cm), the development is complete, and the plate is removed from the chamber and dried.

Because most compounds are colorless, no separation will be noticed after development unless the materials are *visualized*. To accomplish this, the plates are placed under ultraviolet light, revealing those materials that fluoresce as bright spots on a dark background. When a fluorescent dye has been incorporated into the solid phase, nonfluorescent substances appear as dark spots against a fluorescent background when exposed to the ultraviolet light. A second method of visualization is accomplished when the plate is sprayed with a chemical reagent that reacts with the separated substances and causes them to form colored spots. Figure 5-8 shows the chromatogram of a marijuana extract that has been separated into its components by TLC and visualized by having been sprayed with a chemical reagent.

Once the components of a sample have been separated, their identifica-

SOLVENT FRONT —

ORIGIN —

Figure 5-8.   Chromatogram of a marijuana extract.

tion must follow. For this, the questioned sample must be developed alongside an authentic or standard sample on the same TLC plate. If both the standard and the unknown are found to travel the same distances up the plate from their origins, they can tentatively be identified as being the same. For example, a sample suspected of containing heroin and quinine is chromatographed alongside known heroin and quinine standards, as shown in Figure 5-9. A confirmation of the identity of the suspect material is made by comparing the migration distances of the heroin and quinine standards against those of the components of the unknown material. If the distances are the same, a tentative identification can be made. However, it must be cautioned that such an identification cannot be considered definitive, for the possibility always exists that numerous other substances can migrate the same distance

Figure 5-9. Chromatograms of known heroin (1) and quinine (2) standards alongside suspect sample (3).

up the plate when chromatographed under similar conditions. Thus, thin-layer chromatography cannot by itself provide an absolute identification; it must be utilized in conjunction with other testing procedures to prove absolute identity.

The distance a spot has traveled up a thin-layer plate can be assigned a numerical value known as the R_f value. This value is defined as the distance traveled by the component divided by the distance traveled by the moving liquid phase. For example, in Figure 5-9 the moving phase was allowed to travel 10 cm up the plate before the plate was removed from the tank. After visualization, the heroin spot moved 8 cm and thus has an R_f value of 0.8; the quinine migrated 4 cm, and has an R_f value of 0.4.

There are literally thousands of possible combinations of liquid and solid phases that can be chosen from in thin-layer chromatography. Fortunately, years of research have produced much published data relating to the proper selection of TLC conditions for separating and identifying specific classes of substances—e.g., drugs, dyes, and petroleum products. These references, along with the personal experiences of the analyst, will aid in the proper selection of TLC conditions for specific problems.

Thin-layer chromatography is a powerful tool for solving many of the analytical problems presented to the forensic scientist. The method is both rapid and sensitive; moreover, less than 100 micrograms of suspect material are required for the analysis. In addition, the equipment necessary for TLC work has minimal cost and space requirements. And numerous samples can be analyzed simultaneously on one thin-layer plate. The principal application of this technique is the detection and identification of components in complex mixtures.

ELECTROPHORESIS

Electrophoresis is somewhat related to thin-layer chromatography in that it separates materials according to their migration rates on a stationary solid phase. However, it does not utilize a moving-liquid phase to move the material; instead, an electrical potential is placed across the stationary medium. The nature of this medium can vary; most forensic applications call for a starch or agar gel coated onto a glass plate. Under these conditions only substances that possess an electrical charge will migrate across the stationary phase. The technique is particularly useful for separating and identifying complex biochemical mixtures. In forensic science, electrophoresis finds its most successful application in the characterization of proteins in dried blood.

Because many of the substances in blood carry an electrical charge, they can be separated and identified by electrophoresis. Forensic serologists have developed several electrophoretic procedures for characterizing dried blood. Many enzymes present in blood are actually composed of distinct proteins that can be separated by electrophoresis on starch gel. These proteins will migrate on the plate at speeds that vary according to their electrical charge and size. After completion of the electrophoresis run, the separated proteins are stained with a suitable developing agent for visual observation. In this manner, characteristic band patterns are obtained that are related to the enzyme type present in the blood. This technique will be discussed in further detail in Chapter 12.

SPECTROPHOTOMETRY

THEORY OF LIGHT

We have already seen that when white light passes through a glass prism, it is dispersed into a continuous spectrum of colors. This phenomenon demonstrates the fact that white light is not homogeneous but is actually composed of a range of colors that extends from red through violet. Similarly, the observation that a substance has a color is also consistent with this description of white light. For example, when light is passed through a red glass, all the component colors of light are absorbed by the glass except for red, which passes through or is transmitted by the glass. Likewise, one can determine the color of an opaque object by observing its ability to absorb some of the component colors of light while reflecting others back to the eye. Color is thus a visual indication of the fact that objects absorb certain portions of visible light and transmit or reflect others. Scientists have long recognized this phenomenon and have learned to characterize different chemical substances by the type and quantity of light they absorb.

To understand why materials absorb light, one must first comprehend the nature of light. Two simple models have been developed to explain light's behavior. The first model describes light as a continuous wave; the second depicts it as a stream of discrete energy particles. Together, these two very different descriptions can explain all of the observed properties of light; but by itself, no one model can explain all the facets of the behavior of light.

The wave concept depicts light as having an up-and-down motion of a continuous wave, as shown in Figure 5-10. Several terms are used to describe such a wave. The distance between two consecutive crests (or one trough to the next trough) is called the **wavelength**; the Greek letter *lambda* (λ) is used as its symbol, and the unit of nanometers is frequently used to express its value. The number of crests (or troughs) passing any one given point in a unit of time is defined as the **frequency** of the wave. Frequency is normally designated by the letter f, and is expressed in cycles per second (cps). The speed of light in a vacuum is a universal constant at 300,000,000 meters per second, and is designated by the symbol c. Frequency and wavelength are

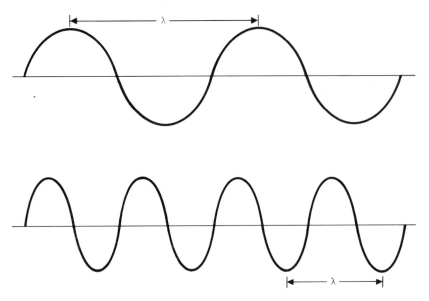

Figure 5-10. The frequency of the lower wave is twice that of the upper wave.

inversely proportional to one another, as shown by the relationship expressed in Equation (5-1).

$$f = \frac{c}{\lambda} \qquad \qquad (5\text{-}1)$$

Actually, visible light is only a small part of a large family of radiation waves known as the **electromagnetic spectrum.** All electromagnetic radiations travel at the speed of light (c) and are only distinguishable from one another by their different wavelengths or frequencies. (Figure 5-11 illustrates the various types of electromagnetic radiations in the order of decreasing frequency.) Hence, the only property that distinguishes X-rays from radio waves is the different frequencies the two types of waves possess. Similarly,

Electromagnetic spectrum

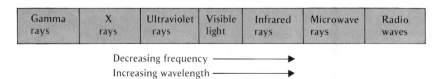

Gamma rays	X rays	Ultraviolet rays	Visible light	Infrared rays	Microwave rays	Radio waves

Decreasing frequency ⟶
Increasing wavelength ⟶

Figure 5-11. Electromagnetic spectrum.

the range of colors that comprise the visible spectrum can be correlated with frequency. For instance, the lowest frequencies of visible light are red in color, with those waves having a somewhat lower frequency falling into the invisible infrared region. The highest frequencies of visible light are violet in color, and those radiations having a somewhat higher frequency extend into the invisible region. No definite boundary exists between any one color or any one region of the electromagnetic spectrum; instead, each region is comprised of a continuous range of frequencies, each blending into the other.

Ordinarily, light in any region of the electromagnetic spectrum is a collection of waves possessing a range of wavelengths. Under normal circumstances this light will be comprised of waves which are all out of step with each other (incoherent light). However, it is now possible for scientists to produce light that has all its waves pulsating in unison (see Figure 5-12). This is called coherent light or a laser (*l*ight *a*mplification by the *s*imulated *e*mission of *r*adiation). Light in this form is very intense and can be focused on a very small area. Laser beams can be focused down to pinpoints that are so intense that they can zap microscopic holes in a diamond.

As long as electromagnetic radiation is moving through space, its behavior can be described as that of a continuous wave; however, once radiation is absorbed by a substance, the model of light as a stream of discrete par-

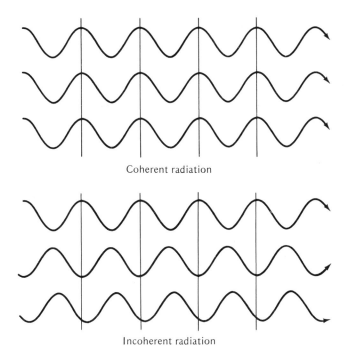

Coherent radiation

Incoherent radiation

Figure 5-12. Coherent and incoherent radiation.

ticles must be invoked to best describe its behavior. Here, light is depicted as consisting of energy particles that are known as **photons**. Each photon has a definite amount of energy associated with its behavior. This energy is related to the frequency of light, as shown by Equation (5-2):

$$E = hf \qquad\qquad (5\text{-}2)$$

E specifies the energy of the photon, f the frequency of radiation, and h is a universal constant called *Planck's constant*. As shown by Equation (5-2), the energy of a photon is directly proportional to its frequency. Therefore, the photons of ultraviolet light will be more energetic than the photons of visible or infrared light, and exposure to the more energetic photons of X-rays presents more danger to human health than exposure to the photons of radio waves.

ABSORPTION OF ELECTROMAGNETIC RADIATION

Just as a substance can absorb visible light to produce color, many of the invisible radiations of the electromagnetic spectrum are likewise absorbed. This absorption phenomenon is the basis for spectrophotometry, an important analytical technique in chemical identification. Spectrophotometry measures the quantity of radiation that a particular material absorbs as a function of wavelength or frequency.

We have already observed in the description of color that an object will not absorb all the visible light it is exposed to; instead, it will selectively absorb some of the component frequencies and will reflect or transmit others. Similarly, the absorption of other types of electromagnetic radiation by chemical substances is also found to be selective. The key questions that must be asked are: Why does a particular substance absorb only at certain frequencies and not at others? And, are these frequencies predictable? The answers are not simple ones. Scientists find it most difficult to predict with certainty all the frequencies at which any one substance will absorb in a particular region of the electromagnetic spectrum. What is known, however, is that a chemical substance will absorb photons of radiation that have a frequency that corresponds to an energy requirement of the substance, as defined by Equation (5-2). Different materials have different energy requirements and therefore absorb at different frequencies. What is most important to the analyst is that these absorbed frequencies are measurable, and they can be used to characterize a material.

The selective absorption of a substance is measured by an instrument called the **spectrophotometer**. It produces a graph or **absorption spectrum** that depicts the absorbance of light as a function of wavelength or frequency. The absorption of ultraviolet (UV), visible, and infrared (IR) radiations is particularly applicable for obtaining qualitative data pertaining to the identification of organic substances.

Absorption at a single wavelength or frequency of light is not 100 percent complete—there will always be some radiation transmitted or reflected by the material. Just how much radiation a substance will absorb is defined by a fundamental relationship known as Beer's Law, Equation (5-3):

$$A = kc \tag{5-3}$$

Here, A symbolizes the absorbance or the quantity of light taken up at a single frequency, c is the concentration of the absorbing material, and k is a proportionality constant. From this relationship, it is seen that the quantity of light absorbed at any frequency is directly proportional to the concentration of the absorbing species; the more material you have, the more radiation it will absorb. By defining the relationship between absorbance and concentration, Beer's Law permits spectrophotometry to be used as a technique for quantitation.

THE SPECTROPHOTOMETER

The spectrophotometer is the instrument used to measure and record the absorption spectrum of a chemical substance. The basic components of a simple spectrophotometer are the same regardless of whether it is designed to measure the absorption of UV, visible, or IR radiation. These components are illustrated diagrammatically in Figure 5-13. They include: (1) a radiation source, (2) a monochromator or frequency selector, (3) a sample holder, (4) a detector to convert electromagnetic radiation into an electrical signal, and (5) a recorder to produce a record of the signal.

The choice of a source will vary with the type of radiation desired. For visible radiation, an ordinary tungsten bulb provides a convenient source of radiation. In the UV region, a hydrogen or deuterium discharge lamp is normally used, and a heated molded rod containing a mixture of rare-earth oxides is a good source of IR light.

Figure 5-13.   Parts of a simple spectrophotometer.

The function of the monochromator is to select a single wavelength or frequency of light from the source. In some inexpensive spectrophotometers this may be accomplished when the light is caused to pass through colored glass filters that will remove all radiation from the beam except for a desired range of wavelengths. More precise spectrophotometers may employ a prism or diffraction grating to disperse radiation into its component wavelengths or frequencies.[2] The desired wavelength is obtained when the dispersed radiation is focused onto a narrow slit that permits only selected radiations to pass through.

Sample preparation varies with the type of radiation being studied. Absorption spectra in the UV and visible regions are usually obtained from samples that have been dissolved in an appropriate solvent. Because the cells holding the solution must be transparent to the light being measured, glass cells are used in the visible region and quartz cells in the ultraviolet region. Practically all substances absorb in some region of the IR spectrum, so sampling techniques must be modified to measure absorption in this spectral region; special cells made out of sodium chloride or potassium bromide are commonly utilized because they will not absorb light over a wide range of the IR portion of the electromagnetic spectrum.

The detector measures the quantity of radiation that passes through the sample by converting it to an electrical signal. UV and visible spectrophotometers employ photoelectric tube detectors. A signal is generated when the photons strike the tube surface to produce a current that is directly proportional to the intensity of the light transmitted through the sample. When this signal is compared to the intensity of light that is transmitted to the detector in the absence of an absorbing material, the absorbance of a substance can be determined at each wavelength or frequency of light selected. The signal from the detection system is then fed into a recorder, which plots absorbance as a function of wavelength or frequency. Modern spectrophotometers are designed to trace an entire absorption spectrum automatically.

ULTRAVIOLET, VISIBLE, AND INFRARED SPECTROPHOTOMETRY

Ultraviolet (UV) and visible spectrophotometry measure the absorbance of UV and visible light as a function of wavelength or frequency. For example, the UV absorption spectrum of heroin shows a maximum absorption band at a wavelength of 278 nanometers (Figure 5-14). From this it can readily

---

[2] Present-day spectrophotometers use diffraction gratings to disperse light into its component wavelengths. A diffraction grating is made by scratching many thousands of parallel lines on a transparent surface such as glass. As light passes through the narrow spacings between the lines, it spreads out and produces a spectrum similar to that formed by a prism.

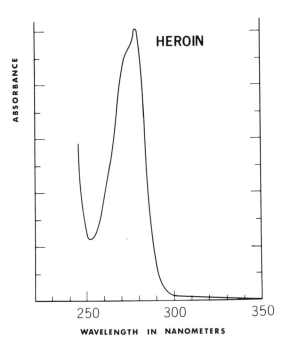

Figure 5-14. Ultraviolet spectrum of heroin.

be seen that the simplicity of a UV spectrum facilitiates its use as a tool for determining a material's probable identity. For instance, a white powder may have a UV spectrum comparable to heroin, and therefore may be tentatively identified as such. (Fortunately, sugar and starch, common diluents of heroin, do not absorb UV light.) However, this technique will not provide for a definitive result; the possibility always exists that there are other drugs or materials that have a UV absorption spectrum similar to that of heroin. But this lack of specificity does not diminish the value of the technique, for the analyst has quickly eliminated thousands of other possible drugs from consideration and can now proceed to conduct other confirmatory tests, such as thin-layer or gas chromatography, to complete the identification.

In contrast to the simplicity of a UV spectrum, absorption in the infrared region provides a far more complex pattern. Figure 5-15 (a) and (b) depicts the IR spectra of heroin and secobarbital. Here the absorption bands are so numerous that each spectrum can provide enough characteristics to specifically identify a substance. Different materials always have distinctively different infrared spectra; each IR spectrum is therefore equivalent to being a "fingerprint" of that substance and no other. This technique is one of the few tests available to the forensic scientist that can be considered specific in itself for identification. The IR spectra of thousands of organic compounds have been collected, indexed, and catalogued to serve as invaluable references for identifying organic substances.

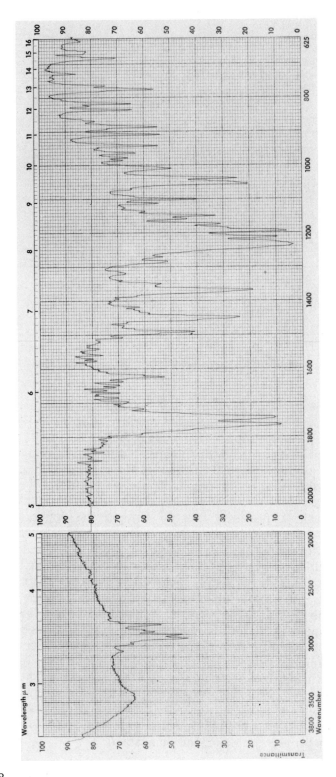

Figure 5-15(a). Infrared spectrum of heroin.

128

Figure 5-15(b). Infrared spectrum of secobarbital.

129

MASS SPECTROMETRY

In a previous section the operation of the gas chromatograph was discussed. This instrument is one of the most important tools to be found in a crime laboratory. Its ability to separate the components of a complex mixture is unsurpassed. However, gas chromatography does suffer one important drawback, that is, its inability to produce a specific identification. A forensic chemist cannot unequivocally state the identification of a substance based solely on a retention time as determined by the gas chromatograph. Fortunately, by coupling the gas chromatograph to a mass spectrometer this problem has largely been overcome.

The separation of a mixture's components is first accomplished on the gas chromatograph. A direct connection between the GC column and the mass spectrometer then allows each component to flow into the spectrometer as it emerges from the gas chromatograph. In the mass spectrometer the material enters a high-vacuum chamber where a beam of high-energy electrons is aimed at the sample molecules. The electrons collide with the molecules causing them to lose electrons and to acquire a positive charge (commonly called *ions*). These positively charged molecules or ions are very unstable or are formed with excess energy and almost instantaneously decompose into numerous smaller fragments. The fragments then pass through an electric or magnetic field where they are separated according to their masses. The unique feature of mass spectrometry is that under carefully controlled conditions no two substances produce the same fragmentation pattern. In essence, one can think of this pattern as a "fingerprint" of the substance being examined.

The technique thus offers itself as a specific means for identifying a chemical structure. It is also sensitive to minute concentrations. At present, mass spectrometry finds its widest application in areas relating to the identification of drugs; however, further research is expected to yield significant applications with respect to the identification of other types of physical evidence. Figure 5-16 illustrates the mass spectrum of heroin; here, each line represents a fragment of a different mass (actually the ratio of mass to charge), and the line height reflects the relative abundance of each fragment.

The combination of the gas chromatograph and mass spectrometer is further enhanced when a computer is added to the system. The integrated gas chromatograph/mass spectrometer/computer system provides the ultimate in speed, accuracy, and sensitivity. With the ability to record and store in its memory several hundred mass spectra, such a system can detect and identify substances present in only one-millionth of a gram quantities. Furthermore, the computer can be programmed to compare an unknown spectrum against a comprehensive library of mass spectra stored in its memory. The advent of personal-size computers and microcircuitry has made it possible to design mass spectrometer systems which can fit on a small table. Such a unit is pictured in Figure 5-17.

Figure 5-16. Mass spectrum of heroin.

Figure 5-17. A table-top mass spectrometer. *Courtesy* Hewlett Packard, Palo Alto, California.

Another variation of mass spectrometry known as **chemical ionization mass spectrometry** has been developed. The major advantage of this approach is that it simplifies the mass spectral fragmentation pattern that is produced by a substance. This is exemplified by the relatively simple chemical ionization mass spectrum of heroin shown in Figure 5-18, as contrasted with its conventional and more complex mass spectrum shown in Figure 5-16. Because chemical ionization patterns are simple and easy to interpret, the forensic scientist can analyze mixtures placed directly into the mass spectrometer without resorting to a prior gas chromatographic separation.

Figure 5-18.   Chemical ionization mass spectrum of heroin.

REVIEW QUESTIONS

1. Anything that has mass and occupies space is defined as _____.
2. The basic building blocks of all substances are the _____.
3. The number of elements known today is _____.
4. An arrangement of elements by similar chemical properties is accomplished in the _____ table.
5. An _____ is the smallest particle of an element that can exist.
6. Substances composed of two or more elements are called _____.
7. A _____ is the smallest unit of a compound formed by the union of two or more atoms.
8. The physical state that retains a definite shape and volume is a _____.
9. A gas (has, has no) definite shape or volume.
10. During the process of _____ solids will go directly to the gaseous state, bypassing the liquid state.
11. The attraction forces between the molecules of a liquid are (more, less) than those in a solid.
12. Different _____ are separated by definite visible boundaries.

13. Carbon-containing substances are classified as _____.
14. _____ substances encompass all noncarbon containing materials.
15. A _____ analysis describes the identity of a material, and a _____ analysis relates to a determination of the quantity of a substance.
16. The study of the absorption of light by chemical substances is known as _____.
17. The separation of a mixture's components can be accomplished utilizing the technique of _____.
18. Henry's Law describes the distribution of a volatile chemical compound between its liquid and gas phases. (True, False)
19. The (higher, lower) the solubility of a gas in a liquid, the greater will be its tendency to remain dissolved in that liquid.
20. In order for chromatography to occur, one phase must be made to move continuously in one direction over a stationary phase. (True, False)
21. A technique that separates mixtures on the basis of their distribution between a stationary liquid phase and a moving gas phase is _____.
22. The time required for a substance to travel through the gas chromatographic column is a useful identifying characteristic known as _____.
23. Solid materials that are not readily dissolved in solvents for injection into the gas chromatograph can be _____ into numerous gaseous products prior to entering the gas chromatograph.
24. A major advantage of high-performance liquid chromatography is that the entire process takes place at _____ temperature.
25. A technique that utilizes a moving liquid phase and a stationary solid phase to separate mixtures is _____.
26. Since most chemical compounds are colorless, the final step of the thin-layer development usually requires that they be _____ by spraying with a chemical reagent.
27. The distance a spot has traveled up a thin-layer plate can be assigned a numerical value known as the _____ value.
28. Thin-layer chromatography yields the positive identification of a material. (True, False)
29. The migration of materials along a stationary phase under the influence of an electrical potential describes the technique of _____.
30. Color is a usual indication that substances selectively absorb light. (True, False)
31. The distance between two successive identical points on a wave is known as _____.
32. Frequency and wavelength are directly proportional to one another. (True, False)

33. Light, X-rays, and radio waves are all members of the _____ spectrum.
34. Red light is (higher, lower) in frequency than violet light.
35. Light that has all its waves pulsating in unison is called a _____.
36. One model of light depicts it as consisting of energy particles known as _____.
37. The energy of a light particle (photon) is directly proportional to its frequency. (True, False)
38. Red light is (more, less) energetic than violet light.
39. The selective absorption of electromagnetic radiation by materials (can, cannot) be used as an aid for identification.
40. The amount of radiation a substance will absorb is directly proportional to its concentration as defined by _____ Law.
41. The _____ is the instrument used to measure and record the absorption spectrum of a chemical substance.
42. The function of the _____ is to select a single frequency of light emanating from the spectrophotometer's source.
43. An (ultraviolet, infrared) absorption spectrum provides a unique "fingerprint" of a chemical substance.
44. The technique of _____ exposes molecules to a beam of high-energy electrons in order to fragment them.

FURTHER REFERENCES

Krishnan, S. S., *An Introduction to Modern Criminal Investigation with Basic Laboratory Techniques*, Springfield, Ill.: Charles C. Thomas, Publisher, 1978.

Midkiff, Charles R., Jr., and Willard D. Washington, "Diamond and Sapphire Cell Infrared Spectroscopy—A Powerful New Tool in the Forensic Science Laboratory," *Journal of Police Science and Administration*, 7 (1979), 426.

Saferstein, Richard, Jew-Ming Chao, and J. Manura, "Identification of Drugs by Chemical Ionization Mass Spectroscopy—Part II," *Journal of Forensic Sciences*, 19, no. 3 (1974), 463.

Saferstein, Richard, "Forensic Applications of Mass Spectrometry," in *Forensic Science Handbook*, R. Saferstein, ed. Englewood Cliffs, N.J.: Prentice-Hall, Inc., 1982.

Smith, R. N., "Forensic Applications of High-Performance Liquid Chromatography," in *Forensic Science Handbook*, R. Saferstein, ed. Englewood Cliffs, N.J.: Prentice-Hall, Inc., 1982.

Stafford, David T., "Forensic Capillary Gas Chromatography," in *Forensic Science Handbook*, Vol. 2, R. Saferstein, ed. Englewood Cliffs, N.J.: Prentice-Hall, Inc., 1987.

AUDIOVISUAL PRESENTATIONS

Colorimetric Analysis (39 35-mm slides and audio tape). Prentice-Hall Media, Tarrytown, N.Y.

Gas Chromatography—Basic Relationships and Instrumentation (43 35-mm slides and audio tape). Prentice-Hall Media, Tarrytown, N.Y.

Use Thin-Layer Chromatography for Simple Separations (39 35-mm slides and audio tape). Prentice-Hall Media, Tarrytown, N.Y.

6

Inorganic Analysis

INTRODUCTION

In the previous chapter, analytical techniques were described for characterizing a class of matter known as organics. Generally, these materials contain the element carbon in their chemical composition. Although organic substances do constitute a substantial portion of the physical evidence submitted to crime laboratories, the element carbon does not appear among the earth's most abundant elements. It is perhaps rather surprising to observe that about three-quarters of the weight of the earth's crust is composed of only two elements—oxygen and silicon. In fact, only ten elements make up approximately 99 percent of the earth's crust (see Table 6-1). The remaining elements may be considered almost as impurities, although exceedingly important ones. Carbon, the element that is a constituent of most chemical compounds, comprises less than 0.1 percent of the earth's crust.

Considering these facts, it is certainly reasonable to expect that noncarbon-containing substances—that is, inorganics—will be encountered as physical evidence at crime scenes. One only has to consider the prevalence of metallic materials, such as iron, steel, copper, and aluminum, in our society to understand the possibilities of finding tools, coins, weapons, and metal scrapings at crime scenes.

Less well-known, but perhaps almost as significant to the criminalist, is the utilization of inorganic chemicals as pigments in paints and dyes, the

Table 6-1.

ELEMENTAL ABUNDANCE AS PERCENTAGES IN THE EARTH'S CRUST

Element	Percentage by Weight
Oxygen	47.3
Silicon	27.7
Aluminum	7.9
Iron	4.5
Calcium	3.5
Sodium	2.5
Potassium	2.5
Magnesium	2.2
Titanium	0.5
Hydrogen	0.2
Other Elements	1.2

incorporation of inorganics into explosive formulations, and the prevalence of inorganic poisons such as mercury, lead, or arsenic.

To appreciate fully the role that inorganic analysis has in forensic science, we must first examine its application to the basic objectives of the crime laboratory—the identification and comparison of physical evidence. The identification of inorganic evidence is exemplified by a typical request to examine an explosive formulation suspected of containing the inorganic chemical potassium chlorate, or perhaps to examine a poisonous powder thought to be arsenic. In each case, the forensic scientist must perform tests that will ultimately determine the specific chemical identity of the suspect materials to the exclusion of all others. Only after tests are completed and their results found to be identical to tests previously recorded for a known potassium chlorate or a known arsenic can a valid conclusion as to the chemical identity of the evidence be reached.

However, in a situation that requires a comparison of two or more objects in order to ascertain their common origin, a different problem is presented to the analyst. For example, a criminalist may be requested to determine whether or not a piece of brass pipe found in the possession of a suspect compares to a broken pipe found at the crime scene. The condition of the two pipes might not allow for their comparison by the physical fitting together of broken edges. Under these circumstances, the only alternative will be to attempt a comparison through chemical analysis. Here, it is not enough for the analyst to conclude that both pipes are alike because they are brass (an alloy of copper and zinc). After all, hundreds of thousands of brass pipes are known to exist, a situation that is hardly conducive to proving that these two particular pipes were at one time a single unit. The examiner must go a step further to try and distinguish these pipes from all others. Although this may not be possible, a comparison of the pipes' trace elements—that is, elements present in small quantities—will provide a meaningful criterion for at least increasing the probability that the two pipes originated from the same source.

Considering the fact that most of our raw materials originate from the earth's crust, it is not surprising to observe that they are rarely obtained in pure form; instead, they include numerous elemental impurities that usually have to be eliminated through industrial processing. However, in most cases it is not economically feasible to completely exclude all such minor impurities, especially in light of the fact that their presence will have no effect on the appearance or performance of the final product. For this reason, we find that many of our manufactured products, and even most natural materials, contain small quantities of elements present in concentrations of less than 1 percent. For the criminalist, the presence of trace elements is particularly useful because they provide "invisible" markers that may establish the source of a material or at least provide additional points for comparison. Table 6-2 illustrates how two types of brass alloys can readily be distinguished by their elemental composition. Similarly, the comparison of trace elements present in paint or other types of metallic specimens may provide particularly meaningful data with respect to source or origin. Currently, forensic investigators are examining the evidential value of trace elements known to be present in hair, soil, fibers, and glass, as well as in all types of metallic objects. One illustrative example of this application occurred with the examination of the bullet and bullet fragments recovered after the assassination of President Kennedy.

Table 6-2.

ELEMENTAL ANALYSIS OF BRASS ALLOYS

Elemental	High-Tensile Brass %	Manganese Brass %
Copper	57.0	58.6
Aluminum	2.8	1.7
Zinc	35.0	33.8
Manganese	2.13	1.06
Iron	1.32	0.90
Nickel	0.48	1.02
Tin	0.64	1.70
Lead	0.17	0.72
Silicon	0.08	Nil

Source: *R. L. Williams, "An Evaluation of the SEM with X-Ray Microanalyzer Accessory for Forensic Work," in* Scanning Electron Microscopy/1971, *O. Johari and I. Corvin, eds. (Chicago: IIT Research Institute, 1971), p. 541.*

EVIDENCE IN THE ASSASSINATION
OF PRESIDENT KENNEDY

Ever since President Kennedy was killed in 1963, questions have lingered on as to whether Lee Harvey Oswald was part of a conspiracy to assassinate the President, or, as the Warren Commission concluded, a lone assassin. In arriving at their conclusions the Warren Commission reconstructed the crime as follows: Oswald fired three shots from behind the President while positioned in the Texas School Book Depository building. The President was struck by two bullets, with one bullet totally missing the President's limousine. One bullet hit the President in the back, exited from his throat, and then went on to strike Governor Connally who was sitting in a jump seat in front of the President. The bullet hit Connally first in his back, then exited from his chest, struck his right wrist, and then temporarily lodged in his left thigh. This bullet was later found in the Governor's stretcher at the hospital. A second bullet fatally wounded the President in the skull.

In a room at the Texas School Book Depository was found a 6.5-mm Mannlicher-Carcano military rifle with Oswald's palm print on it. Also found were three spent 6.5-mm Western Cartridge Co./Mannlicher-Carcano (WCC/MC) cartridge cases. Oswald, an employee of the Book Depository, had been sent there that morning and also a few minutes after the assassination, disappearing soon thereafter. He was apprehended a few miles away from the Depository nearly two hours after the shooting.

Critics of the Warren Commission have long argued that evidence exists for proving Oswald did not act alone. Eyewitness accounts and acoustical data interpreted by some experts have been used to advocate the contention that someone else fired at the President from a region in front of the limousine (the so-called "grassy knoll"). Furthermore, it is argued, that the Warren Commission's reconstruction of the crime relied on the assumption that only one bullet caused both the President's throat and Connally's back wounds. Critics contend that such damage would have deformed and mutilated a bullet. Instead, the recovered bullet showed some flattening, no deformity, and only about a 1 percent weight loss.

In 1977, at the request of the U.S. House of Representatives Select Committee on Assassinations, the bullet taken from Connally's stretcher along with bullet fragments recovered from the car and various wound areas were examined for trace element levels.

Lead alloys used for the manufacture of bullets contain an assortment of trace elements. For example, antimony is often added to lead as a hardening agent; copper, bismuth, and silver are other trace elements commonly found in bullet lead. In this case, the bullet and bullet fragments were compared for their antimony and silver content. Previous studies had amply demonstrated that the levels of these two elements are particularly important for characterizing WCC/MC bullets. Bullet lead from this type of ammunition ranges in antimony concentration from 20 to 1200 parts per million (ppm) and 5 to 15 ppm in silver content.

As can be seen in Table 6-3, the samples designated Q1 and Q9 (the Connally stretcher bullet and fragments from Connally's wrist, respectively) are indistinguishable from one another in antimony and silver content. The samples Q2, Q4, 5, and Q14 (Q4, 5 being fragments from Kennedy's brain, and Q2 and Q14 being fragments recovered from two different areas in the car) also are indistinguishable in antimony and silver content but are different from Q1 and Q9.

The conclusions derived from studying these results are:

1. There is evidence of only two bullets—one of a composition of 815 ppm antimony and 9.3 ppm silver, the other of a composition of 622 ppm antimony and 8.1 ppm silver.
2. Both bullets have a composition highly consistent with WCC/MC bullet lead, although other sources cannot entirely be ruled out.
3. The bullet found in the Connally stretcher also damaged Connally's wrist. The absence of bullet fragments from the back wounds of Kennedy and Connally prevented any effort at linking these wounds to the stretcher bullet.

None of the above conclusions can totally verify the Warren Commission's reconstruction of the assassination, but the results are at least consistent with the Commission's findings.

Table 6-3.

ANTIMONY AND SILVER CONCENTRATIONS IN THE KENNEDY
ASSASSINATION BULLETS

Sample	Silver (parts per million)*	Antimony (parts per million)	Sample Description
Q1	8.8 ± 0.5	833 ± 9	Connally stretcher bullet
Q9	9.8 ± 0.5	797 ± 7	Fragments from Connally's wrist
Q2	8.1 ± 0.6	602 ± 4	Large fragment from car
Q4, 5	7.9 ± 0.3	621 ± 4	Fragment from Kennedy's brain
Q14	8.2 ± 0.4	642 ± 6	Small fragments found in car

Reprinted *with permission from V. P. Guinn, "JFK Assassination: Bullet Analyses,"* Analytical Chemistry, *51 (1979), 484A. Copyright 1979, American Chemical Society.* *One part per million equals 0.0001%.*

The analyses on the Kennedy assassination bullets were performed by the technique of neutron activation analysis. The remainder of this chapter will be devoted to describing this and other techniques currently used for the examination of inorganic physical evidence.

THE EMISSION SPECTRUM OF ELEMENTS

We have already observed that organic molecules can readily be characterized by their selective absorption of ultraviolet, visible, or infrared radiations. Equally significant to the analytical chemist is the knowledge that the elements will also selectively absorb and emit light. These observations form the basis of two important analytical techniques designed to determine the elemental composition of materials—emission spectroscopy and atomic absorption spectrophotometry.

The statement that elements emit light should not come as a total surprise, for one need only observe the common tungsten incandescent light bulb or the glow of a neon light to confirm this observation. When the light emitted from a bulb or from any other light source is passed through a prism, it is separated into its component colors or frequencies. The resulting display of colors is called an emission spectrum.

When sunlight or the light from an incandescent bulb is passed through a prism, we have already observed that a range of rainbow colors is produced. This emission spectrum is called a continuous spectrum because all the colors merge or blend into one another to form a continuous band. However, not all light sources produce such a spectrum. For example, if the light from a sodium lamp or a mercury arc lamp or a neon light was passed through a prism, the resultant spectrum would consist not of a continuous band but of several individual colored lines separated by dark spaces. Here, each line represents a definite wavelength or frequency of light that is separate and distinct from all others present in the spectrum. This type of spectrum is called a line spectrum. Figure 6-1 shows the line spectra of several elements.

It is important to realize that heated matter in a solid or liquid state produces a continuous spectrum that is not very indicative of its composition. However, if this same matter is vaporized and "excited" by exposure to high temperature, each element present will emit light that is composed of select frequencies that are characteristic of the element. This spectrum is in essence a "fingerprint" of an element and offers itself as a very practical method of identification. Sodium vapor, for example, always shows the same line spectrum, which differs from the spectrum of all other elements.

An emission spectrograph is an instrument used to obtain and record the line spectra of elements. Essentially, this instrument requires a means for vaporizing and exciting the atoms of elements so that they emit light, a means for separating this light into its component frequencies, and a means

Hydrogen

Helium

Mercury

Figure 6-1. Some characteristic emission spectra.

of recording the resultant spectrum. A simple emission spectrograph is depicted in Figure 6-2.

Excitation of the specimen under investigation is accomplished when it is inserted between two carbon electrodes through which a direct current arc is passed. The arc produces a sufficient amount of heat to vaporize and excite the specimen's atoms. The resultant emitted light is collected by a lens and is focused onto a prism that disperses it into component frequencies. The separated frequencies are then directed toward a photographic plate where they are recorded as line images. Normally, a specimen consists of numerous elements; hence, the typical emission spectrum contains many lines. Each element present in the spectrum can be identified when it is compared to a standard chart that shows the position of the principal spectral lines of all the elements. However, the more common situation in forensic analysis

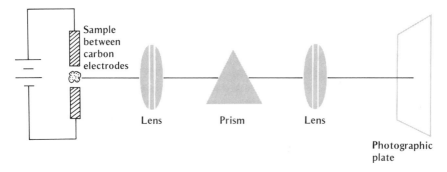

Sample between carbon electrodes

Lens

Prism

Lens

Photographic plate

Figure 6-2. Parts of a simple emission spectrograph.

simply requires a rapid comparison of the elemental composition of two or more specimens. This can readily be accomplished when the emission spectra are matched line for line, an approach illustrated in Figure 6-3. Here the emission spectra of two paint chips are shown to be comparable.

A recent advancement in emission spectroscopy has been the utilization of a laser beam to vaporize a small portion of the specimen. The laser beam is focused through a microscope onto a selected area of the specimen. The intense energy of laser radiation is sufficient to vaporize the specimen, causing it to rise between two carbon electrodes situated just above the sample. As the vapor passes between the electrodes, it triggers an electrical discharge that excites the atoms and causes them to emit light (see Figure 6-4). In this manner it is possible to determine the elemental composition of a specimen that is no larger than the size of the period at the end of this sentence. Trace elements present in concentrations of 0.1 to 0.01 percent are readily detected by this procedure.

Figure 6-3. A comparison of paint chips 1 and 2 by emission spectrographic analysis. A line-for-line comparison shows both paints have the same elemental composition.

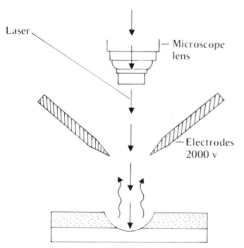

Figure 6-4.   Laser microprobe.

ATOMIC ABSORPTION SPECTROPHOTOMETRY

When an atom is vaporized, it will absorb many of the same frequencies of light that it emits in an excited state. The selective absorption of light by atoms is the basis for a technique known as **atomic absorption spectrophotometry**. A simple atomic absorption spectrophotometer is illustrated in Figure 6-5.

In atomic absorption spectrophotometry the specimen is heated to a temperature that is hot enough to vaporize its atoms while leaving a substantial number of atoms in an unexcited state. Normally, the specimen is inserted into an air-acetylene flame to achieve this temperature. The vaporized atoms are then exposed to radiation emitted from a light source. In practice, the technique achieves great specificity by using as its radiation source a discharge tube made of the very same element being analyzed in the specimen. When the discharge lamp is turned on, it emits only those frequencies of light that are present in the emission spectrum of the element. Likewise, the sample will only absorb these frequencies when it contains this very same element. Therefore, if one wanted to determine the presence of the element antimony in a specimen, the atomic absorption spectrophotometer would have to be fitted with a discharge lamp that is constructed of antimony. Under these conditions the sample will only absorb light when it contains antimony.

Once the radiation has passed through the sample, a monochromator, consisting of a prism or a diffraction grating and a slit, isolates the desired radiation frequency and transmits it to a detector. The detector converts the light into an electrical signal, the intensity of which is recorded on a stripchart recorder.

The absorption of light by the element of interest is the phenomenon that is being measured in atomic absorption spectrophotometry. The concentration of the absorbing element will be directly proportional to the

Figure 6-5. Parts of a simple flame atomic absorption spectrophotometer.

quantity of the light absorbed. The higher the concentration of the element, the more light absorbed. For this reason, atomic absorption spectroscopy has its most useful application in providing an accurate determination of an element's concentration in a sample. Furthermore, the technique is sufficiently sensitive as to find wide application in detecting and quantitating elements that are present at trace levels. However, the technique does have one drawback, in that the analyst can only determine one element at a time, each time having to select the proper lamp to match the particular element under investigation.

Although atomic absorption spectrophotometry has been utilized for chemical analysis since 1955, it has not yet found wide application for solving forensic problems. However, a modification in the design of the instrument promises to change this situation. By substituting a heated graphite furnace or a heated strip of metal (tantalum) for the flame, analysts have succeeded in achieving a more efficient means of atomic volatilization and as a result have produced a substantial increase in the sensitivity of the technique. Many elements can now be detected at levels that approach one-trillionth of a gram.

The high sensitivity of "flameless" atomic absorption now equals or surpasses that of any known analytical procedure. Considering the relative simplicity and low cost of the technique, atomic absorption spectrophotometry has become an attractive method for detecting and measuring the smallest levels of trace elements present in physical evidence.

THE ORIGIN OF EMISSION AND ABSORPTION SPECTRA

Any proposed theory that attempts to explain the origin of emission and absorption spectra must relate to the fundamental structure of the element—the atom. Scientists now know that the atom is composed of even more elementary particles that are collectively known as *subatomic particles*. The most important subatomic particles are the **proton, electron,** and **neutron.** The masses of the proton and neutron are each about 1837 times the mass of an electron. The proton is a particle with a positive electrical charge; the electron has a negative charge equal in magnitude to that of the proton; and the neutron is a neutral particle having neither a positive nor a negative charge. The properties of the electron, proton, and neutron are summarized below:

Particle	Symbol	Relative Mass	Electrical Charge
Proton	P	1	+1
Neutron	n	1	0
Electron	e	1/1837	−1

A popular descriptive model of the atom, and the one that will be adopted for the purpose of this discussion, pictures an atom as consisting of electrons orbiting around a central nucleus—an image that is analogous to our solar system, in which the planets revolve around the sun.[1] The nucleus of the atom is comprised of positively charged protons and neutrons that have no charge. Because the atom has no net electrical charge, the number of protons must always be equal to the number of negatively charged electrons in orbit around the nucleus.

With this knowledge, we can now begin to describe the atomic structure of the elements; for example, hydrogen has a nucleus consisting of one proton and no neutrons, and it has one orbiting electron. Helium has a nucleus comprised of two protons and two neutrons with two electrons in orbit around the nucleus (see Figure 6-6).

The behavior and properties that distinguish one element from another must be related to those differences that exist in the atomic structure of each element. One such distinction resides in the fact that each element possesses a different number of protons. This number is called the **atomic number** of the element. As we look back at the periodic table, illustrated in Figure 5-1, we see that the elements are numbered consecutively from 1 to 106. This number represents the atomic number or number of protons associated with each element. **An element is therefore a collection of atoms, all having the same number of protons.** Thus, each atom of hydrogen has 1 and only 1 proton, each atom of helium has 2 protons, each atom of silver has 47 protons, and each atom of lead has 82 protons in its nucleus.

To explain the origin of atomic spectra, our attention must now focus on the orbiting electrons of the atom. As electrons move around the nucleus they are confined to a path of flight from which they cannot stray. This orbital path is associated with a definite amount of energy and is therefore called an *energy level*. Each element has its own set of characteristic energy levels located at varying distances from the nucleus. Some of these levels are occupied by electrons; others are empty.

An atom will be in its most stable state when all of its electrons are

Hydrogen   Helium

Figure 6-6. The atomic structure of hydrogen and helium.

---

[1] Actually, the electrons are moving so rapidly around the nucleus as to be best visualized as being in the form of an electron cloud spread out over the surface of the atom.

positioned in their lowest possible energy orbitals in the atom. When an atom absorbs energy, such as heat or light, its electrons are pushed into higher energy orbitals. In this condition the atom is in an **excited state**. However, because energy levels have fixed values, only a definite amount of energy can be absorbed in moving an electron from one level to another. This is a most important observation, for it means that atoms will absorb only a definite value of energy, and all other energy values will be excluded. In atomic absorption spectrophotometry, a photon of light interacts with an electron, causing it to jump into a higher orbital as shown in Figure 6-7(a). A specific frequency of light is required to effect this transition, and its energy must correspond to the exact energy difference between the two orbitals involved in the transition. This energy difference is expressed by the relationship $E = hf$, where E represents the energy difference between the two orbitals, f is the frequency of absorbed light, and h is a universal constant called Planck's constant. Any energy value that is more or less than this difference will not affect the transition. Hence, an element is selective in the frequency of light it will absorb, and this selectivity is determined by the electron energy levels each element possesses.

In the same manner, if atoms are exposed to intense heat, enough energy will be generated to push electrons into higher unoccupied energy orbitals. Normally, the electron will not remain in this excited state for long, and it will quickly fall back to its original energy level. As the electron falls back, it will have to release energy. An emission spectrum testifies to the fact that this energy loss comes about in the form of light emission; see Figure 6-7(b). The frequency of light emitted will again be determined by the relationship $E = hf$, where E is the energy difference between the upper and lower energy levels, and f is the frequency of emitted light. Because each element has its own characteristic set of energy levels, each will emit a unique set of frequency values. The emission spectrum thus provides us with a "picture" of the energy levels that surround the nucleus of each element.

Thus, we see that as far as atoms are concerned, energy is a two-way street. Energy can be put into the atom while at the same time energy is given off; what goes in must come out. The chemist has the option of studying the atom using either approach. Atomic absorption spectrophotometry carefully measures the value and amount of light energy going into the atom; emission spectroscopy collects and measures the various light energies given off. The end result is the same; atoms are identified by the existence of characteristic energy levels.

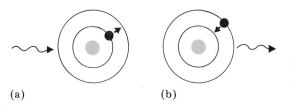

(a)   (b)

Figure 6-7. (a) The absorption of light by an atom causing an electron to jump into a higher orbital. (b) The emission of light by an atom caused by an electron falling back to a lower orbital.

NEUTRON ACTIVATION ANALYSIS

Once scientists realized that it was possible to change the number of sub-atomic particles in the atom's nucleus, the unleashing of a new source of energy—nuclear energy—was inevitable. This energy has proven so awesome in its power that the very survival of civilization will depend on man's ability to refrain from using its destructive forces. Today, of course, this threat does not obscure the fact that controlled nuclear energy promises to be a source of power capable of relieving our dependency on earth's dwindling reserves of fossil fuels. For the chemist, nuclear chemistry offers itself as a new tool for identifying and quantitating the elements.

Until now, our discussion of subatomic particles has been limited to the proton and electron. However, in order to understand the principles of nuclear chemistry we must look at the other important subatomic particle, the neutron. Although the atoms of a single element must have the same number of protons, there is nothing to prevent them from having different numbers of neutrons. The total number of protons and neutrons in a nucleus is known as the **atomic mass number**. Atoms having the same number of protons but differing solely in the number of neutrons they possess are called **isotopes**. For example, the element hydrogen actually consists of three isotopes; besides ordinary hydrogen, which has one proton and no neutrons in its nucleus, two other isotopes exist, deuterium and tritium. Deuterium (or heavy hydrogen) also has one proton but contains one neutron as well. Tritium has one proton and two neutrons in its nucleus. The atomic structures of these isotopes are shown in Figure 6-8. Therefore, all the isotopes of hydrogen have an atomic number of one but differ in their **atomic mass numbers**. Hydrogen has an atomic mass of one, deuterium a mass of two, and tritium a mass of three. Ordinary hydrogen makes up 99.98 percent of all the hydrogen atoms found in nature.

Like hydrogen, most elements are known to have two or more isotopes. The element tin, for example, has as many as ten isotopes. Many of these isotopes are quite stable and for all intents and purposes, the isotopes of any one element have indistinguishable properties. Others, however, are not as stable and will decompose with time by a process known as **radioactive decay**. Radioactivity is the emission of radiation that accompanies the spontaneous disintegration of unstable nuclei. Radioactivity is actually comprised of three types of radiation: **alpha rays**, **beta rays**, and **gamma rays**.

Figure 6-8. Isotopes of hydrogen.

Alpha rays have proven to be positively charged particles, each having a mass approximately four times that of a hydrogen atom. These particles are known to be helium atoms stripped of their orbiting electrons. Beta rays are actually electrons, and the gamma rays are electromagnetic radiations similar to X-rays but of a higher frequency and energy (refer to the electromagnetic spectrum in Figure 5-11). Fortunately, the vast majority of naturally occurring isotopes are not radioactive, and those that do exist—i.e., radium, uranium, and thorium—are found in such small quantities in the earth's crust that their radioactivity presents no hazard to human survival.

The existence of isotopes would be of little importance to the forensic chemist were it not for the fact that scientists have mastered the techniques for synthesizing radioactive isotopes. If the only distinction between isotopes of an element is the number of neutrons each possesses, is it not reasonable to assume that by bombarding atoms with neutrons, some neutrons will be captured to make new isotopes? This is exactly what takes place in a nuclear reactor. A nuclear reactor is simply a source of neutrons that can be used for bombarding the atoms of a specimen, thereby creating radioactive isotopes. When a neutron is captured by the nucleus of an atom, a new isotope is formed with one additional neutron. In this state the nuclei are said to be activated, and many will immediately begin to decompose by emitting radioactivity.

To identify the activated isotope it is necessary to measure the energy of the gamma rays emitted as radioactivity. The gamma rays of each element can be associated with a characteristic energy value. Furthermore, once the element has been identified, its concentration can be measured by the intensity of its gamma ray radiation; intensity is directly proportional to the concentration of the element in a specimen. The technique of bombarding specimens with neutrons and measuring the resultant gamma ray radioactivity is known as **neutron activation analysis**. The process is depicted in Figure 6-9.

The major advantage of neutron activation analysis is that it offers itself as a nondestructive method for identifying and quantitating trace elements. A median detection sensitivity of one-billionth of a gram (one nanogram) makes neutron activation analysis one of the most sensitive methods available today for the quantitative detection of many elements. Further, neutron activation has the capability to perform a simultaneous analysis for 20 to 30 elements. A major drawback to the technique is its expense. Only a handful of crime laboratories have access to a nuclear reactor; in addition, sophisticated analyzers are needed to detect and discriminate gamma ray emissions.

As far as forensic analysis is concerned, neutron activation has been employed for characterizing the trace elements present in metals, drugs, paint, soil, gunpowder residues, and hair. A typical illustration of its application occurred during the investigation of a theft of copper telegraphic wires in Canada. Four lengths of copper wire (A_1, A_2, A_3, A_4) found at the scene of the theft were compared by neutron activation with a length of copper wire

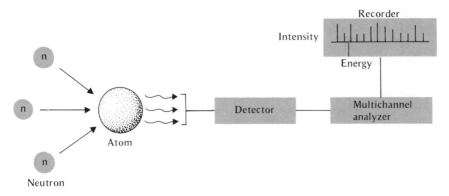

Figure 6-9. The neutron activation process requires the capture of a neutron by the nucleus of an atom. The new atom is now radioactive and emits gamma rays. A detector permits the identification of the radioactive atoms present by measuring the energies and intensities of the gamma rays emitted.

(B) seized at a scrap yard and suspected of being stolen. All were bare, single-stranded wire with the same general physical appearance and a diameter of 0.28 cm. Prior experiments had revealed that significant variations could be expected in the concentration levels of the trace elements selenium, gold, antimony, and silver for wires originating from different sources. A comparison of these elements present in the wire involved in the theft was undertaken. After exposing the wires to neutrons in a nuclear reactor, neutron activation analysis revealed a match between A_1 and B that was well within experimental error (see Table 6-4). The findings suggested a common origin of control and suspect wires.

Table 6-4.

CONCENTRATION OF TRACE ELEMENTS IN COPPER WIRE

	Selenium	*Gold*	*Antimony*	*Silver*
Control Wire				
A_1	2.4	0.047	0.16	12.7
A_2	3.5	0.064	0.27	17.2
A_3	2.6	0.050	0.20	13.3
A_4	1.9	0.034	0.21	12.6
Suspect Wire				
B	2.3	0.042	0.15	13.0

Source: *R. K. H. Chan, "Identification of Single-Stranded Copper Wires by Nondestructive Neutron Activation Analysis,"* Journal of Forensic Sciences, *17 (1972), 93. Reprinted by permission of the American Society for Testing and Materials, copyright 1972.*
Note: *Average concentration measured in part per million.*

X-RAY DIFFRACTION

Up until now we have discussed methods for detecting and identifying the elements. Emission spectroscopy, atomic absorption, and neutron activation analysis tell us what elements are present in a particular substance, but they do not provide any information as to how the elements are combined into compounds. One way of eliciting this information is to aim a beam of X-rays at a crystal and to study how the X-rays interact with the atoms that comprise the substance under investigation. This technique is known as **X-ray diffraction**.

X-ray diffraction can only be applied to the study of solid, crystalline materials, that is, solids having a definite and orderly arrangement of their atoms. For example, sodium chloride (common table salt), pictured in Figure 4-7, is crystalline. Fortunately, many substances, including 95 percent of all inorganic compounds, are crystalline in nature and hence are identifiable by X-ray diffraction analysis. The atoms in a crystal can be thought of as being comprised of a series of parallel planes. As the X-rays penetrate the crystal, a portion of the beam is reflected by each of the atomic planes. As the reflected beams leave the crystal's planes they combine with one another to form a series of light and dark bands known as a **diffraction pattern**. Every compound is known to produce its own unique diffraction pattern, thus giving analysts a means for "fingerprinting" compounds.

A diagram depicting the X-ray diffraction process is illustrated in Figure 6-10. Diffraction patterns for potassium nitrate and potassium chlorate, two common constituents of homemade explosives, are shown in Figure 6-11 (a) and (b). A comparison of a questioned specimen with a known X-ray pattern is a rapid and specific way of proving chemical identity.

One drawback to the X-ray diffraction is its lack of sensitivity. The technique is suitable for identifying the major constituents of a mixture, but often fails to detect the presence of substances comprising less than 5 percent of a mixture. For this reason, the forensic chemist must resort to

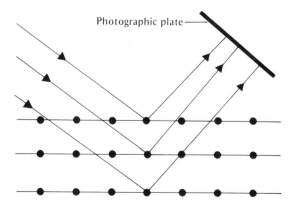

Photographic plate

Figure 6-10. A beam of X-rays being reflected off the atomic planes of a crystal. The diffraction patterns that are formed are recorded on photographic film. These patterns are unique for each crystalline substance.

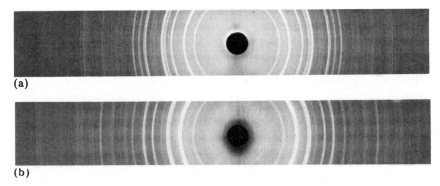

(a)

(b)

Figure 6-11. (a) X-ray diffraction pattern for potassium nitrate. (b) X-ray diffraction pattern for potassium chlorate.

more sensitive techniques—i.e., emission spectroscopy, atomic absorption, and neutron activation analysis—if there is a need to identify the trace elements that may be present.

REVIEW QUESTIONS

1. The elements _____ and _____ make up 75 percent of the weight of the earth's crust.
2. Only _____ elements make up about 99 percent of the weight of the earth's crust.
3. The presence of _____ elements in materials provides useful "invisible" markers when comparing physical evidence.
4. The knowledge that elements selectively _____ and _____ light provides the basis for important analytical techniques designed to detect the presence of elements in materials.
5. An _____ is a display of colors or frequencies emitted from a light source.
6. A continuous spectrum consists of a blending of colors. (True, False)
7. A _____ spectrum shows distinct frequencies or wavelengths of light.
8. A line spectrum of an element (is, is not) characteristic of the element.
9. Matter in a solid or liquid state will produce an emission spectrum that is characteristic of its composition. (True, False)
10. The _____ is an instrument used to obtain and record the line spectrum of elements.
11. A recent development in emission spectroscopy utilizes a _____ _____ in combination with an emission spectrograph.

12. The selective absorption of light by atoms is the basis for a technique known as _____.
13. The composition of the discharge lamp (does, does not) have to be taken into consideration when performing an analysis by atomic absorption for a particular element.
14. One advantage of atomic absorption analysis is that it can simultaneously detect 20–30 elements. (True, False)
15. Three important subatomic particles of the atom are the _____, _____, and _____.
16. The proton and electron (are, are not) of approximately equal mass.
17. A proton imparts the nucleus of an atom with a _____ charge.
18. The number of protons (is, is not) always equal to the number of electrons in orbit around the nucleus of an atom.
19. Each atom of the same element always has the same number of _____ in its nucleus.
20. The number of protons in the nucleus of an atom is called the _____.
21. Each element has its own characteristic set of energy levels. (True, False)
22. To move an electron from one energy level to the next requires a definite amount of energy. (True, False)
23. As an electron falls back from a higher to lower energy level, it emits _____.
24. The total number of protons and neutrons present in a nucleus is known as the _____.
25. Atoms differing only in the number of neutrons present in their nuclei are called _____.
26. Deuterium has the greatest number of protons of all the isotopes of hydrogen. (True, False)
27. Radioactivity is composed of the following emissions: _____, _____, and _____.
28. Beta particles are identical to _____.
29. Electromagnetic radiations similar to X-rays but of a higher energy are _____.
30. A nuclear reactor is a source of _____.
31. The technique of bombarding specimens with neutrons and measuring the resultant gamma ray emissions is known as _____.
32. As X-rays are reflected off a material's surface, they will form a series of light and dark bands known as a _____.
33. X-ray diffraction patterns are obtained from (crystalline, amorphous) substances.

FURTHER REFERENCES

Krishnan, S. S., "Merits and Demerits of Forensic Activation Analysis when Compared to Other Analysis Methods," *Journal of Radioanalytical Chemistry*, 15 (1973), 165–72.

———, *An Introduction to Modern Criminal Investigation with Basic Laboratory Techniques*. Springfield, Ill.: Charles C. Thomas, Publisher, 1978.

Singhal, S. P., "Atomic Absorption Spectroscopy in Forensic Chemistry," *The Canadian Society of Forensic Science Journal*, 7 (1974), 7.

Walls, H. J., *Forensic Science*, 2nd ed. New York: Praeger, 1974.

Willard, H. H., L. L. Merritt, J. A. Dean, and F. A. Settle, Jr., *Instrumental Methods of Analysis*, 6th ed. New York: D. Van Nostrand Co., 1981.

AUDIOVISUAL PRESENTATIONS

Basic Atomic Absorption Spectroscopy—Principles of Atomic Absorption (37 35-mm slides and audio tape). Prentice-Hall Media, Tarrytown, N.Y.

7

The Microscope

A microscope is an optical instrument that uses a lens or a combination of lenses to magnify and resolve the fine details of an object. The earliest methods for examining physical evidence in crime laboratories relied almost solely on the microscope to study the structure and composition of matter. Even the advent of modern analytical instrumentation and techniques in recent years has done little to diminish the usefulness of the microscope for forensic analysis. If anything, the development of the powerful scanning electron microscope promises to add a new dimension to forensic science heretofore unattainable within the limits of the ordinary light microscope.

The earliest and simplest microscope was the single lens commonly referred to as a *magnifying glass*. The hand-held magnifying glass makes things appear larger than they are because of the way light rays are refracted, or bent, in passing from the air into the glass and back into the air. The magnified image is observed by looking through the lens as shown in Figure 7-1. Such an image is known as a virtual image; it can only be seen by looking through a lens and cannot be viewed directly. This is distinguished from a real image, which can be seen directly, like the image that is projected onto a motion picture screen.

The ordinary magnifying glass can achieve a magnification of about five to ten times. Higher magnifying power is obtainable only with a **compound microscope** constructed of two lenses mounted at each end of a hollow tube. The object to be magnified is placed under the lower lens, called the **objective lens**, and the magnified image is viewed through the upper lens, known as the

155

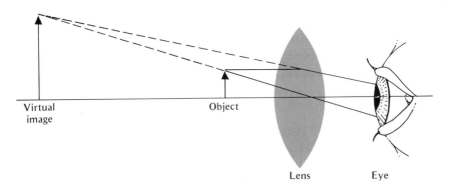

Figure 7-1. The passage of light through a lens showing how magnification is obtained.

eyepiece lens. As shown in Figure 7-2, the objective lens forms a real, inverted, and magnified image of the object. The eyepiece, acting just like a simple magnifying glass, further magnifies this image into a virtual image, which is what is seen by the eye. The combined magnifying power of both lenses can produce an image magnified up to 1500 times.

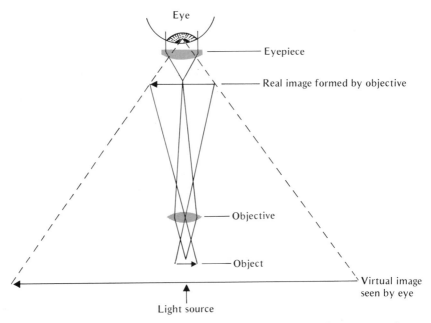

Figure 7-2. The principle of the compound microscope. The passage of light through two lenses forms the virtual image of the object seen by the eye.

The optical principles of the compound microscope are incorporated into the basic design of different types of light microscopes. Those microscopes found most applicable for examining forensic specimens are:

1. The compound microscope
2. The comparison microscope
3. The stereoscopic microscope
4. The polarizing microscope
5. The microspectrophotometer

After a description of these five microscopes, we will talk about a completely different approach to microscopy, the scanning electron microscope (SEM). This instrument focuses a beam of electrons instead of visible light onto the specimen to produce a magnified image. The principle and design of this microscope permit magnifying powers as high as 100,000 times.

THE COMPOUND MICROSCOPE

The parts that collectively comprise the compound microscope are illustrated in Figure 7-3(a). Basically, this microscope consists of a mechanical system, which supports the microscope, and an optical system. The latter illuminates the object under investigation and passes the light through a series of lenses to form an image of the specimen on the retina of the eye. The optical path of light through a compound microscope is shown in Figure 7-3(b).

The mechanical system is composed of six parts:

Base. The support upon which the instrument rests.

Arm. A C-shaped upright structure hinged to the base that supports the microscope and acts as a handle for carrying.

Stage. The horizontal plate upon which the specimens are placed for study. The specimens are normally mounted on glass slides that are held firmly in place on the stage by means of spring clips.

Body Tube. A cylindrical hollow tube on which the objective and eyepiece lenses are mounted at opposite ends. This tube merely serves as a corridor through which light passes from one lens to another.

Coarse Adjustment. This knob serves to focus the microscope lenses on the specimen by raising and lowering the body tube.

Fine Adjustment. The movements effected by this knob are similar to those of the coarse adjustment but are of a much smaller magnitude.

Figure 7-3(a). Parts of the compound microscope: (1) base, (2) arm, (3) stage, (4) body tube, (5) coarse adjust, (6) fine adjust, (7) illuminator, (8) condenser, (9) objective lens, and (10) eyepiece lens. *Courtesy* E. Leitz, Inc., Rockleigh, New Jersey.

The optical system is made up of four parts:

Illuminator. Most modern microscopes use artificial light supplied by a light bulb to illuminate the specimen being examined. If the specimen is transparent, the light is directed up toward and through the specimen stage from an illuminator built into the base of the microscope. This is known as **transmitted illumination.** When the object is opaque—that is, not transparent—the light source must be placed above the specimen so that it can be reflected off the specimen's surface and into the lens system of the microscope. This type of illumination is known as **vertical** or **reflected illumination.**

Condenser. The condenser collects light rays from the base illuminator and concentrates them on the specimen. The simplest condenser is

DIALUX

Figure 7-3(b). Optics of the compound microscope. *Courtesy* E. Leitz, Inc., Rockleigh, New Jersey.

known as the **Abbé condenser.** It consists of two lenses held together in a metal mount. The condenser also includes an iris diaphragm that can be opened or closed to control the amount of light passing into the condenser.

Objective Lens. This is the lens positioned closest to the specimen. To facilitate changing from one objective lens to another, several objectives are mounted on a revolving nosepiece or turret located above the specimen. Most microscopes are **parfocal,** meaning that when the microscope is focused with one objective in position, the other objective can be rotated into place by revolving the nosepiece while the specimen remains very nearly in correct focus.

Eyepiece or Ocular Lens. This is the lens closest to the eye. A microscope having only one eyepiece is **monocular;** one constructed with two eyepieces (one for each eye) is **binocular.**

Each microscope lens is inscribed with a number signifying its magnifying power. The image that is viewed by the microscopist will have a total magnification that is equal to the product of the magnifying power of the objective and eyepiece lenses. For example, an eyepiece lens with a magnification of 10 times (10X) used in combination with an objective lens of 10 times will have a total magnification power of 100 times (100X). Most forensic work will require a 10X eyepiece in combination with either a 4X, 10X, 20X, or 45X objective. The respective magnifications will be 40X, 100X, 200X, and 450X.

In addition, each objective lens is inscribed with its numerical aperture (N.A.). The ability of an objective lens to resolve details into separate images instead of one blurred image is directly proportional to the numerical aperture value of the objective lens. For example, an objective lens of N.A. 1.30 can separate details that are twice as close as compared to a lens with a N.A. of 0.65. The maximum useful magnification of a compound microscope is approximately 1000 times the N.A. of the objective being used. This magnification is sufficient to permit the eye to see all the detail that can be resolved. Any effort to increase the total magnification beyond this figure will yield no additional detail and is referred to as *empty magnification*.

Although a new student of the microscope may be tempted to immediately choose the highest magnifying power available to view a specimen, the experienced microscopist realizes that a number of important factors must be weighed before the selection of magnifying power is made. A first consideration must be the size of the specimen area, or the **field of view**, that the examiner wishes to study. As magnifying power increases, the field of view decreases. Thus, it is best to first select a low magnification in which a good general overall view of the specimen is seen, and to later switch to a higher power in which a smaller portion of the specimen can be viewed in more detail.

The **depth of focus** is also a function of magnifying power. After a focus has been achieved on a specimen, the depth of focus defines the thickness of that specimen. Areas lying above and below this region will be blurred and can only be viewed when the focus is readjusted. Depth of focus decreases as magnifying power increases.

THE COMPARISON MICROSCOPE

Forensic microscopy often requires a side-by-side comparison of specimens. This kind of examination can best be performed with a comparison microscope such as the one pictured in Figure 7-4. Basically, the comparison microscope is two compound microscopes combined into one unit. The unique feature of its design is that it uses a bridge incorporating a series of

Figure 7-4. The comparison microscope. Two independent objective lenses joined together by an optical bridge. *Courtesy* E. Leitz, Inc., Rockleigh, New Jersey.

mirrors and lenses to join two independent objective lenses into a single binocular unit. When a viewer looks through the eyepiece lenses of the comparison microscope, a circular field equally divided into two parts by a fine line is observed. The specimen mounted under the left-hand objective is seen in the left half of the field, and the specimen under the right-hand objective is observed in the right half of the field. It is important that the optical characteristics of the objective lenses be closely matched to assure that each specimen is seen at equal magnification and with minimal but identical lens distortions.

Figure 7-5 shows the striation markings on two bullets that have been placed under the objective lenses of a comparison microscope. Modern firearms examination began with the introduction of the comparison microscope with its ability to give the firearms examiner a side-by-side magnified view of bullets. Bullets that are fired through the same rifle barrel will display comparable rifling markings on their surfaces. By matching the majority of striations present on each bullet, a conclusion that both bullets traveled through the same barrel is justified.

Figure 7-5. Photomicrograph taken through a comparison microscope. On the left are the striation markings on the test-fired bullet, fired through the suspect weapon. On the right are the markings of the crime-scene bullet. *Courtesy* Laboratoire de L'Identité Judicaire, Paris.

THE STEREOSCOPIC MICROSCOPE

The details that characterize the structure of many types of physical evidence do not always require examination under very high magnifications. For such specimens the stereoscopic microscope has proven quite adequate, providing magnifying powers that range from 10X to 125X. This microscope has the advantage of presenting a distinctive three-dimensional image of an object. Also, whereas the image formed by a compound microscope is inverted, the stereoscopic microscope is made more convenient for use by the placement of erecting prisms in its light path, permitting the formation of a right-side-up image. The stereoscopic microscope, shown in Figure 7-6, is actually two monocular compound microscopes properly spaced and aligned to present a three-dimensional image of a specimen to the viewer who looks through both eyepiece lenses.

The stereoscopic microscope is undoubtedly the most frequently used and versatile microscope found in the crime laboratory. Its wide field of view and great depth of focus make it an ideal instrument for locating trace evidence that may be present in debris, garments, weapons, or tools. Furthermore, its potentially large working distance (the distance between the objective lens and the specimen) makes it quite applicable for the microscopic examination of big, bulky items. When fitted with vertical illumination, the stereoscopic microscope becomes the primary tool for characterizing physical evidence as diverse as paint, soil, gunpowder residues, and marijuana.

Figure 7-6. A schematic diagram of a stereoscopic microscope. This microscope is actually two separate monocular microscopes, each having its own set of lenses except for the lowest objective lens, which is common to both microscopes. *Courtesy* Wild Heerbrugg Ltd., Switzerland.

THE POLARIZING MICROSCOPE

It will be recalled from the discussion in Chapter 5 that light's wavelike motion in space can be invoked to explain many facets of its behavior. The waves that comprise a beam of light can be pictured as vibrating in all directions perpendicular to the direction in which the light is traveling. However, it is a familiar observation that when a beam of light passes through certain types of specially fabricated crystalline substances, it emerges vibrating in only one plane. Light that is confined to a single plane of vibration is said to be **plane-polarized**. The device that polarizes light in this manner is called a **polarizer**. A common example of this phenomenon is the passage of sunlight through polaroid sunglasses. By transmitting light vibrating in the vertical plane only, these sunglasses will have the effect of eliminating or reducing light glare. Most glare consists of partially polarized light that has been reflected off horizontal surfaces and thus is vibrating in a horizontal plane.

Because polarized light appears no different to the eye than ordinary light, special means must be devised for detecting it. This is simply accomplished by placing a second polarizing crystal, called an **analyzer**, in the path of the polarized beam. As shown in Figure 7-7, if the polarizer and analyzer are aligned parallel to each other, the polarized light will pass through and be seen by the eye. If, on the other hand, the polarizer and analyzer are set perpendicular to one another, or are "crossed," no light will penetrate, and the result will be total darkness or extinction.

In this manner the design of a compound or stereoscopic microscope can be modified to be outfitted with a polarizer and analyzer so as to be capable of allowing the viewer to detect polarized light. Such a microscope is known as a **polarizing microscope**. Essentially, the polarizer is placed between the light source and the sample stage to polarize the light before it passes through the specimen. The polarized light penetrating the specimen must then pass through an analyzer before it reaches the eyepiece and finally the eye. Normally, the polarizer and analyzer are "crossed" so that when no specimen is in place, the field appears dark. However, the effect of introducing a specimen that polarizes light will be to reorient the polarized light, allowing it to pass through the analyzer. This result produces vivid colors and intensity contrasts that make the specimen readily distinguishable.

The most obvious and important applications of this microscope relate to studying materials that polarize light. For example, as we learned in Chap-

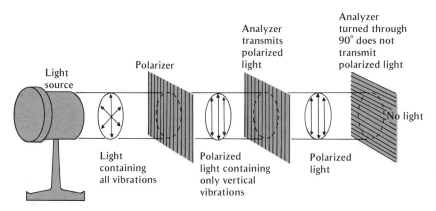

Figure 7-7. Polarization of light.

ter 4 (see page 84), many crystalline substances are birefringent; that is, they will split a beam of light into two light-ray components of different refractive index values. What makes this observation particularly relevant to our discussion of the polarizing microscope is that both light beams are polarized at right angles to one another. With this knowledge, polarizing microscopy has found wide application for the examination of birefringent minerals present in soil. By utilizing the immersion method (see page 87) and selecting the proper immersion liquids, a refractive index corresponding to each plane of polarized light can be determined. Thus, when a mineral is viewed under polarized light in a liquid that matches one of its refractive indices, the Becke line will no longer be visible. This information plus observations on crystal color, and form, etc., makes it possible for the microscopist to identify the mineral. Similarly, criminalists take advantage of the fact that many synthetic fibers are birefringent in order to characterize them with a polarizing microscope.

THE MICROSPECTROPHOTOMETER

From a practical point of view, few instruments present in a crime laboratory can match the versatility of the microscope. The microscope's magnifying power is an indispensable necessity for searching and locating minute traces of physical evidence. Once located, many items of physical evidence may be characterized by a microscopic examination of their morphological features. Likewise, the microscope can be used to study how light interacts with the material under investigation, or it can be used to observe the effects that other chemical substances are having on such evidence. Each of these features will allow an examiner to better characterize and identify physical evidence. Recently, by linking it to a computerized spectrophotometer, a new dimension has been added to the capability of the microscope. This combination has given rise to a new instrument called the **microspectrophotometer**.

In many respects this is an ideal marriage from the forensic scientist's viewpoint. In Chapter 5 we saw how a chemist can take advantage of the selective absorption of light by materials in order to characterize them. In particular, light in the ultraviolet, visible, and infrared regions of the electromagnetic spectrum have proved most helpful for this purpose. Unfortunately, in the past, forensic chemists were unable to take full advantage of the capabilities of spectrophotometry for examining trace evidence as most spectrophotometers are not well suited for examining the very small particles frequently encountered as evidence. However, with the development of the microspectrophotometer, a forensic analyst can now view a particle under a microscope while, at the same time, a beam of light is directed at the particle in order to obtain its absorption spectrum. Depending on the type of light employed, an examiner can acquire either a visible or an IR spectral pattern of a substance being viewed under the microscope. The obvious advantage of this approach is to provide the forensic scientist with added information that will characterize trace quantities of evidence. A microspectrophotometer designed to measure the uptake of visible light by materials is shown in Figure 7-8.

The visual comparison of color is usually one of the first steps in examining paint, fiber, and ink evidence. Such comparisons are easily obtained using a comparison microscope. Now with the use of the microspectrophotometer, not only can the color of materials be compared visually but at the same time an absorption spectrum can be plotted for each item under examination to display the exact wavelengths at which it absorbs in the visible light spectrum. Occasionally, colors that appear similar by visual examination will show significant differences in their absorption spectra. An example of this approach is shown in Figure 7-9 where the microspectrophotometer is utilized to distinguish counterfeit and authentic currency by comparing the spectral patterns of inked lines on currency.

Another emerging technique in forensic science is the utilization of the infrared microspectrophotometer for the examination of fibers and paints. The "fingerprint" IR spectrum (see pp. 127–129) is unique for each chemical substance. Therefore, if such a spectrum can be obtained from either a fiber or a paint chip, it will allow the analyst to better identify and compare the type of chemicals from which these materials are manufactured. With a microspectrophotometer, a forensic analyst can view a substance through the

Figure 7-8. A visible light microspectrophotometer. *Courtesy* Nanometrics Inc., Sunnyvale, California.

Figure 7-9. Two $50 bills are shown above; one is genuine and the other
is counterfeit. Below each bill is a microphotograph of an inked line
present on each bill. Each line was examined under a visible light microspectrophotometer. As shown, the visible absorption spectrum of each line
is readily differentiated, thus allowing the examiner to distinguish a counterfeit bill from the genuine currency. *Courtesy* Peter W. Pfefferli, forensic
scientist, Lausanne, Switzerland.

microscope and at the same time have the instrument plot the infrared absorption spectrum for that material.

THE SCANNING ELECTRON MICROSCOPE (SEM)

All the microscopes described thus far utilize light coming off the specimen to produce a magnified image. The scanning electron microscope is, however, a special case in the family of microscopes. Here, the image formation is produced by aiming a beam of electrons onto the specimen and studying electron emissions on a closed TV circuit. The beam of electrons is emitted from a hot tungsten filament and is focused by means of electromagnets onto the surface of the specimen. This primary electron beam causes the emission of electrons from the elements that make up the upper layers

Figure 7-10.   The cystolithic hairs of the marijuana leaf as viewed with a scanning electron microscope (800✕). *Courtesy* Jeff Albright.

of the specimen. The emitted electrons are collected, and the amplified signal is displayed on a cathode ray or TV tube. By scanning the primary electron beam across the specimen's surface in synchronization with the cathode ray tube, it is possible to convert the emitted electrons into an image of the specimen for display on the cathode tube.

The major attractions of the SEM image are its high magnification, high resolution, and great depth of focus. In its usual mode the SEM has a magnification that ranges from 10X to 100,000X. Its depth of focus is some 300 times better than optical systems at similar magnifications, and the resultant picture is almost stereoscopic in appearance. Its great depth of field and magnification are exemplified by the magnification of cystolithic hair on the marijuana leaf, as shown in Figure 7-10.

Undoubtedly, as the SEM becomes available at lower cost, the technique will rapidly become accepted as a routine instrument in the crime laboratory. Already, some manufacturers are offering SEMs that are small compact table models at relatively attractive prices (see Figure 7-11).

Another facet of scanning electron microscopy has been the use of X-ray production as a means of determining the elemental composition of the specimen under examination. X-rays are generated when the electron beam of the scanning electron microscope strikes a target. When the SEM is coupled

Figure 7-11. Scanning electron microscope. *Courtesy* International Scientific Instruments, Mountain View, California.

to an X-ray analyzer, the emitted X-rays can be sorted according to their energy values and used to build up a picture of the elemental distribution in the specimen. Because each element emits X-rays of characteristic energy values, the X-ray analyzer can identify the elements present in a specimen. Furthermore, the element's concentration can be determined by measuring the intensity of the X-ray emission.

A relatively new application of scanning electron microscopy has been as a tool for determining whether or not a suspect recently has fired a gun. In this case, an attempt is made to remove any gunshot particles that may be remaining on a shooter's hands by lifting them off with a piece of adhesive tape. The tape is then examined under the SEM for the presence of particles that may have originated from the bullet primer. These particles can be characterized by their size, shape, and elemental composition. As shown in Figure 7-12, when the sample of gunshot residue is exposed to a beam of electrons from the scanning electron microscope, X-rays are emitted. These

Figure 7-12. A schematic diagram of a scanning electron microscope displaying the image of a gunshot residue particle. Simultaneously, an X-ray analyzer detects and displays X-ray emissions from the elements lead (Pb), antimony (Sb), and barium (Ba) present in the particle. *Courtesy* Aerospace Corp., El Segundo, California.

X-rays are passed into a detector where they are converted into electrical signals. These signals are sorted and displayed according to the energies of the emitted X-rays. Through the use of this technique, the elements lead, antimony, and barium, frequently found in most primers, can be rapidly detected and identified.

REVIEW QUESTIONS

1. A microscope uses a combination of _____ to magnify an image.
2. A type of image that cannot be viewed directly is called a _____ image.
3. A _____ microscope consists of two lenses mounted at each end of a hollow tube.
4. The lens closest to the specimen is called the _____.
5. The lens nearest the viewer's eye is called the _____.
6. The image seen through a compound microscope is (virtual, real).
7. The coarse and fine adjustments are part of the microscope's mechanical system. (True, False)
8. A transparent specimen is viewed through a microscope using _____ light.
9. An opaque object requires _____ illumination for viewing with a microscope.
10. A _____ collects light rays from the base illuminator and concentrates them on the specimen.
11. A microscope that remains in focus regardless of which objective lens is rotated into place is _____.
12. A microscope having only one eyepiece is monocular; one having two eyepieces is _____.
13. Each microscope lens is inscribed with a number signifying its _____.
14. An eyepiece lens of 10× used in combination with an objective lens of 20× will have a total magnification power of _____.
15. The ability of an objective lens to resolve details into separate images is directly proportional to its _____.
16. The size of the specimen area in view is known as the _____.
17. As magnification increases, the field of view (increases, decreases).
18. The thickness of a specimen in view is known as the _____.
19. The depth of focus (increases, decreases) with increasing magnification.
20. A side-by-side view of two specimens is best obtained with the _____ microscope.
21. A bridge is used to join two independent objective lenses into a single binocular unit to form a comparison microscope. (True, False)

22. Two monocular compound microscopes properly spaced and aligned describe the _____ microscope.
23. The stereoscopic microscope is the least frequently used microscope in a typical crime laboratory. (True, False)
24. The stereoscopic microscope offers a large _____ between the objective lens and the specimen.
25. Light confined to a single plane of vibration is said to be _____.
26. If a polarizer and analyzer are placed (perpendicular, parallel) to each other, no light will penetrate.
27. The _____ microscope allows a viewer to detect polarized light.
28. Crystals that are _____ will produce two planes of polarized light each perpendicular to the other.
29. By utilizing a _____ one can view a particle under a microscope while at the same time a beam of light is directed at the particle in order to obtain its absorption spectrum.
30. The _____ microscope focuses a beam of electrons on a specimen to produce an image.
31. When a beam of electrons strikes a specimen, _____ are emitted whose energies correspond to elements present in the specimen.

FURTHER REFERENCES

De Forest, Peter R., "Foundations of Forensic Microscopy," in *Forensic Science Handbook*, R. Saferstein, ed. Englewood Cliffs, N.J.: Prentice-Hall, Inc., 1982.

McCrone, W. C., "Forensic Microscopy," in *Forensic Science*, 2nd ed., G. Davies, ed. Washington, D.C., American Chemical Society, 1986.

McCrone, Walter C., and John G. Delly, *The Particle Atlas*, Vol. 1, 2nd ed. Ann Arbor, Mich.: Ann Arbor Science Publishers, 1973.

McCrone, Walter C., Lucy B. McCrone, and John G. Delly, *Polarized Light Microscopy*. Ann Arbor, Mich: Ann Arbor Science Publishers, 1978.

Schlueter, Gene E., and Walter E. Gumpertz, "The Stereomicroscope-Instrumentation and Techniques," *American Laboratory*, 8 (1979), 61.

Taylor, M. E., "Scanning Electron Microscopy in Forensic Science," *Journal of the Forensic Science Society*, 13 (1973), 269.

AUDIOVISUAL PRESENTATIONS

An Introduction to the Design and Use of the Simple Student Microscope (57 35-mm slides and audio tape). Prentice-Hall Media, Tarrytown, N.Y.

How to Use and Maintain a Stereoscopic Microscope (48 35-mm slides and audio tape). Prentice-Hall Media, Tarrytown, N.Y.

Laboratory Instrumentation (filmstrips and audio tape). Robert J. Brady Co., Bowie, Md.

CASE READING

MICROSCOPIC TRACE EVIDENCE—THE OVERLOOKED CLUE

Arthur Koehler—Wood Detective

Skip Palenik

Walter C. McCrone Associates Inc.

. . . Arthur Koehler . . . wood technologist and chief of the division of silvicultural relations at the U.S. Forest Products Laboratory in Madison, Wisconsin, . . . was born on June 4, 1885 in Mishicot, Wisconsin. His father was a carpenter and young Koehler grew up on a farm with a love of both wood and fine tools. This love naturally led him into forestry and he received a B.S. degree in the subject from the University of Michigan in 1911. . . . Upon graduation he went to work for the U.S. Forest Service in Washington, D.C., and three years later obtained a post at the U.S. Forest Products Laboratory where he served in various capacities until his retirement.

Although his primary responsibilities lay in wood identification and the correlation of microscopic wood structure and end use, Koehler also began to build a reputation as a wood detective after his success in obtaining evidence from wood fragments which were submitted to the laboratory in several cases of local importance. . . . The case which thrust Koehler into the limelight of international publicity, however, was the Lindbergh kidnapping case in which he, by the most painstaking work, traced the kidnap ladder back to the lumberyard from which its constituent parts had been purchased.

Sometime between the hours of 8 and 10 P.M. on the night of March 1, 1932 a kidnapper climbed into the nursery of the newly completed home of Charles and Anne Lindbergh in Hopewell, New Jersey, and abducted their infant son. The only clues left behind were a few indistinct muddy foot-

---

prints, a ransom note in the nursery, a homemade ladder and a chisel found a short distance from the house. Scarcely two months later, on May 12, the dead body of the child was found, half buried in the woods, about a mile from the Lindbergh home. One of the most intensive manhunts in U.S. history ensued, but failed to uncover any trace of the kidnapper or the ransom money which had been paid.[1]

Shortly after the news of the kidnapping broke in the press Koehler wrote a letter to Colonel Lindbergh offering his services to help with the investigation of the ladder. He never received a reply (which was not surprising considering the flood of mail which arrived at the Lindbergh home in the weeks following the kidnap). He was not entirely surprised though when his boss, Carlyle P. Winslow, placed before him some slivers of the ladder with the request that the wood be accurately identified.[2] This Koehler did, noting in his report the presence of golden brown, white and black wool fibers which he speculated might be from clothing worn by the kidnapper. That was the last he heard about the ladder for almost a year. During this time it was carried around the country (carefully wrapped in a wool blanket) to various experts including specialists at the National Bureau of Standards.[3] However, after a year of investigation the authorities were no closer to arresting a suspect than they were the day after the crime.

It was almost a year after the kidnapping when Koehler was asked by the head of the U.S. Forest Service, Major Robert Y. Stuart, to travel to Trenton to give the ladder an in-depth examination. Discussions between Colonel Norman Schwarzkopf, who headed the New Jersey State Police (and the kidnap investigation), and Major Stuart had convinced Colonel Schwarzkopf that the ladder might still yield clues about its maker if Koehler were given a chance to examine it thoroughly. Schwarzkopf wasn't too certain about Koehler's ability ("Wasn't he the one who identified the blanket fibers on the wood we sent him," he asked) but felt he had nothing to lose.

For the first time, Koehler saw the ladder (Figure 1). He was immediately struck by the fact that, although it was cleverly contrived, it was shamefully constructed. Instead of rungs it had cleats, which had been carelessly mortised with a dull chisel. A dull hand plane had been used needlessly in some places and a handsaw had been drawn carelessly across some of the boards.

Alone for four days, Koehler studied the ladder in the police training school in Wilburtha. He then returned to the Forest Products Laboratory with the ladder and closed himself up in a private laboratory with the best optical equipment available.[4] He began by completely dissecting the ladder into its component parts. Each piece was numbered. The cleats were labeled 1 (bottom) through 11 (top). The rails were numbered starting from 12 (bottom left) to 17 (right-hand top). . . . Each mark was noted and indexed. After probing with microscopes, calipers and a variety of lighting and photographic techniques, the ladder slowly began to give up its secrets.

The sheer number of observations, facts and deductions about the

Figure 1. The ladder used in the kidnapping of the Lindbergh baby.

origin of the ladder (and its producer) made by Koehler are truly staggering. We are concerned here only with those facts and observations which (1) allowed the parts to be traced and (2) described the carpenter and the previous environment of the ladder. The results were presented not as the subject of a single report but of daily letters to the director of the laboratory. As certain aspects were revealed they were pursued until the object could be traced no further. The most pertinent observations and deductions are listed and described below.

1. Microscopical examination showed four types of wood were used (Table 1). North Carolina pine is a trade name for wood from the southern yellow pine group which grows in commercial stands in the Southern U.S. along the Gulf of Mexico and along the Eastern Seaboard

up into New Jersey and southern New York.[5] Douglas fir and Ponderosa pine grow in the Western U.S. and Birch is found throughout the country.[6]

Table I

Woods Used in Kidnap Ladder

CLEATS
    1-10 Ponderosa pine
           1 X 6 inch boards ripped lengthwise into strips
           2-3/4 inches wide to make cleats.

    11   Douglas fir
           Grain matched bottom of rail 15.

SIDE RAILS
    12, 13 — North Carolina pine. Second growth. Cut from one board originally 14 feet long. Dressed to 3-3/4 inches in width. Both dressed on same planer.

    14, 15 — Douglas fir
           Dressed on two different planers.

      16 — North Carolina pine
           Narrowed from a wider board as indicated by handsaw and hand-planer marks on edges.

      17 — Douglas fir
           Dressed on different planers than 14 and 15.

DOWEL PINS
        Birch

---

2. Rails 12 and 13 showed faint marks which gave information about the planer in the mill where the wood was dressed. . . . [Figure 2 shows] the operation of a mill planer in diagramatic form. Defects in the cutters allowed the number of knives in the cutters to be determined by counting cutter marks between defect marks. Eight cutter heads dressed the wide surface and six heads the edges. . . .

The lumber went through the planer at a rate of 0.93 inches per complete revolution of the top and bottom cutter heads and 0.86 inches per revolution of the cutter heads that dressed the edges. This was determined by the distance of identical cuts made by a defective knife on each surface. . . .[7] Using the fact that the cutters in mill planers

Figure 2. Detail of a cutter head illustrating how a defect allowed the number of knives to be determined.

are usually driven at 3600 revolutions per minute it was possible to calculate the speed at which the wood passed into the planer as 258 feet per minute for the edge and 279 feet per minute for the board surfaces. The difference in the speed of the horizontal and vertical heads indicated that the planer was belt driven.

3. Rail 16 had four nail holes made by old fashioned square cut 8-penny nails. The holes had no connection with the construction of the ladder and therefore indicated prior use. The nail holes were clean and free from rust indicating inside use. This was confirmed by the general appearance of the rail which, although sapwood, showed no sign of exposure to the weather for any length of time since it was bright and unchecked. Therefore, it must have been nailed down indoors. Since it was low-grade lumber it would not have been used for finish purposes, but for rough construction. The spacing of the nails at 16 and 32 inches was considered significant and the suggestion was made that the rail came from the interior of a barn, garage or attic.

After an initial, futile attempt to trace the birch dowels, Koehler set out to try and trace the North Carolina rails (numbers 12 and 13). Although North Carolina pine grew in a large region it would not be profitable to ship it far, and since the ladder had turned up in New Jersey he felt certain that it had been milled somewhere in the Atlantic States. Using the Southern Lumberman's Directory, a list of 1598 planing mills from Alabama to New York was compiled. A confidential letter from Colonel Schwarzkopf and a two-page description written by Koehler were sent off to all of the mills on the list.

Of all the letters sent, only 25 mills reported having planers which matched the specifications outlined in the letter. Two were immediately excluded since they didn't dress lumber of the requisite size. Samples of 1 × 4 inch wood were requested from each of the remaining 23 mills. A sample received from the M. G. and J. J. Dorn mill of McCormick, South Carolina, showed exactly the marks Koehler was looking for.

A visit to the mill showed that the particular spacing was due to a pulley which had been purchased in September of 1929. The records of the mill showed that forty-six carloads of 1 × 4 had been shipped north of the Potomac River in the time between the purchase of the pulley and the kidnapping. . . . After personally visiting the final destination of each of the shipments, Koehler and Detective Bornmann finally arrived at a Bronx firm, the National Lumber and Millwork Company. Although the entire shipment had long before been sold, the foreman remembered that some storage bins had been built from some of the wood. The wood matched that from the ladder perfectly (Figures 3 and 4). Examination of wood from shipments before and after the Bronx carload showed that the belt on the planer had been changed and the knife sharpened. This meant that this shipment was the only one from which the two particular rails from the attic could have come. Whoever built the ladder had purchased part of the wood here!

Koehler was unprepared for the foreman's answer to his request to see the sales records. They had none. They had started selling cash and carry sometime before the Dorn shipment arrived and had no records. Although he had failed to come up with the carpenter's name, the authorities at least now knew the region where the kidnapper lived and bought his wood for the ladder.

Figure 3. Comparison of knife marks from mill planer on edges of 1 × 4 inch pine from two shipments from the Dorn mill and a ladder rail.

Ladder
rail

From Bronx
yard

M 23450 F

Figure 4. Comparison of knife marks on upper surface of ladder rail and North Carolina pine board located in shipment to the National Lumber and Millwork Company.

Koehler went back to his laboratory and, undaunted, started tracing the Douglas fir rails. At the time a suspect was arrested, he had succeeded in tracing one of the boards to a mill in Bend, Oregon, and another to Spokane, Washington. With the arrest of Richard Hauptmann on September 19, 1934. . . , his role in the case changed from an investigative to a comparative one. In Hauptmann's garage a variety of tools were found whose markings could be compared with those from the ladder. Comparative micrographs of marks made with Hauptmann's plane and plane marks on the ladder showed that his plane was used to plane the cleats (Figure 5). Finally, one of the investigators searching the attic of the suspect's home found that a board had been sawed out of the floor (Figure 6). Koehler's examination showed that the nail holes in the floor joists and the ladder rail (No. 16)

Edge of rung
No. 1

Lumber planed
by Arthur Koehler
with Hauptmann's
plane

Edge of rung
No. 6

Lumber planed
by Arthur Koehler
with Hauptmann's
plane

Edge of rung
No. 10

Figure 5. Comparison of defect marks in Hauptman's hand plane with marks on cleats (runs) from the ladder.

Figure 6. Rail 16 fitted into its original position in Hauptman's attic.

aligned perfectly. A detailed analysis of the grain and wood itself showed that rail 16 and the section of board remaining in the attic were originally all one piece (Figures 7 and 8).

Richard Bruno Hauptmann was convicted and sentenced to death in

Figure 7. Composite photograph by Koehler showing comparison of end grain (growth rings) in board from attic and rail 16.

Figure 8. Construction by Koehler showing probable grain pattern of missing piece between attic board and rail 16.

a sensational trial. Although, in retrospect, there may have been many errors and a good deal of prejudice in the trial itself, the professionalism and objectiveness of Arthur Koehler still stand as an example of science at its best in the service of the law. . . .

Acknowledgement

The author gratefully acknowledges the invaluable assistance of Dr. Regis Miller and Donna Christensen of the Forest Products Laboratory in Madison, Wisconsin, for making available documents and photographs which were necessary to this article. Additional thanks are due James Gerakaris of McCrone Associates for preparing the drawings of the ladder and mill planer.

References

1. Waller, George. Kidnap; The Story of the Lindbergh Case. Dial Press, New York, 1961.
2. Koehler, Arthur. "Who Made That Ladder?" as told to Boyden Sparkes. The Saturday Evening Post **297**. 42, p. 10, April 20, 1935.
3. Saylor, Charles, Proffer. Optical Microscopy as Used in Unorthodox Ways, SPIE, **104**, Multi-disciplinary Microscopy, 31–33, 1977.
4. Koehler, Arthur. The Saturday Evening Post **297**, p. 84, April 20. 1935.
5. Isenberg, Irving. Pulpwoods of the United States and Canada, Institute of Paper Chemistry, Appleton, pp. 19–22, 1951.
6. Christensen, Donna. Wood Technology and the Lindbergh Kidnap Case. Report, May 1971.
7. Koehler, Arthur. Techniques Used in Tracing the Lindbergh Kidnapping Ladder, Am. J. Police Science **27**, 5 (1937).

8

Hairs, Fibers, and Paint

The trace evidence that is transferred between individuals and objects during the commission of a crime will, if recovered, often corroborate other evidence developed during the course of an investigation. Although in most cases, physical evidence cannot by itself provide for a positive identification of a suspect, laboratory examination may narrow the origin of such evidence to a group that includes the suspect. Utilizing many of the instruments and techniques described in the previous three chapters, the crime laboratory has developed a variety of procedures for comparing and tracing the origins of physical evidence. It will be the purpose of this and forthcoming chapters to apply these techniques to the analysis of the types of physical evidence most often encountered at crime scenes. We will begin with a discussion of hairs, fibers, and paint.

MORPHOLOGY OF HAIR

Hair is encountered as physical evidence in a wide variety of crimes. However, any review of the forensic aspects of hair examination must start with the observation that it is not yet possible to individualize a human hair to any single head or body. Over the years, criminalists have tried in vain to find a way to isolate the physical and chemical properties of hair that could serve as individual characteristics of identity. One by one these efforts have repeatedly failed to uncover any one property that remains consistent with

183

time and is uniform throughout the head or body. It is a testimony to hair's reluctance to yield distinctive chemical properties that its color and structure, or morphology, still remain its most characteristic forensic features.

This is not to imply that hair has no value as physical evidence. On the contrary, when it is properly collected at the crime scene and its submission to the laboratory is accompanied by an adequate number of controls, hair can provide strong corroborative evidence for placing an individual at a crime site.

Hair is an appendage of the skin that grows out of an organ known as the *hair follicle*. The length of a hair extends from its root or bulb embedded in the follicle, continues into a shaft, and terminates at a tip end. It is the shaft, which is composed of three layers—the **cuticle, cortex,** and **medulla**—that is subjected to the most intense examination by the forensic scientist (see Figure 8-1).

Cuticle. Two of the features that make hair a good subject for establishing individual identity are its resistance to chemical decomposition and its ability to retain structural features over a long period of time. Much of

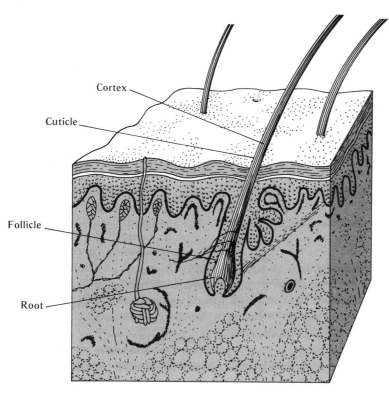

Figure 8-1.

this resistance and stability is attributed to the cuticle or outside covering of the hair. The cuticle is formed by overlapping scales that always point toward the tip end of each hair. The scales are formed from specialized cells that have hardened (kerantinized) and flattened in progressing from the follicle. The scales of most animal hair can best be described as having the appearance of shingles on a roof. Although the scale pattern is not a useful characteristic for individualizing human hair, the variety of patterns formed by animal hair makes it an important feature for species identification. Figure 8-2 shows the scale patterns of some animal hairs and of a human hair as

(a)   (b)   (c)

(d)   (e)   (f)

Figure 8-2. Scale patterns of various types of hair. **(a)** Human head hair (600X); **(b)** dog (1250X); **(c)** deer (120X); **(d)** rabbit (300X); **(e)** cat (2000X); **(f)** horse (450X). *Courtesy* International Scientific Instruments, Mountain View, California, and New Jersey State Police.

viewed by the scanning electron microscope. Another method of studying the scale pattern of hair is to make a cast of its surface. This is readily done by embedding the hair in a soft medium, such as clear nail polish or softened vinyl. When the medium has hardened, the hair is removed, and there remains a clear, distinct impression of the hair's cuticle, ideal for examination with a compound microscope.

Cortex. Contained within the protective layer of the cuticle is the cortex. The cortex is actually made up of spindle-shaped cortical cells that are aligned in a regular array, parallel to the length of the hair. The cortex derives its major forensic importance from the fact that it is embedded with the pigment granules that impart hair with color. It is the color and distribution of these granules that provide the criminalist with important points of comparison between the hair of different individuals.

The structural features of the cortex are examined microscopically after the hair has been mounted in a liquid medium that has a refractive index closely matched to that of the hair; usually, Canadian balsam is used. Under these conditions the amount of light reflected off the hair's surface is minimized, and the amount of light penetrating the hair is optimized.

Medulla. The medulla is a collection of cells having the appearance of a central canal running through a hair. In many animals this canal is a most predominant feature, occupying more than half of the hair's diameter. The **medullary index** measures the diameter of the medulla relative to the diameter of the hair shaft, and is normally expressed as a fraction. For humans the index generally has a value less than $1/3$; for most other animals the value is $1/2$ or greater.

It is important to stress that the presence and appearance of the medulla vary from individual to individual, and even between hairs of a given individual. Not all hairs have medullae, and when they do exist, the degree of medullation can vary. In this respect, medullae may be classified as being continuous, interrupted, fragmented, or absent (see Figure 8-3). Human head hairs generally exhibit no medullae or have fragmented ones; they rarely show continuous medullation. One noted exception is the Mongoloid race

Continuous   Interrupted

Fragmented   **Figure 8-3.** Medulla patterns.

who usually have head hairs with continuous medullae. Also, most animals have medullae that are either continuous or interrupted.

Another interesting feature of the medulla is its shape. Humans, as well as many animals, have medullae that give a nearly cylindrical appearance. Other animals exhibit medullae that have a patterned shape. For example, the medulla of a cat can best be described as resembling a string of pearls, whereas members of the deer family show a medullary structure consisting of spherical cells occupying the entire hair shaft. Figure 8-4 illustrates medullary sizes and forms for a number of common animal hairs and a human head hair.

IDENTIFICATION AND COMPARISON OF HAIR

Most often when hair evidence is present in a criminal case, the prime purpose for its examination in a crime laboratory is to establish whether the hair is human or animal in origin, or to determine whether human hair retrieved at a crime scene compares with hair that is known to have come from a particular individual. Although the distinction of animal hair from human hair can normally be accomplished with little difficulty, the problem of human hair comparisons is one that must be undertaken with extreme caution and with an awareness of hair's tendency to exhibit variable morphological characteristics not only from one person to another but also within a single individual.

A careful microscopic examination of hair will reveal morphological features that can distinguish human hair from the hair of animals. The hair of various animals also differs in structure to such an extent that the examiner may often be able to identify the species of animal from which the hair originated. It is important, however, that before such a conclusion is reached the examiner has access to a comprehensive collection of reference standards and the accumulated experience of hundreds of prior hair examinations. Scale structure, medullary index, and medullary shape are features that are particularly important in hair identification.

The most common request that is made of the laboratory when hair is used as forensic evidence is to determine whether or not hair recovered at the crime scene compares to hair removed from a suspect. In most cases, such a comparison relates to hair obtained from the scalp or pubic area. Ultimately, the evidential value of the comparison will depend on the degree of probability with which the examiner can associate the questioned hair to a particular individual.

In making a hair comparison, a comparison microscope is an invaluable tool that allows the examiner to view the questioned and known hair together side by side. Any variations in the microscopic characteristics will thus be readily observed. Because hair from any part of the body exhibits a range of characteristics, it is necessary to have an adequate number of known hairs that are representative of all its features when making a comparison.

(a)   (b)   (c)

(d)   (e)   (f)

Figure 8-4. Medulla patterns for various types of hair. (a) Human head hair (450X). (b) dog (450X). (c) deer (100X). (d) rabbit (450X). (e) cat (450X). (f) mouse (450X). All *courtesy* Linda Jankowski.

In comparing hair, the criminalist is particularly interested in matching the color, length, and diameter. Other important features are the presence or absence of a medulla, and the distribution and color intensity of the pigment granules present in the cortex. A microscopic examination may also be able to distinguish dyed or bleached hair from natural hair. A dyed color will often be present in the cuticle as well as throughout the cortex. Bleaching, on the other hand, tends to remove pigment from the hair and to give it a yellowish tint. If there has been a growth of hair since it was last bleached or dyed, the natural-end portion will be quite distinct in color. An estimate of the time since dying or bleaching can be made because hair is known to grow at a rate of approximately one centimeter per month. Other significant but less frequent features may be observed in hair. For example, morphological abnormalities may be present due to certain diseases or deficiencies. Also the presence of fungal and nit infections can serve to further link a hair specimen to a particular individual.

Hair is class evidence and thus it is not possible, except in rare instances, to determine that a questioned hair sample came from a particular individual to the exclusion of all others. In seeking to define how closely a particular hair can be associated with an individual, the examiner must to a large extent rely on experience. Each case will have to be evaluated on its own merits. A recent study conducted by the laboratory of the Royal Canadian Mounted Police offers an interesting insight into the evidential value of a hair comparison.[1] One hundred different individuals were asked to submit a sample of 80 to 100 hairs randomly selected from various regions of the scalp. From these, depending on the homogeneity of the sample, 6 to 11 mutually dissimilar hairs were selected to represent the range of length, coarseness, and color present in the 80 to 100 hairs. The representative hairs were then mounted individually on glass slides and compared to one another, utilizing a comparison microscope. A total of 861 hairs from the 100 individuals were compared in this manner.

By use of a card coding system it was possible to record 366,630 hair comparisons between the 861 hairs. As a result, it was estimated that if one human head hair found at the scene of a crime is found to be similar to a representative hair from a suspect's head, the odds against it originating from another person are about 4500 to 1. Another study conducted along the same lines revealed that the odds against two similar pubic hairs originating from two different individuals are about 800 to 1.[2] Because Negroid and Mongoloid hairs exhibit less variation in many of their characteristics, it is

---

[1] B. D. Gaudette and E. S. Keeping, "An Attempt at Determing Probabilities in Human Scalp Hair Comparison," *Journal of Forensic Sciences*, 19 (1974), 599.

[2] B. D. Gaudette, "Probabilities and Human Pubic Hair Comparisons," *Journal of Forensic Sciences*, 21 (1976), 514.

expected that these odds would be somewhat less for persons of these racial origins.

Until more definitive probability data are acquired, a final assessment of the significance of any hair comparison will depend almost entirely on the experience and judgment of the examiner. However, these initial studies have confirmed what many forensic scientists have long suspected—hair, when accompanied by a thorough collection of control specimens, can be highly distinctive evidence for personal identification.

A number of questions may be asked to further ascertain the present status of forensic hair examinations.

Can the body area of a hair be determined? Normally, little difficulty is experienced in ascertaining the body area of those hairs commonly submitted to crime laboratories. For example, scalp hairs generally show little diameter variation and have a more uniform distribution of pigment color when compared to other body hairs. Pubic hairs are short and curly with wide variations in shaft diameter and usually have continuous medullae. Beard hairs are coarse, normally triangular in cross section, and have blunt tips acquired from cutting or shaving.

Can the racial origin of hair be determined? In many instances the examiner can distinguish hair originating from members of different races; this is especially true of Caucasian and Negroid head hair. Negroid hairs are normally kinky, containing dense, unevenly distributed pigments. Caucasian hairs are usually straight or wavy with very fine to coarse pigments that are more evenly distributed when compared to Negroid hair. Sometimes a cross-sectional examination of hair may aid in the identification of race. Cross sections of hair from Caucasians are oval to round in shape, whereas cross sections of Negroid hair are flat to oval in shape. However, it must be emphasized that all of these observations are general in nature, with many possible exceptions. The criminalist must approach the determination of race from hair with caution and a good deal of experience.

Can the age and sex of a hair be determined? The age of an individual cannot be learned from a hair examination with any degree of certainty except with infant hair. Infant hairs are fine, short in length, have fine pigment, and are rudimentary in character. Although the presence of dye or bleach on the hair may offer some clue to sex, present hair styles make these characteristics less valuable than they were in the past. Currently, a number of researchers are making good progress in studies aimed at determining the sex origin of human hair. Most of this research has concentrated on using techniques for identifying genetic substances in human cells. However, at this time sexual discrimination of hair cells is not considered to be a routine forensic technique.

Is it possible to determine if hair was forcibly removed from the body? A microscopic examination of the hair root *may* establish whether the hair has fallen out or has been pulled out of the skin. A hair root found to have follicular tissue (root sheath cells) adhering to it, as shown in Figure 8-5, is indicative of a hair that has been pulled out either by another person or by brushing or combing. Hair naturally falling off the body will show a bulbous-shaped root free of any adhering tissue. However, the absence of sheath cells cannot always be relied upon for correctly judging whether or not hair has been forcibly pulled from the body. It has been demonstrated that in some cases the root of a hair may be devoid of any adhering tissue even when it has been pulled from the body. Apparently, an important consideration is how quickly the hair is pulled out of the head. Hairs pulled quickly from the head are much more likely to have sheath cells as compared to hairs which have been removed slowly from the scalp.[3]

Are efforts being made to individualize human hair? At the present time, there is a widespread interest among forensic scientists in the possibilities of individualizing human hair through trace elemental content. The neutron activation analysis of hair has been found to be quite sensitive. However, a lot more research remains to be conducted before the technique can be judged valid for forensic comparisons. The variation of the hair's elements over an individual's head, its possible variation with time, and the influence of environment and diet are all aspects of the problem that require considerable research efforts before any forensic significance can be assigned to the

Figure 8-5. Head hair forcibly removed with follicular tissue attached. *Courtesy* New Jersey State Police.

---

[3] L. A. King, R. Wigmore and J. M. Twibell, "The Morphology and Occurrence of Human Hair Sheath Cells," *Journal of the Forensic Science Society*, 22 (1982), 267.

elemental composition of hair. A more fruitful approach for associating hair to a particular individual has been the determination of blood factors in sheath cells which may be attached to a human hair root.[4] These factors will be discussed in greater detail in Chapter 12. At this point a case analyzed in the author's laboratory will serve to illustrate the utility of this approach, as described below.

> White and brown head hairs were found adhering to the vehicle of an individual believed to have been involved in a hit-and-run fatality. The brown hair compared microscopically to the victim's brown hair control. The white hair offered minimal physical characteristics; however, sufficient follicular tissue was present on the hair root to identify the following blood factors: EsD 1, PGM 2-1, and GLOI-1. These factors, present in approximately 4 percent of the population, were also found in the victim's control hair tissue.

THE COLLECTION OF HAIR EVIDENCE

When questioned hairs are submitted to a forensic laboratory for examination, they must always be accompanied by an adequate number of control samples from the victim of the crime and from individuals suspected of having deposited hair at the crime scene. We have learned that hair from different parts of the body varies significantly in its physical characteristics. Likewise, hair from any one area of the body also can have a wide range of characteristics. For this reason, it is imperative that the questioned and control hairs come from the same area of the body; one cannot, for instance, compare head hair to pubic hair. It is also important that the collection of control hair be carried out in a way to ensure a representative sampling of hair from any one area of the body.

As a general rule, forensic hair comparisons involve either head hair or pubic hair. The collection of fifty full-length hairs from all areas of the scalp will normally ensure a representative sampling of head hair. Likewise, a minimum collection of two dozen full-length pubic hairs should cover the range of characteristics present in this portion of the body. In rape cases, care must first be taken to comb the pubic area with a clean comb to remove all loose foreign hair present before the victim is sampled for control hair. The comb is to be packaged in a separate envelope.

Because a hair may show variation in color and other morphological features over its entire length, the entire hair length is collected. This requirement is best accomplished by either pulling the hair out of the skin or clipping it at the skin line.

---

[4] D. Montgomery and B. W-H. Jay, "Multiple Enzyme Systems Grouping of Human Root Sheaths," *The Canadian Society of Forensic Science Journal*, 15 (1982), 1.

As a matter of routine, hair samples are collected from the victim(s) of suspicious deaths during an autopsy. As the autopsy may occur early in an investigation, the need for hair controls may not always be apparent. However, one should never rule out the possible involvement of hair evidence in subsequent investigative findings. Failure to make this simple collection at an opportune time may result in complicated legal problems at a later date.

TYPES OF FIBERS

Just as hair left at a crime scene can serve as identification, the same logic can reasonably be extended to the fibers that comprise our fabrics and garments. Fibers may become important evidence in incidents that involve personal contact—such as homicide, assault, or sexual offenses—in which cross-transfers may occur between the clothing of suspect and victim. Similarly, it is not uncommon to find that the force of impact between a hit-and-run victim and a vehicle leaves fibers, threads, or even whole pieces of clothing adhering to parts of the vehicle. Fibers may also become fixed in screens or glass broken in the course of a breaking-and-entering attempt.

Regardless of where and under what conditions fibers are recovered, their ultimate value as forensic evidence will depend on the criminalist's ability to narrow their origin to a limited number of sources or even to a single source. Unfortunately, the mass production of our garments and fabrics has served to limit the value of fiber evidence in this respect, and it is only under the most unusual circumstances that the recovery of fibers at a crime scene will provide individual identification with a high degree of certainty.

For centuries man was dependent on the source and forces of nature for textile fibers. Early in the twentieth century the first manufactured fiber—rayon—became a practical reality, followed in the 1920s by the introduction of cellulose acetate. Since the late 1930s, scientists have produced literally dozens of new fibers. In fact, the development of fibers, fabrics, finishes, and other textile-processing techniques have made greater advances since 1900 than in the four to five thousand years of recorded history before the twentieth century. Today, such varied things as clothing, carpeting, drapes, wigs, and even artificial turf attest to the predominant role that manufactured fibers have come to play in our culture and environment.

For the purpose of discussing the forensic examination of fibers, it will be convenient to classify them into two broad groups: natural and man-made.

NATURAL FIBERS

Natural fibers are derived in whole from animal or plant sources. Animal fibers comprise the majority of the natural fibers encountered in crime laboratory examinations. These include hair coverings from such animals as sheep (wool), goats (mohair, cashmere), camels, llamas, alpacas, and vicuñas; fur fibers include those obtained from animals such as mink, rabbit, beaver, and muskrat.

Any discussion of the forensic examination of animal fibers will merely restate procedures developed in the previous section for the forensic examination of animal hairs. The identification and comparison of such hairs will rely solely on a microscopic examination of color and morphological characteristics. Again, a sufficient number of control specimens must be examined to establish the range of fiber characteristics that comprise the suspect fabric.

By far the most prevalent plant fiber is cotton. However, the wide use of undyed white cotton fibers in clothing and other fabrics has made its evidential value almost meaningless, although the presence of dyed cotton in a combination of colors has, in some cases, served to enhance its evidential significance. The microscopic view of cotton fiber, shown in Figure 8-6, reveals its most distinguishing feature—a ribbonlike shape with twists at irregular intervals.

MAN-MADE FIBERS

Beginning with the introduction of rayon in 1911 and the development of nylon in 1939, man-made fibers have increasingly replaced natural fibers in garments and fabrics. Today such fibers are marketed under hundreds of different trademark names. To reduce consumer confusion, the U.S. Federal

Figure 8-6. Photomicrograph of cotton fiber (450X). *Courtesy* Linda Jankowski.

Trade Commission has approved the following "generic" or family names for the grouping of all man-made fibers:

Acetate	Metallic	Rayon
Acrylic	Modacrylic	Rubber
Anidex	Novoloid	Saran
Aramid	Nylon	Spandex
Azlon	Nytril	Triacetate
Glass	Olefin	Vinal
Lastrile	Polyester	Vinyon

Many of these generic classes are produced by several manufacturers and are sold under a confusing variety of trademark names. For example, in the United States, polyesters and marketed under names that include: Dacron®, Fortrel®, and Kodel®. In England, polyesters are called Terylene®.

The first machine-made fibers were manufactured from raw materials that were derived from cotton or wood pulp. These materials are processed, and pure cellulose is extracted from them. Depending on the type of fiber that is desired, the cellulose may be chemically treated and dissolved in an appropriate solvent before it is forced through the small holes of a spinning jet or spinnerette to produce the fiber. Fibers manufactured from natural raw materials in this manner are classified as **regenerated** fibers and commonly include rayon, acetate, and triacetate, all of which are produced from regenerated cellulose.

Most of the fibers presently manufactured are produced solely from synthetic chemicals and are therefore classified as **synthetic fibers**. These include nylons, polyesters, and acrylics. The creation of synthetic fibers became a reality only when scientists developed a method of synthesizing long-chained molecules called **polymers**.

In 1930, chemists discovered an unusual characteristic of one of the polymers under investigation. It was found that when a glass rod in contact with viscous material in a beaker was slowly pulled away, the substance adhered to the rod and formed a fine filament that hardened as soon as it entered the cool air. Furthermore, it was observed that the cold filaments could be stretched several times their extended length to produce a flexible, strong, and attractive fiber. The first synthetic fiber was to be improved upon and marketed as nylon. Since then, fiber chemists have successfully synthesized new polymers and have developed more efficient methods for manufacturing them. These efforts have produced a multitude of synthetic fibers.

THE POLYMER

The polymer is the basic chemical substance of all synthetic fibers. Indeed, an almost unbelievable array of household, industrial, and recreational products are manufactured from polymers; these include plastics, paints, adhesives, and synthetic rubber. Polymers exist in countless forms and varieties and with the proper treatment can be made to assume different chemical and physical properties.

As we have already observed, chemical substances are composed from basic structural units called **molecules**. The molecules of most materials are comprised of just a few atoms; for example, water, H_2O, has 2 atoms of hydrogen and 1 atom of oxygen. The heroin molecule, $C_{21}H_{23}O_5N$, contains 21 atoms of carbon, 23 of hydrogen, 5 atoms of oxygen, and 1 atom of nitrogen. Polymers, on the other hand, are formed by linking together a large number of molecules, so that it is not unusual for a polymer to contain thousands or even millions of atoms. This is why polymers are often referred to as **macromolecules**, or "big" molecules.

Simply, a polymer can be pictured as resembling a long repeating chain, with each link representing the basic structure of the polymer (see Figure 8-7). The repeating molecular units in the polymer, called **monomers**, are joined together end to end, so that on a greatly enlarged scale, thousands upon thousands are linked together to form a long chain. What makes polymer chemistry so fascinating is the countless varieties of possibilities that exist for linking different molecules together. By simply varying the chemical structure of the basic molecules, or monomers, and by devising numerous ways to weave them together, chemists have created polymers that exhibit different properties. It is this versatility that enables polymer chemists to synthesize glues, plastics, paints, and fibers.

Monomer

Figure 8-7. The chain-link model of a segment of a polymer molecule. The actual molecule may contain as many as several million monomer units or links.

It would be a mistake to give the impression that all polymers are synthesized in the chemical laboratory. Indeed, this is far from true, for nature has produced polymers that man has not yet been able to copy. For example, the proteins that form the basic structure of animal hairs, as well as of all living matter, are polymers, composed of thousands of amino acids linked together in a highly organized arrangement and sequence. Similarly, cellulose, the basic ingredient of wood and cotton, and starch are both natural polymers built by the combination of several thousand carbohydrate monomers, as shown in Figure 8-8. Hence, the synthesis of man-made fibers merely represents an extension of chemical principles that nature has successfully utilized to produce hair and vegetable fibers.

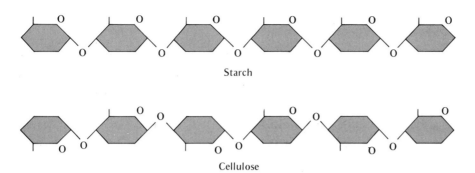

Starch

Cellulose

Figure 8-8. Starch and cellulose are natural carbohydrate polymers consisting of a large number of repeating units or monomers.

IDENTIFICATION AND COMPARISON OF MAN-MADE FIBERS

The evidential value of fibers is related to the criminalist's ability to trace their origin. Obviously, if the examiner is presented with fabrics that can be exactly fitted together at their torn edges, it is a virtual certainty that the fabrics were of common origin. Such a fit is demonstrated in Figure 8-9 for a piece of fabric that was removed from a vehicle suspected of involvement in a hit-and-run fatality. The exact fit with the remains of the victim's trousers resulted in the direct implication of the car's driver in the incident.

However, a more common case finds the criminalist presented with a very limited number of fibers for identification and comparison. Generally, in these situations, the possibilities for obtaining a physical match are nonexistent, and the examiner must resort to a side-by-side comparison of the control and crime-scene fibers.

The first and most important step in the examination will be a microscopic comparison for color and diameter. Unless there is agreement between these two characteristics, there would be little reason to suspect a comparison. Other morphological features that could be present to aid in the comparison are lengthwise striations on the surface of some fibers and the pitting of the fiber's surface with delustering particles (usually titanium dioxide) added in the manufacturing process to reduce shine (Figure 8-10). The shape of a fiber through a cross-sectional view may also assist in characterizing the fiber. In the previously discussed Wayne Williams case (pp. 59 to 73), it was unusually shaped yellow-green fibers discovered on a number of the murder victims which ultimately were linked to a carpet in the home of Wayne Williams. This fiber proved to be a key element in proving the guilt of Williams. A photomicrograph of this unusually shaped fiber is shown in Figure 8-11 (p. 200).

Figure 8-9. A piece of fabric found on a suspect hit-and-run vehicle inserted into the torn trousers of the victim. *Courtesy* New Jersey State Police.

Although two fibers may seem to have the same color when they are viewed under the microscope, there may actually exist compositional differences in the dyes that were applied to them during their manufacture. In fact, most textile fibers are impregnated with a mixture of dyes selected to obtain a desired shade or color. The significance of a fiber comparison is enhanced when the forensic examiner can show that the questioned and control fibers actually have the same dye composition. The microspectrophotometer (p. 165) is a convenient way for analysts to compare the colors of fibers through spectral patterns. This technique is not limited by sample size as a fiber as small as 1 millimeter or less in length can be examined by this type of microscope. The examination is nondestructive and is carried out on fibers simply mounted on a microscope slide. A more detailed analysis of the fiber's dye composition can be obtained through a chromatographic separation of the dye constituents. To accomplish this, small strands of fibers are compared for dye content by first extracting the dye off each fiber with a suitable solvent and then spotting the dye solution onto a thin-layer chromatography

(a)   (b)

Figure 8-10. Photomicrographs of synthetic fibers. **(a)** Cellulose triacetate
(450X). **(b)** Nylon embedded with titanium dioxide particles (450X).
Courtesy Linda Jankowski.

plate. The dye components of the questioned and control fibers are separated on the thin-layer plate and compared side by side for similarity.[5]

Once this phase of the analysis is complete, and before any conclusion can be reached that two or more fibers compare, each must be shown to have the same chemical composition. In this respect, tests are performed to confirm that all the fibers involved belong to the same broad generic class. Additionally, the comparison will be substantially enhanced if it can be demonstrated that all the fibers belong to the same subclassification within their generic class. For example, when we speak of nylon, we must remember that there are at least five different types of nylon available in commercial and consumer markets. These include nylon 6, nylon 6-10, nylon 11, nylon 6-6, and Quiana®. Although all types of nylon have many properties

---

[5] R. Resua, "A Semi-Micro Technique for the Extraction and Comparison of Dyes in Textile Fibers," *Journal of Forensic Sciences*, 25 (1980), 168.

Figure 8-11. A scanning electron photomicrograph of the cross section of a nylon fiber removed from a sheet used to transport the body of a murder victim. The fiber, associated with a carpet in Wayne Williams's home, was manufactured in 1971 in relatively small quantities. *Courtesy* Federal Bureau of Investigation, Washington, D.C.

in common, each may differ in physical shape, appearance, and dyeability owing to modifications in basic chemical structure. Similarly, a study of 40 different brand-name acrylic fibers revealed that they could actually be divided into 25 distinguishable groups on the basis of their polymeric structure and physical characteristics.[6]

Textile chemists have devised numerous tests for determining the class of a fiber. However, unlike the textile chemist, the criminalist frequently does not have the luxury of having a substantial quantity of fabric to work with and must therefore select those tests that will yield the most information with the least amount of material. Only a single fiber may be available for analysis, and often this may amount to no more than a minute strand recovered from a fingernail scraping of a homicide or rape victim.

A most useful physical property of fibers, from the criminalist's point of view, arises out of the knowledge that many manufactured fibers exhibit double refraction or birefringence (see page 84). Synthetic fibers are manufactured by melting a polymeric substance or dissolving it in a solvent and then forcing it through the very fine holes of a spinnerette. The polymer emerges as a very fine filament with its molecules aligned parallel to the length of the filament (see Figure 8-12). Just as the regular arrangement of atoms

[6] K. W. Smalldon, "The Identification of Acrylic Fibers by Polymer Composition as Determined by Infrared Spectroscopy and Physical Characteristics," *Journal of Forensic Sciences*, 18 (1973), 69.

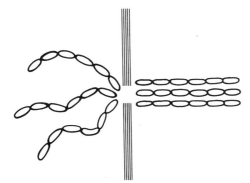

Figure 8-12. In the production of man-made fibers, the bulk polymer is forced through small holes to form a filament in which all the polymers are aligned in the same direction.

produces a crystal, so will the regular arrangement of the fiber's polymers cause crystallinity in the finished fiber. It is the crystallinity that makes a fiber stiff and strong and is responsible for its exhibiting the optical property of double refraction.

Light passing through a synthetic fiber emerges polarized, perpendicular and parallel to the length of the fiber. Depending on the class of fiber, each polarized plane of light will have a characteristic index of refraction. This value can be determined by immersing the fiber in a fluid that has a comparable refractive index and observing the disappearance of the Becke line under a polarizing microscope. Table 8-1 lists the two refractive indices of some common classes of fibers, along with their birefringence. The virtue of this

Table 8-1.
REFRACTIVE INDICES OF COMMON TEXTILE FIBERS

| Fiber | Refractive Index | | Birefringence |
	Parallel	Perpendicular	
Acetate	1.478	1.477	0.001
Triacetate	1.472	1.471	0.001
Acrylic	1.524	1.520	0.004
Nylon			
Nylon 6	1.568	1.515	0.053
Nylon 6-6	1.582	1.519	0.063
Polyester			
Dacron	1.710	1.535	0.175
Kodel	1.642	1.540	0.102
Modacrylic	1.536	1.531	0.005
Rayon			
Cuprammonium rayon	1.552	1.520	0.032
Viscose rayon	1.544	1.520	0.024

Note: *The listed values are for specific fibers, which explains the highly precise values given. In identification work such precision is not practical: values within 0.02 or 0.03 of those listed will suffice.*

Figure 8-13(a). Infrared spectrum of Orlon 42.

202

Figure 8-13(b).   Infrared spectrum of Acrilan 16.

technique is that a single fiber, microscopic in size, can be analyzed in a nondestructive manner.

The polymers that comprise a man-made fiber, just as in any other organic substance, will selectively absorb infrared light in a characteristic pattern. Infrared spectrophotometry thus provides a rapid and reliable method for identifying the generic class, and in some cases the subclasses, of a very small quantity of fibers.[7] The infrared spectra of two types of acrylic fibers are shown in Figure 8-13 (a) and (b).

The technique of pyrolysis gas chromatography also has the ability to characterize small quantities of polymers, such as those that comprise synthetic fibers, plastics, or paints. Here, as shown in Figure 8-14, the polymer chain is decomposed by a heated filament, and the resultant products are swept into and through a gas chromatograph column. What emerge and are recorded are the separated decomposition products of the polymer. It is the pattern of this chromatogram or "pyrogram" that distinguishes one polymer from another. Figure 8-15 illustrates how pyrogram patterns distinguish various members of the acrylic class of fibers.

Once it has been determined that there is a fiber match, the question of the significance of such a finding is bound to be raised. In reality, there is no

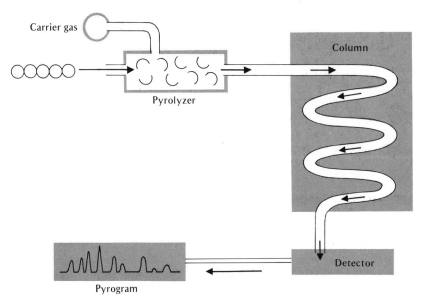

Figure 8-14. Schematic diagram of pyrolysis gas chromatography.

[7]R. Cook and M. D. Paterson, "New Techniques for the Identification of Microscopic Samples of Textile Fibers by Infrared Spectroscopy," *Forensic Science International*, 12 (1978), 237.

VELICREN

TIME (MINUTES)

(a)

ZEFRAN TYPE 1207

TIME (MINUTES)

(b)

Figure 8-15. Pyrograms of two acrylic fibers. *Courtesy* Varian Instruments, California.

205

analytical technique which will permit the criminalist to associate a fiber strand definitively to any single garment. Furthermore, except in the most unusual of circumstances, there are no statistical data bases available for determining the probability of a fiber's origin. Considering the mass distribution of synthetic fibers and the constantly changing fashion tastes of our society, it is highly unlikely that such data will be available in the foreseeable future. Nevertheless, one should not discount or minimize the significance of a fiber association. In our society there exists an enormous variety of fibers. By simply looking around at individuals whom we randomly come in contact with on a daily basis, it becomes obvious how unlikely it is to find two different people wearing identically colored fabrics (with the exception of blue denim materials or white cottons). There are literally thousands of different colored fibers in our environment. Combine this fact with the knowledge that forensic scientists compare not only the color of fibers but also their size, shape, microscopic appearance, chemical composition, and dye content and one can now begin to appreciate how unlikely it is to find two indistinguishable colored fibers emanating from randomly selected sources. Furthermore, the significance of a fiber association will increase dramatically if the analyst is able to link two or more distinctly different fibers to the same object. Likewise, the associative value of fiber evidence will be dramatically enhanced if it's accompanied by other types of physical evidence linking a person or object to a crime.

As is the case with most class evidence, the decision for determining how significant a fiber comparison is will ultimately be dictated by the circumstances of the cases, by the location, number, and nature of the fibers examined, and most important of all, by the judgment of an experienced examiner.

Case Reading

On a cold winter's day. . . ., a female was found in the alleyway of an east Harlem tenement. In close proximity to the body was a California florist flower box and a plastic liner. The decedent was identified as a member of a well-known church. She was known to have been selling church literature in the buildings that surround the alley in which the body was discovered. The detectives investigating the case forwarded the flower box, plastic liner, and the decedent's clothing to the forensic science laboratory. On the box and liner were found tan wool fibers, red acrylic fibers, and navy blue wool fibers (all identified by polarized light microscopy). The three types of questioned fibers were compared microscopically with the decedent's clothing. All three were found to be consistent in all respects to the textile fibers composing the decedent's clothing (tan wool overcoat, navy blue wool/polyester blend slacks, and red acrylic sweater), thereby associating the woman with the flower box and liner. In addition, light blue nylon rug fibers and several brown-colored rabbit hairs were found on the box and liner. Similar light blue nylon rug fibers and rabbit hairs, as well as red colored nylon rug fibers, were found on the decedent's tan wool overcoat. Neither the rabbit hairs, nor the nylon rug fibers, could be associated with the victim's environment (her clothing or residence).

All this information was conveyed to the field investigators. Upon further inquiry in the neighborhood, the investigating officers learned the identification of a man who had, the day after the body was discovered, sold a full length, brown-colored, rabbit hair coat to a local man. The investigators obtained the rabbit hair coat from the purchaser. The hair composing the coat was compared microscopically to the questioned rabbit hairs found on the victim's wool coat, and the flower box liner. The specimens of questioned rabbit hair were found to be consistent in all physical and microscopic characteristics to the rabbit hair composing the suspect's coat. Armed with this information, the police now had probable cause to obtain a search warrant for the suspect's apartment.

In the suspect's apartment two rugs were found. One was colored light blue and the other was red in color; both rugs were composed of nylon fibers. Samples of each rug were collected by the crime scene unit and forwarded to the forensic science laboratory for comparison with the questioned rug fibers found on the victim's clothing, the flower box, and plastic liner. Both the questioned and known rug fibers were found to be consistent in all respects. The presence of light blue nylon rug fibers, red nylon rug fibers, and brown-colored rabbit hairs on the flower box, plastic liner, and woman's clothing enabled the author to make associations between the woman, flower box, and liner found in the alleyway with the suspect and his apartment. . . .

Further inquiry about the suspect was made in the neighborhood by the investigating officers. A witness was located who stated he saw the suspect carrying a large California flower box a day or two before the body was discovered.

From the evidence it was theorized that the woman was killed in the suspect's apartment, placed in the flower box, brought up to the roof of the building in which the defendant resided, and thrown off the building into the alley below. On the basis of all of this evidence, the suspect was arrested, indicted, and tried for murder in the second degree. After two trials, at which extensive testimony (three days) about the trace evidence was given by the author, the defendant was found guilty of murder in the second degree, and subsequently sentenced to life imprisonment.[8]

---

[8] Reprinted in part by permission of the American Society of Testing and Materials from N. Petraco, "Trace Evidence—The Invisible Witness," *Journal of Forensic Sciences*, 31 (1986), 321. Copyright 1986.

THE COLLECTION OF FIBER EVIDENCE

As criminal investigators have become more aware of the potential contribution of trace physical evidence to the success of their investigation, they have placed greater emphasis on conducting thorough crime-scene searches for evidence of forensic value. Their skill and determination at carrying out these tasks will be tested when it comes to the collection of fiber-related evidence. Fiber evidence can be associated with virtually any type of crime. It's the kind of evidence that will not usually be seen with the naked eye and thus can be easily overlooked by someone not specifically looking for it. For the investigator committed to optimizing the laboratory's chances for locating minute strands of fibers, the task becomes one of identifying and preserving potential "carriers" of fiber evidence. Relevant articles of clothing should be packaged carefully in paper bags. Each article must be placed in a separate bag to avoid the possibility of cross-contamination of evidence. Scrupulous care must be taken to prevent articles of clothing from different people or from different locations from coming into contact. Such articles must not even be placed on the same surface prior to their packaging. Likewise, carpets, rugs, and bedding are to be folded carefully to protect areas suspected of containing fibers. Car seats should be carefully covered with polyethylene sheets to protect fiber evidence, and knife blades should be covered to protect adhering fibers. If a body is thought to have been wrapped at one time in a blanket or carpet, adhesive tape lifts of exposed body areas may reveal fiber strands.

Occasionally, it may be necessary for the field investigator to remove a fiber from an object, particularly if the possibility exists that loosely adhering fibrous material will be lost in transit to the laboratory. These fibers must be removed with a clean forcep and placed in a small sheet of paper, which, after folding and labeling, can be placed inside another container. Again, scrupulous care must be taken to avoid fibers collected from different objects or from different locations from coming into contact.

In the laboratory the search for fiber evidence on clothing and other relevant objects as well as in debris is a time-consuming and tedious process. The search will test the skill and patience of the examiner. The crime-scene investigator can reduce this task to manageable proportions by collecting only relevant items for examination. It is essential from the onset of an investigation that the crime-scene investigator pinpoint areas where a likely transfer of fiber evidence occurred and then take necessary measures to ensure the proper collection and preservation of these materials.

THE FORENSIC EXAMINATION OF PAINT

Our environment is literally surrounded with millions of objects whose surfaces are painted. Thus, it is not surprising to observe that paint, in one form or another, is one of the most prevalent types of physical evidence received by the crime laboratory. Paint as physical evidence is perhaps most frequently encountered in hit-and-run and burglary cases. For example, a chip of dried paint or a paint smear may be transferred to the clothing of a hit-and-run victim on impact with an automobile, or paint smears could be transferred onto a tool during the commission of a burglary. Obviously, there exist numerous possibilities and situations under which a transfer of paint from one surface to another could impart an object with an identifiable forensic characteristic.

In most circumstances the criminalist will be required to compare two or more paints for the ultimate purpose of establishing their common origin. Through such a comparison it may be possible, for example, to associate an individual or a vehicle with the crime site. However, the criminalist need not be confined to comparisons alone. Crime laboratories can often provide valuable assistance in identifying the color, make, and model of an automobile by examining small quantities of paint recovered at an accident scene. Such requests, normally made in connection with hit-and-run cases, can lead to the apprehension of the responsible vehicle.

Paint, when spread onto a surface, will dry into a hard film that can best be described as consisting of pigments suspended in a binder. Pigments impart color to paint and are usually mixtures of different inorganic compounds added to the paint by the manufacturer to produce specific colors. The binder provides the support medium for the pigments and is a polymeric substance. Paint is thus comprised of a binder and pigments, as well as other materials added for bulk, all dissolved in a suitable solvent. After the paint has been applied to a surface, the solvent evaporates, leaving behind a hard polymeric binder and any pigments that were suspended in it.

The microscope has traditionally been and remains the most important instrument for locating and comparing paint specimens. When one considers the thousands upon thousands of paint colors and shades that are known to exist, it is quite understandable why color, more than any other property, imparts paint with its most distinctive forensic characteristics. Questioned and known specimens are best compared side by side under a stereoscopic microscope for color, surface texture, and color layer sequence.

The importance of layer structure for evaluating the evidential significance of paint evidence cannot be overemphasized. When paint specimens possess colored layers that match with respect to number and sequence of colors, the examiner can begin to confidently think in terms of relating the paints to a common origin. How many layers must be matched before the criminalist can conclude that the paints come from the same source? There is no one accepted criterion. Much depends on the uniqueness of each layer with respect to its color and texture, as well as the frequency with which the particular combination of colors under investigation is observed to occur. Because there are at present no books or journals that have compiled this type of information, the criminalist is left to his own experience and knowledge when making this decision.

Unfortunately, the vast majority of the paint specimens presented to the criminalist will not have a layer structure of sufficient complexity to allow them to be individualized to a single source, nor is it common to have paint chips that can be physically fitted together to prove common origin, as shown in Figure 8-16. However, the diverse chemical composition of modern paints does provide for additional points of comparison between specimens. Specifically, a thorough comparison of paint must include a chemical analysis of either the paint's pigments or its binder composition, or both.

The wide variation in binder formulations provides particularly significant information with respect to the forensic comparison of automobile finishes. At present, automobile finishes can be classified into three broad classes:

1. Acrylic Lacquers. The polymers that comprise the acrylic lacquer binders typically have long chains with few, if any, chemical bonds acting as cross-links between adjacent chains. This is shown schematically in Figure 8-17(a). Such binders, when heated, become soft and more or less fluid. This is preferred by some manufacturers because local surface irregularities are smoothed out in the process. Currently, most vehicles made by General Motors have a topcoat of acrylic lacquer paint; however, General Motors is planning to utilize acrylic enamel finishes. For the most part, these changes are planned to coincide with the introduction of new model vehicles.

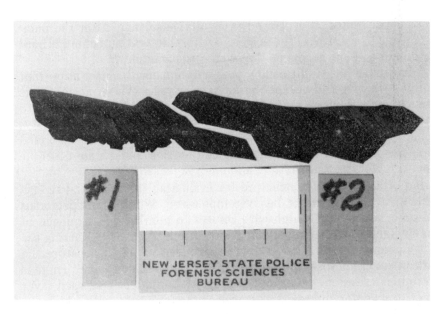

Figure 8-16. Paint chip no. 1 was recovered from the scene of a hit-and-run. Paint chip no. 2 was obtained from the suspect vehicle. *Courtesy* New Jersey State Police.

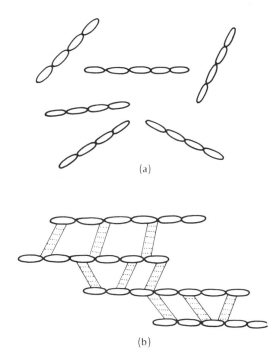

Figure 8-17. Schematic representation of (a) an uncross-linked polymer and (b) a highly cross-linked polymer.

2. Acrylic Enamels. Acrylic enamels are polymers, which, when heated, form an extensively cross-linked network that becomes extremely hard and resistant to attack by solvents. A schematic representation of a highly cross-linked polymer using chemical bonds between adjacent polymer chains is shown in Figure 8-17(b). American Motors, Ford, Chrysler, and most imported brands use acrylic enamel paints as topcoat finishes on their cars.

3. Alkyd Enamels. The polymers that comprise the alkyd enamels also produce an extensively cross-linked surface when heated. Some cars imported to the United States have alkyd enamel finishes.

Fortunately, acrylic lacquer paints can readily be distinguished from other classes by their solubility in acetone. Thus, a paint chip found to be soluble in acetone is immediately associated with a General Motors vehicle. However, just knowing the type of automobile finish contributes very little to the individuality of the paint. What is more important is the knowledge that paint manufacturers make each of the above three classes of automobile finishes in hundreds of varieties; this is most helpful to the criminalist who is trying to associate a paint chip to one car as distinguished from the thousands of similar models that have been produced in any one year. For instance, there are over 100 automobile production plants in the United States. Each has the option of using one paint supplier for a particular color or varying its paint suppliers during a model year. Although a paint supplier is obligated to maintain strict quality control over a paint's color, the batch formulation of any paint binder can vary depending on the availability and cost of basic ingredients.

Pyrolysis gas chromatography has proven to be a particularly invaluable technique for distinguishing most of these formulations. Here, paint chips as small as 20 micrograms are decomposed by heat into numerous gaseous products and are sent through a gas chromatograph. What results is a pyrogram that is sufficiently detailed to reflect chemical makeup of the binder. Figure 8-18 illustrates how the patterns produced by paint pyrograms can differentiate acrylic enamel paints removed from two different automobiles.

The elements that comprise the inorganic pigments of paints can be identified by any one of a variety of techniques—i.e., emission spectroscopy, neutron activation analysis, X-ray diffraction, and X-ray spectroscopy (pp. 169-170). The emission spectrograph, for instance, can simultaneously detect 15 to 20 elements in most automobile paints. Some of these elements are relatively common to all paints and have little forensic value; others are less frequently encountered and provide excellent points of comparison between paint specimens (see Figure 6-3).

Infrared spectrophotometry is still another analytical technique used to provide the analyst with information about both the binder and pigment composition of paint.[9] Both of these components will selectively absorb infrared radiation to yield a spectrum that is highly characteristic of a paint specimen.

Once a paint comparison is completed, the task of assessing the significance of the finding begins. How certain can one be that two similar paints did indeed come from the same surface? For instance, to a casual observer countless identically colored automobiles are seen on our roads and streets. If this is the case, what value is a comparison of a paint chip from a hit-and-run scene to paint removed from a suspect car? From previous discussions it should be apparent that far more is involved in a paint comparison than matching surface paint colors. Paint layers present beneath a surface layer offer valuable points of comparison. Furthermore, forensic analysts are capable of detecting subtle differences in paint binder formulations, as well as major or minor differences in the elemental composition of paint. Obviously, to the naked eye these properties cannot be discerned.

The significance of a paint comparison was convincingly demonstrated from data recently gathered at the author's laboratory. Paint chips, randomly taken from 500 vehicles located in a local wreck yard, were compared by layer structure, solvent tests, pyrolysis gas chromatography, and X-ray spec-

---

[9] P. G. Rodgers et al., "The Classification of Automobile Paint by Diamond Window Infrared Spectrophotometry, Part I: Binders and Pigments," *The Canadian Society of Forensic Science Journal*, 9 (1976), 1.

(a)   TIME (MINUTES)

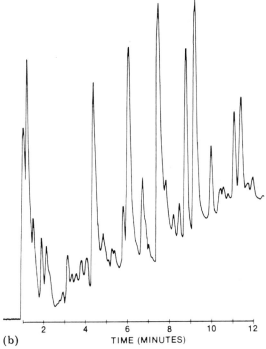

(b)   TIME (MINUTES)

Figure 8-18. Paint pyrograms of acrylic enamel paints. **(a)** Paint from a Ford model. **(b)** Paint from a Chrysler model. *Courtesy* Varian Instruments, California.

troscopy. All were distinguishable except for 8 pairs. In statistical terms these results signify that if a crime-scene paint and a paint control removed from a suspect car compare by the above tests, the odds against the crime-scene paint originating from another randomly chosen vehicle are approximately 16,000 to 1. Obviously, this type of evidence is bound to forge a strong link between the suspect car and the crime scene.

It is often requested of crime laboratories to identify the make and model of a car from a very small amount of paint left behind at a crime scene. Such information is frequently of use in a search for an unknown car involved in a hit-and-run incident. Often, the questioned paint can be identified when its color is compared to color chips representing the various makes and models of manufactured cars. However, in many cases, it is not possible to state the exact make or model of the car in question since any one paint color can be found on more than one car model. For instance, General Motors may use the same paint color for several production years on cars in their Cadillac, Buick, Oldsmobile, Pontiac, and Chevrolet lines.

Color charts for automobile finishes are available from various paint manufacturers and refinishers. Starting with the 1974 model year, the Law Enforcement Standards Laboratory at the National Bureau of Standards collected and disseminated to crime laboratories auto paint color samples from U.S. domestic passenger cars. This collection, now distributed by Collaborative Testing Services, McLean, Va., promises to further enhance the ability of the criminalist to match an unknown paint chip to a particular vehicle model.

Case Reading

In the early morning hours . . . . atop a lonely roof garage on the westside of Manhattan, three men were found murdered. Each man had been shot once in the back of the head. A light-colored van was seen speeding away from the scene. Hours later, in a secluded alley street on the lower eastside of Manhattan, the body of a fully clothed woman was found lying face down by two dog walkers. The woman had been killed in the same manner as the men on the roof garage.

The condition of the woman's body, and other evidence, made it apparent that she had been shot at the garage, and then transported to the alley.

An eyewitness to the incident stated that he saw a man shoot a woman and place her in a light-colored van. The gunman then chased down the three men who were coming to the woman's aid, and shot each one of them. Days later, the prime suspect to the killings was arrested in Kentucky, in a black-colored van.

Numerous items of evidence (over 100) were collected from the van, and forwarded to the New York City police laboratory for examination. Among the items of evidence forwarded were three sets of vacuum sweepings from the van's interior.

An autopsy of the woman produced several items of trace evidence that were removed from the victim and forwarded to the author for microscopic examination. The woman's clothing was also received by the author for trace analysis.

A prime question that arose during the investigation was: could the woman's body, which had been placed in a light-colored van at the garage, and later left in an alley on the lower eastside, be associated with the black van recovered over 1000 km (600 miles) away from the scene? Microscopic analysis and comparison of the trace evidential materials found on the victim and inside the van made this association possible.

Listed in Table 1 are all the items of similar trace materials that both the victim and the van had in common.

Microscopic comparisons of the questioned human head hair present on the victim's clothing were made with known samples. Ten of the brown-colored and gray-colored caucasian head hairs from the victim's blazer were consistent in microscopic characteristics to the defendant's known head hair sample. One chemically treated head hair found on the victim was consistent

Table I

ITEMS OF SIMILAR TRACE EVIDENCE THAT WERE RECOVERED FROM
BOTH THE VICTIM AND THE VAN'S INTERIOR

	Source	
Trace Evidence	*Victim*	*Van*
White seed	mouth	sweepings
Paint chips gray metallic/black	hair and wool blazer	sweepings and floor
Sawdust	hair, blazer, and sheet	sweepings and misc. items
Glass fragments clear amber green	wool blazer and sheet	sweepings and misc. items
Cellophane	wool blazer	floor
Urethane foam	wool blazer	sweepings, misc. items, and foam mattress
Blue olefin plastic	skirt	floor
Dog hair brown/white white	wool blazer	sweeping and misc. items
Human hair brown gray	wool blazer	hair brush, sweepings, and misc. items

in microscopic characteristics to the known head hair sample obtained from the defendant's wife. One forcibly removed, brown-colored, caucasian head hair that was found on the rear door of the van's interior by the Kentucky state police was found to be consistent in all characteristics with the decedent's known head hair sample.

Microscopic comparisons of the white- and brown/white-colored dog hair from the victim's clothing, and the van's interior, were made with known samples of dog hair obtained from a dog owned by the defendant's nephew, the van's previous owner. The questioned dog hairs were found to be consistent with the hair from the nephew's dog.

The white seed that was recovered from the victim's mouth by the medical examiner, and the white seed that was found in the van's sweepings by the author, were forwarded to an internationally known botanist for identification and comparison. During the trial, the botanist testified that the two seeds were identical in all respects, and that although he could not identify the seed, both were either from the same species of plant, *if not the same plant*, probably a rare wild flower.

Sixteen gray metallic/black-colored paint chips from the victim and her clothing were compared to the gray metallic/black-colored paint removed from the van. Samples from the questioned and known sources were examined and compared by microscopic, chemical, and instrumental means. All of the paint specimens from the van and from the victim were found to be similar in all respects.

The remaining items of trace evidence from the victim and the van were examined and compared microscopically, and where necessary, by chemical and instrumental methods. Each of the remaining types of trace evidence from the victim was found to be similar to its counterpart from the van.

Blue- and black-colored flakes of acrylic paint were found in the van's sweepings, and on the suspect's sneakers. No blue- or black-colored paint flakes were found on the victim or her clothing. During a crime scene search of the defendant's residence in New Jersey, a large quantity of blue- and black-colored acrylic paint was found in the garage. It was apparent from the evidence present in the defendant's garage that a large rectangular shaped object had recently been painted with blue- and black-colored paint. The blue and black paint flakes from all the sources and the known blue (undercoat) and black (topcoat) paint from the van were compared by microscopic, chemical, and instrumental means. All the samples of paint were found to be consistent in every respect.

At the trial, extensive testimony concerning the collection, examination, identification, and comparison of the trace evidence from the victim and the van was given by the author, over a two-day period. When questioned about the source of the trace evidence found on the victim and her clothing, the author stated unequivocally that the trace evidence on the victim was from the defendant's van. On the basis of this evidence and other circumstantial evidence, the defendant was found guilty of all charges and sentenced to 100 years in prison.[10]

COLLECTION AND PRESERVATION OF PAINT EVIDENCE

As has already been noted, paint chips are most likely to be found on or near persons or objects involved in hit-and-run incidents. The recovery of loose paint chips from a garment or from the road surface must be done with the utmost care to keep the paint chip intact. Paint chips may be picked up with a tweezers or scooped up with a piece of paper. Paper druggist folds and glass or plastic vials make excellent containers for paint. If the paint is smeared or imbedded in garments or objects, the investigator should not attempt to remove it; instead, it is best to package the whole item carefully and send it on to the laboratory for examination.

When a transfer of paint occurs in hit-and-run situations, such as to the clothing of a pedestrian victim, uncontaminated control paint must always be collected from an undamaged area of the vehicle for comparison in the laboratory. It is particularly important that the collected paint be close to the area of the car that was suspected of being in contact with the victim. This is necessary because other portions of the car may have faded or been repainted. Control samples are always removed so as to include all the paint layers down to the bare metal. This is best accomplished by removing a painted section with a clean scalpel or knife blade. Samples 1/4 inch square are sufficient for laboratory examination. Each paint sample should be separately packaged and marked as to the exact location of its recovery. When a cross-transfer of paint occurs between two vehicles, again all the layers, including the foreign as well as the underlying original paints, must be removed from each vehicle. A control sample from an adjacent undamaged area of each vehicle must also be taken in such cases. Carefully wipe the blade of any knife or scraping tool used before collecting each sample. This step will avoid cross-contamination of paints.

Tools used to gain entry into buildings or safes often contain traces of paints as well as other substances such as wood, safe insulation, etc. Care must be taken that this type of trace evidence is not lost. It is preferable that the scene investigator avoid making any attempt to remove the paint, choosing instead to package the tool for laboratory examination. Control paint should be collected from all surfaces suspected of having been in contact with the tool. Again, all layers of paint must be included in the sample.

---

[10] Reprinted, by permission of the American Society of Testing and Materials from N. Petraco, "Trace Evidence—The Invisible Witness," *Journal of Forensic Sciences*, 31 (1986), 321. Copyright 1986.

In some cases in which the tool has left its impression on a surface, control paint is collected from an uncontaminated area adjacent to the impression. No attempt is to be made to collect the paint from the impression itself. If this is done, the impression may be permanently altered and its evidential value lost.

REVIEW QUESTIONS

1. Hair is an appendage of the skin, growing out of an organ known as the _____.
2. The three layers that comprise the hair shaft are _____, _____, and _____.
3. The scales of most animal hairs can be described as having the appearance of shingles on a roof. (True, False)
4. The _____ contains the pigment granules that impart color to hair.
5. The central canal running through many hairs is known as the _____.
6. The diameter of the medulla relative to the diameter of the hair shaft is the _____.
7. Human hair generally has a medullary index of less than a _____; the hair of most animals has an index of _____ or greater.
8. Human head hairs generally exhibit (continuous, absent) medullae.
9. If a medulla exhibits a patterned shape, the hair is (human, animal) in origin.
10. A single hair (can, cannot) be individualized to one person.
11. In making hair comparisons it is best to view the hairs side by side under a _____ microscope.
12. _____ hairs are short and curly with wide variation in shaft diameter.
13. It (is, is not) possible to determine the time when hair was last bleached or dyed.
14. The age and sex of hair can be determined through an examination of its morphological features. (True, False)
15. Hair forcibly removed from the body (always, often) has follicular tissue adhering to its root.
16. The elemental composition of hair can be determined by a technique known as _____.
17. A minimum collection of _____ full-length hairs will normally ensure a representative sampling of head hair.
18. A minimum collection of _____ full-length pubic hairs is recom-

mended to cover the range of characteristics present in this region of the body.

19. _____ fibers are derived totally from animal or plant sources.

20. The most prevalent natural plant fiber is _____.

21. Regenerated fibers, such as rayon and acetate, are manufactured by chemically treating cellulose and passing it through a spinnerette. (True, False)

22. Fibers manufactured solely from synthetic chemicals are classified as _____.

23. Polyester was the first synthetic fiber. (True, False)

24. _____ are composed of a large number of atoms arranged in repeating units.

25. The basic unit of the polymer is called the _____.

26. _____ are polymers composed of thousands of amino acids linked together in a highly organized arrangement and sequence.

27. A first step in the forensic examination of fibers will be the comparison of color and diameter. (True, False)

28. The dye components removed from fibers can be separated and compared by _____ chromatography.

29. Synthetic fibers possess the physical property of _____ because they are crystalline.

30. The technique of _____ characterizes a fiber by decomposing its polymer chain and separating the resultant gaseous products.

31. Normally, fibers possess (individual, class) characteristics.

32. The two most important components of dried paint from the criminalist's point of view are the _____ and the _____.

33. The most important physical property of paint relating to a forensic comparison is _____.

34. Paints can be individualized to a single source only when they have a sufficiently detailed _____.

35. The polymeric paint binder used primarily by General Motors is _____.

36. A highly cross-linked polymer binder used by most American automobile manufacturers is _____.

37. Acrylic enamels are readily dissolved by the solvent acetone. (True, False)

38. Pyrolysis gas chromatography is a particularly valuable technique for characterizing paint's (binder, pigments).

39. Emission spectroscopy can be used to identify the (inorganic, organic) components of paint's pigments.

40. Paint samples removed for examination must always include all the paint layers. (True, False)

FURTHER REFERENCES

Appleyard, H. M., "Fibre Identification and Analysis of Fibre Blends," *Analyst*, 101 (1976), 595.

Bisbing, R. E., "The Forensic Identification and Association of Human Hair," in *Forensic Science Handbook*, R. Saferstein, ed. Englewood Cliffs, N.J.: Prentice-Hall, Inc., 1982.

Crown, David A., *The Forensic Examination of Paints and Pigments*. Springfield, Ill.: Charles C. Thomas, Publisher, 1968.

"Don't Miss a Hair," *FBI Law Enforcement Bulletin*, May 1976, p. 9.

Gaudette, B. D., "Some Further Thoughts on Probabilities and Human Hair Comparisons," *Journal of Forensic Sciences*, 23 (1978), 758.

_____, "Strong Negative Conclusions in Hair Comparison—A Rare Event," *The Canadian Society of Forensic Science Journal*, 18 (1985), 32.

_____, "The Forensic Aspects of Textile Fiber Examination," in *Forensic Science Handbook, Vol. 2*, R. Saferstein, ed. Englewood Cliffs, N.J.: Prentice-Hall, Inc., 1987.

Grieve, M. C., "The Role of Fibers in Forensic Science Examinations," *Journal of Forensic Sciences*, 28 (1983), 877.

Hicks, J. W., *Microscopy of Hair, A Practical Guide and Manual*. Washington, D.C.: U.S. Government Printing Office, 1977.

Manura, John J., and Richard Saferstein, "Examination of Automobile Paints by Laser Beam Emission Spectroscopy," *Journal of the Association of Official Analytical Chemists*, 56 (1973), 1227.

Nielsen, H. K. R., "Forensic Analysis of Coatings," *Journal of Coatings Technology*, 56 (1984), 21.

Porter, J., and C. Fouweather, "An Appraisal of Human Head Hair as Forensic Evidence," *Journal of the Society of Cosmetic Chemists*, 26 (1975), 299.

Saferstein, R., "Forensic Aspects of Analytical Pyrolysis," in *Pyrolysis and GC in Polymer Analysis*, S. A. Lieberman and E. J. Levy, eds. New York: Marcel Dekker, 1985.

The Textile Institute, *Identification of Textile Materials*, 7th ed. Manchester, England: The Textile Institute, 1975.

Thornton, J. I., "Forensic Paint Examination," in *Forensic Science Handbook*, R. Saferstein, ed. Englewood Cliffs, N.J.: Prentice-Hall, Inc., 1982.

9

Drugs

A drug can be defined as a natural or synthetic substance that is used to produce physiological or psychological effects in man or other higher-order animals. However, this colorless clinical definition does not really tell us what drugs are; in their modern context, drugs mean something different to each person. To some, drugs are a necessity for sustaining and prolonging life; to others, drugs provide an escape from the pressures of life; and to some, they are a means of ending it.

Considering the wide application and acceptance of drugs in our society, it was perhaps inevitable that a segment of our population would abuse their use. During the 1960s, succeeding waves of hallucinogens, amphetamines, and barbiturates found their way out of laboratories, pharmacies, and medicine chests into the streets. During this decade, marijuana became the most widely used illicit drug in the United States, and alcohol consumption continued to rise—today 90 million Americans drink alcohol regularly and 10 million of these are hopelessly addicted or have severe problems in coping with their drinking habits.

Drug abuse has grown from a problem generally associated with members of the lower end of the social economic ladder to one that cuts across all social and ethnic classes of society. There are now millions of people addicted to alcohol, barbiturates, and heroin. In addition, there are millions more illegally using drugs such as marijuana, amphetamines, LSD, and cocaine.

In the United States, the epidemic proportions of illegal drug use has produced a situation that finds more than 75 percent of the evidence now being evaluated in crime laboratories to be drug-related. The deluge of drug specimens has forced the expansion of existing crime laboratories and the creation of new ones. For many concerned forensic scientists, the crime laboratory's preoccupation with drug evidence represents a serious distraction from time that could be devoted to the evaluation of evidence related to homicides and other types of serious crimes. However, few can deny that the increasing caseloads associated with drug evidence have provided the major, and often the sole, justification for the expansion of forensic laboratory services. Unquestionably, this expansion has had the effect of increasing the overall analytical capabilities of crime laboratories.

DRUG DEPENDENCE

In assessing the potential danger of drugs, society has become particularly conscious of their affects on human behavior. In fact, the first drugs to be regulated by law in the early years of the twentieth century were those deemed to have "habit-forming" properties. The early laws were aimed primarily at controlling opium and its derivatives, cocaine, and later marijuana. Today, it is known that the ability of a drug to induce dependence after repeated use is submerged in a complex array of physiological and social factors.

Dependence on drugs exists in numerous patterns and in all degrees of intensity, depending on the nature of the drug, the route of administration, the dose, the frequency of administration, and the individual's rate of metabolism. Furthermore, nondrug factors play an equally crucial role in determining the behavioral patterns associated with drug use. The personal characteristics of the user, his expectations about the drug experience, society's attitudes and possible responses, as well as the setting in which the drug is used, are all major determinants of drug dependence.

The question of how to define and measure a drug's influence on the individual and the danger it poses for society is difficult to assess. To this end, the nature and significance of drug dependence must be considered from two overlapping points of view: one relates to the interaction of the drug with the individual, and the second has to do with the drug's impact on society. It will be useful when discussing the nature of the drug experience to approach the problem from two distinctly different aspects of human behavior—psychological **dependency** and physical **dependency**.

The common denominator that characterizes all types of repeated drug use is the creation of a **psychological dependence** for continued use of the drug. In this context it is important to discard the unrealistic image that all drug users are hopeless "addicts" who are social dropouts. The fact is that most users present quite a normal appearance and remain both socially and economically integrated in the life of the community.

The reasons why some people abstain from drugs while others become moderately or heavily involved are difficult if not impossible to answer. Unquestionably, psychological needs arise from numerous personal and social factors that inevitably stem from the individual's desires to create a sense of well-being and to escape from reality. In some cases, the individual may be seeking relief from personal problems or stressful situations, or he or she may be trying to sustain a physical and emotional state that permits an improved level of performance. Whatever the reasons, it is the existence of underlying psychological needs and the desire to fulfill them that create a conditioned pattern of drug use.

The intensity of the psychological dependence associated with a drug's use is difficult to define and to a large extent depends on the nature of the drug used. For drugs such as alcohol, heroin, amphetamines, barbiturates, and cocaine there is a significant likelihood that continued use will result in a high degree of involvement. Others such as marijuana and codeine appear to have a considerably lower potential for the development of psychological dependence. However, this is not to imply that the repeated abuse of drugs deemed to have a low potential for psychological dependency is safe or will always produce low psychological dependence. The fact is that we have no precise way of measuring or predicting the impact of drug abuse on the individual. Even if a system could be devised for controlling the many possible variables affecting a user's response, the unpredictability of the human personality would still have to be contended with; for it is the personal inadequacies of the drug user that represent the underlying motivation for drug use.

Our general knowledge of alcohol consumption should warn us of the fallacy of generalizing when attempting to describe the danger of drug abuse. Obviously, not all drinkers of alcohol are psychologically addicted to the drug; most are "social" drinkers who drink in reasonable amounts and on an irregular basis. Certainly there are many who have progressed beyond this stage and who consider alcohol a necessary crutch for dealing with life's stresses and anxieties. However, a wide range of behavioral patterns does exist among alcohol abusers, and to a large extent the determination of the degree of psychological dependency must be made on an individual basis. Likewise, it would be fallacious to generalize that all users of marijuana can at worst develop a low degree of dependency on the drug. A wide range of factors also influence marijuana's effect, and heavy users of the drug do expose themselves to the danger of developing a high degree of psychological dependency.

Where emotional well-being is the primary motive leading to repeated and intensive use of a drug, certain drugs, when taken in sufficient dose and frequency, are capable of producing physiological changes that encourage their continued use. Once the user abstains from such a drug, severe physical illness follows. It is the desire to avoid this withdrawal sickness or abstinence syndrome that ultimately causes **physical dependence** or addiction. Hence, for the addict who is accustomed to receiving large doses of heroin, the thought of abstaining and encountering body chills, vomiting, stomach cramps, convulsions, insomnia, pain, and hallucinations serves as a powerful inducement for continued drug use.

Interestingly, some of the more widely abused drugs have little or no potential for creating physical dependence. Drugs such as marijuana, LSD, and cocaine do create strong anxieties when their repeated use is discontinued; however, no medical evidence exists to attribute these discomforts to physiological reactions that accompany withdrawal sickness. On the other hand, the use of alcohol, heroin, and barbiturates can result in the development of physical dependency.

Physical dependency develops only when the drug user adheres to a regular schedule of drug intake; that is, the interval between doses must be short enough so that the effects of the drug never wear off completely. For example, the interval between injections of heroin for the drug addict probably does not exceed six to eight hours. Beyond this time the addict begins to experience the uncomfortable symptoms of withdrawal. It is well known that many users of heroin avoid taking the drug on a regular basis for fear of becoming physically addicted to its use. Similarly, the risk of developing physical dependence on alcohol becomes greatest when the consumption is characterized by a continuing pattern of daily use in large quantities.

Table 9-1 categorizes some of the more commonly abused drugs according to their effect on the body, and summarizes their tendency to produce psychological dependency and to induce physical dependency with repeated use.

The social impact of drug dependence is directly related to the extent with which the user has become preoccupied with the drug. Here, the most important element to consider is the extent to which drug use has become interwoven in the fabric of the user's life. The more frequently the drug satisfies the person's need, the greater is the likelihood of his or her preoccupation with its use, with a consequent neglect of individual and social responsibilities. Personal health, economic relationships, and family obligations may all suffer as the drug-seeking behavior increases in frequency and intensity and dominates the individual's life. The extreme of drug dependence may lead to behavior that has serious implications for the public's safety, health, and welfare.

Drug dependence in its broadest sense involves much of the world's population. As a result there must be a complex array of individual, social, cultural, legal, and medical factors that ultimately influence society's decision to prohibit or to impose strict controls on a drug's distribution and use. Invariably, society must weigh the beneficial aspects of the drug against the ultimate harm its abuse will do to the individual and to society as a whole. Obviously, there are many forms of drug dependence that do not carry adverse social consequences, as illustrated by the widespread use of such drug-containing substances as tobacco and coffee. Although the heavy and pro-

Table 9-1.

THE POTENTIAL OF SOME COMMONLY ABUSED DRUGS TO PRODUCE
DEPENDENCY WITH REGULAR USE

Drug	*Psychological Dependence*	*Physical Dependence*
Narcotics		
Morphine	High	Yes
Heroin	High	Yes
Methadone	High	Yes
Codeine	Low	Yes
Depressants		
Barbiturates (short-acting)	High	Yes
Barbiturates (long-acting)	Low	Yes
Alcohol	High	Yes
Methaqualone (Quaalude)	High	Yes
Meprobamate (Miltown, Equanil)	Moderate	Yes
Diazepam (Valium)	Moderate	Yes
Chlordiazepoxide (Librium)	Moderate	Yes
Stimulants		
Amphetamines	High	?
Cocaine	High	No
Caffeine	Low	No
Nicotine	High	No
Hallucinogens		
Marijuana	Low	No
LSD	Low	No
Phencyclidine (PCP)	High	No

longed use of these drugs may eventually damage body organs and result in injury to an individual's health, there is no evidence that they induce physical dependence or result in antisocial behavior even upon prolonged or excessive use. Hence, society is willing to accept the widespread use of these substances.

We are certainly all aware of the disastrous failure in the United States to prohibit the use of alcohol during the 1920s and the current intensive debate on whether or not marijuana should be legalized. Each of these issues emphasizes that the balance between individual desires and needs and society's concern with the consequences of drug abuse is a delicate one; moreover, it is one that is continuously subject to change and reevaluation.

NARCOTIC DRUGS

The term *narcotic* is derived from the Greek word *narkotikos*, which implies a state of lethargy or sluggishness. Pharmacologists actually classify narcotic drugs as substances that bring relief from pain and produce sleep. Unfortunately, "narcotic" has come to be popularly associated with any drug that is socially unacceptable. As a consequence of this incorrect usage, many drugs are improperly called *narcotics*. Furthermore, this confusion has produced legal definitions that are at variance with the pharmacological actions of many drugs. For example, until the early 1970s most drug laws in the United States incorrectly designated marijuana as a narcotic substance; even at the present time many drug-control laws in the United States, including the federal law, classify cocaine as a narcotic drug. Pharmacologically, cocaine is actually a powerful central nervous system stimulant possessing properties opposite to those normally associated with the depressant effects of a narcotic.

Narcotic drugs are analgesics—that is, they relieve pain by exerting a depressing action on the central nervous system. The regular use of a narcotic drug will invariably lead to physical dependence with all its dire consequences. The source of most analgesic narcotics is opium, a gummy, milky juice exuded through a cut made in the unripe pod of the poppy (*Papaver somniferium*), a plant grown mostly in parts of Asia. Opium is brownish in color and has a morphine content that can range from 4 to 21 percent.

Although morphine is readily extracted from opium, for reasons that are not totally known most addicts prefer to use one of its derivatives, heroin. Heroin is made rather simply by reacting morphine with acetic anhydride or acetyl chloride (see Figure 9-1). Heroin's high solubility in

Figure 9-1. The opium poppy and its derivatives. Shown are the poppy plant, crude and smoking opium, codein, heroin, and morphine. *Courtesy* Drug Enforcement Administration, Washington, D.C.

water makes its street preparation for intravenous administration rather simple, for it is only by injection that heroin's effects are almost instantaneously felt and with maximum sensitivity. To prepare the drug for injection, the addict frequently dissolves it in a small quantity of water in a spoon. The process can be speeded up by heating the spoon over a candle or several matches. The solution is then drawn into a syringe or eyedropper for injection beneath the skin. Figure 9-2 shows some of the paraphernalia typically associated with heroin's street administration.

Besides being a powerful analgesic, heroin produces a "high" that is accompanied by drowsiness and a deep sense of well-being; however, the effect is of short duration, generally lasting only three to four hours.

The content of a typical heroin bag is an excellent example of the uncertainty attached to buying illicit drugs. For many years into the 1960s and early 1970s, the average bag contained 15 to 20 percent heroin; however, vigorous law enforcement has slowly reduced the drug's concentration to a level somewhere between 2 to 5 percent. The addict rarely knows or cares what comprises the other 95 percent or so of the material. Traditionally, quinine has been the most common diluent of heroin. Like heroin, it has a bitter taste and was probably originally used to obscure the actual

Figure 9-2.   Heroin paraphernalia. *Courtesy* New Jersey State Police.

potency of a heroin preparation for those who wished to taste-test the material before buying it. Other diluents commonly added to heroin are starch, lactose, procaine (Novacaine), and mannitol.

Codeine is also present in opium, but it is usually prepared synthetically from morphine. It is commonly used as a cough suppressant in cough syrup. Codeine, being only one-sixth as strong as morphine, is not an attractive street drug for addicts.

There are a number of narcotic drugs that are not derived from opium or morphine. However, because they too have the same physiological effects on the body as the opium narcotics, they are commonly referred to as "opiates." Methadone is perhaps the best known of the synthetic opiates. In the 1960s, scientists discovered that a person receiving methadone periodically in oral doses of 80 to 120 milligrams a day would not get high if he then took heroin or morphine. Clearly, although methadone is a narcotic pharmacologically related to heroin, its administration appears to eliminate the addict's desire for heroin while producing minimal side effects. Critics of the controversial methadone maintenance programs claim that methadone is just substituting one narcotic drug for another, and supporters argue that this is the only known treatment for keeping the addict off heroin and offering some hope for eventual abstention from narcotics.

Another synthetic narcotic beginning to receive close scrutiny by legal authorities is propoxyphene, first marketed in 1957 under the trade name of Darvon. This drug is normally prescribed for the relief of moderate pain; however, evidence of its abuse and increasing incidences of propoxyphene overdoses have sparked investigations regarding the drug's usefulness and whether steps are warranted to restrict its availability as a prescription drug.

HALLUCINOGENS

Hallucinogens are drugs that can cause marked alterations in normal thought processes, perceptions, and moods. Perhaps the most popular and controversial member of this class of drugs is marijuana.

MARIJUANA

Marijuana easily qualifies as the most widely used illicit drug in the United States today. For instance, more than 43 million Americans have tried marijuana according to the latest surveys, and almost half that number may be regular users. Marijuana refers to a preparation derived from the plant *Cannabis*. Most botanists believe there is only one species of the plant, *Cannabis sativa L.* The marijuana preparation normally consists of crushed leaves mixed in varying proportions with the plant's flower, stem, and seed. The plant secretes a sticky resin that is known as *hashish*. The resinous material can also be extracted from the plant by soaking in a solvent such as alcohol. On the illicit drug market, hashish usually appears in the form of compressed vegetation containing a high percentage of resin. A potent form of marijuana is known as *sinsemilla*. This is made from the unfertilized flowering tops of the female *Cannabis* plants. This is attained by removal of all male plants from the growing field at the first sign of their appearance. It follows that the production of sinsemilla requires a great deal of attention and care, and the plant is therefore cultivated on small plots.

Marijuana and its related products have been in use legally and illegally for almost three thousand years. The first reference to the medical use of marijuana is in a pharmacy book written about 2737 B.C. by the Chinese Emperor Shen Nung, who recommended it for "female weakness, gout, rheumatism, malaria, beriberi, constipation and absentmindedness." In China, at that time and even today, the marijuana or hemp plant was also a major source of fiber for the production of rope. Marijuana's mood-altering powers probably did not receive wide attention until about 1000 B.C., when it became an integral part of Hindu culture in India. After A.D. 500, marijuana began creeping westward, and references to it began to appear in the Persian and Arabian literature.

The plant was probably brought to Europe by Napoleon's soldiers returning from Egypt in the early years of the nineteenth century. In Europe the drug excited the interests of many physicians who foresaw its application for the treatment of a wide range of ailments. At this time it also found some use as a pain-killer and mild sedative. In later years these applications were to be either forgotten or ignored.

Marijuana was first introduced into the United States around 1920. The weed was smuggled by Mexican laborers across the border into Texas. American soldiers also brought the plant in from the ports of Havana, Tampico, and Veracruz. Although its use was confined to a small segment of the population, its popularity quickly spread from the border and Gulf states into most of the major U.S. cities. By 1937, 46 states and the federal government had laws prohibiting the use or possession of marijuana. Under most of these laws, marijuana was subject to the same rigorous penalties applicable to morphine, heroin, and cocaine, and was often erroneously designated a "narcotic."

Marijuana is a weed that grows wild under most climatic conditions. The plant grows to a height of 5 to 15 feet and is characterized by an odd number of leaflets on each leaf. Normally, each leaf contains five to nine leaflets, all having serrated or saw-tooth edges, as shown in Figure 9-3.

It wasn't until 1964 that scientists isolated the chemical substance largely responsible for the hallucinogenic properties of marijuana. This substance is known as *tetrahydrocannabinol*, or *THC*. Its discovery has allowed researchers to measure the potency of marijuana preparations and has permitted studies related to measuring the effect of marijuana's potency on man. It has also been found that the THC content of *Cannabis* varies in dif-

Figure 9-3. The marijuana leaf. *Courtesy* Drug Enforcement Administration, Washington, D.C.

ferent parts of the plant, generally decreasing in the following sequence: resin, flowers, and leaves. Little THC is found in the stem, roots, or seeds. The potency and resulting effect of the drug fluctuate, depending on the relative proportion of these plant parts in the marijuana mixture.

The potency of marijuana will depend on its form. Marijuana in the form of loose vegetation has an average THC content of about 1.5 percent. The more potent sinsemilla form averages about 3.5–4 percent in THC content, while hashish preparations average about 3.5 percent. Another form of hashish is known as "liquid hashish" or "hashish oil." Hashish in this form is normally a viscous substance, dark green in color and having the consistency of tar (see Figure 9-4). Liquid hashish is produced by efficiently extracting the THC-rich resin from the marijuana plant with an appropriate solvent. The liquid hashish so far discovered has varied between 20 and 65 percent in THC content. Because of its extraordinary potency, one drop of the material can make a "high." Ordinarily, a drop is placed on a regular cigarette or on a marijuana cigarette before smoking.

Any study that relates to marijuana's effect on man must take the potency of the marijuana preparation into consideration. An interesting in-

Figure 9-4. Top to bottom: marijuana vegetation, hashish, and liquid hashish. *Courtesy Drug Enforcement Administration, Washington, D.C.*

sight into the relationship between dosage level and marijuana's pharmacological effect was presented in the first report of the National Commission of Marijuana and Drug Abuse:

> At low, usual "social" doses the user may experience an increased sense of well-being; initial restlessness and hilarity followed by a dreamy, carefree state of relaxation; alteration of sensory perceptions including expansion of space and time; and a more vivid sense of touch, sight, smell, taste and sound; a feeling of hunger, especially a craving for sweets; and subtle changes in thought formation and expression. To an unknowing observer, an individual in this state of consciousness would not appear noticeably different from his normal state.
>
> At higher, moderate doses these same reactions are intensified but the changes in the individual would still be scarcely noticeable to an observer. . . . At very high doses, psychotomimetic phenomena may be experienced. These include distortion of body image, loss of personal identity, sensory and mental illusions, fantasies and hallucinations.[1]

---

[1] *Marihuana—a Signal of Misunderstanding* (Washington, D.C.: U.S. Government Printing Office, 1972), p. 56.

There is no current evidence that experimental or intermittent use causes physical or psychological harm. Marijuana does not cause physical dependency. However, the risk of harm lies instead in the heavy, long-term use of the drug, particularly of the more potent preparations. The heavy user can develop a strong psychological dependence on the drug. Marijuana's long-term effects on the health of people who use it are still largely unknown.

There is accumulating evidence that marijuana has potential medical uses. Two promising areas of research are marijuana's reduction of excessive eye pressure in glaucoma and the lessening of nausea caused by powerful anticancer drugs. There are also suggestions that marijuana might be useful as a muscle relaxant.

OTHER HALLUCINOGENS

There are a substantial number of substances of widely varying chemical compositions that have become part of the drug culture because of their hallucinogenic properties. These include lysergic acid diethylamide (LSD), dimethoxymethylamphetamine (STP), dimethyltryptamine (DMT), mescaline, phencyclidine (PCP), and psilocybin. Of this family of drugs, LSD is the most potent and differs little from the other drugs except for the greater intensity of its induced reactions and side effects.

LSD is synthesized from lysergic acid, a substance derived from ergot, which is a type of fungus that attacks certain grasses and grains. Its hallucinogenic effects were first described by the Swiss chemist Albert Hofmann after he accidentally ingested some of the material in his laboratory in 1943. The drug is very potent; as little as 25 micrograms is enough to start vivid visual hallucinations that may last for about 12 hours. The drug also produces marked changes in mood, leading to laughing or crying at the slightest provocation. Feelings of anxiety and tension almost always accompany LSD's use. Although physical dependence does not develop with continued use, the individual user may be prone to flashbacks and psychotic reactions even after use is discontinued.

The possibility of LSD causing chromosome damage in the children of users has been explored. At present, there is no medical evidence to substantiate this claim; however, this issue has received so much publicity that undoubtedly many have stopped experimenting with the drug for fear of maiming future offspring.

In recent years, abuse of phencyclidine, commonly called PCP, has grown to alarming proportions. Because this drug can be synthesized by rather simple chemical processes, it is manufactured surreptitiously for the illicit market in so-called clandestine laboratories (see Figure 9-5). These laboratories range from large sophisticated operations to small labs located

Figure 9-5. Scene from a clandestine drug laboratory. *Courtesy* Drug Enforcement Administration, Washington, D.C.

in an individual's garage or bathroom. Small-time operators normally have little or no training in chemistry and employ "cookbook" methods to synthesize the drug. Some of the more knowledgeable and experienced operators have been able to achieve clandestine production levels that approach a commercial level of operation.

Phencyclidine is often mixed with other drugs, such as LSD or amphetamine, and is sold as a powder ("Angel Dust"), capsule, tablet, or as a liquid sprayed on plant leaves. The drug is smoked, ingested, or sniffed.

Following oral intake of moderate doses (1–6 milligrams), the user first experiences feelings of strength and invulnerability along with a dreamy sense of detachment. However, the user soon becomes unresponsive, confused, and agitated. Depression, irritability, feelings of isolation, audio and visual hallucinations, and sometimes paranoia accompany PCP's use. Severe depression, tendencies toward violence, and suicide accompany long-term daily use of the drug. In some cases, the PCP user will experience sudden schizophrenic behavior days after the drug has been taken.

DEPRESSANTS

ALCOHOL (ETHYL ALCOHOL)

Many people tend to overlook the fact that alcohol is a drug; as such, its major behavioral effects derive from its depressant action on the central nervous system. In the United States the alcohol industry annually produces over one billion gallons of spirits, wine, and beer for which 90 million consumers pay nearly $40 billion. Unquestionably, these and other statistics support the fact that alcohol is the most widely used and abused drug in the world today.

The behavioral patterns of alcohol intoxication are varied and depend in part on such factors as social setting, amount consumed, and the personal expectation of the individual with regard to alcohol. When alcohol enters the body's bloodstream, it quickly travels to the brain where it acts to suppress the brain's control of thought processes and muscle coordination.

Low doses of alcohol tend to inhibit the mental processes of judgment, memory, and concentration. The drinker's personality becomes expansive and he or she exudes confidence. When taken in moderate doses, alcohol has been found to reduce coordination substantially, inhibit orderly thought processes and speech patterns, and slow down reaction times. Under these conditions, the ability to walk or drive becomes noticeably impaired. In the next chapter we will examine in greater detail the relationship between alcohol blood levels and driving ability. Higher doses of alcohol may cause the user to become highly irritable and emotional; displays of anger and crying are not uncommon. Extremely high doses may cause an individual to lapse into unconsciousness or even into a comatose state that may be a prelude to a fatal depression of circulatory and respiratory functions.

BARBITURATES

Barbiturates are commonly referred to as "downers" because they relax, create a feeling of well-being, and produce sleep. Like alcohol, barbiturates act on the central nervous system to suppress its vital functions. Collectively, barbiturates can be described as derivatives of barbituric acid, which was first synthesized by a German chemist, Adolf Von Bayer, over 100 years ago. Twenty-five barbiturate derivatives are currently used in medical practice in the United States; however, only five—amobarbital, secobarbital, phenobarbital, pentobarbital, and butabarbital—seemingly suffice for most present-day medical applications. Slang terms for "barbs" usually stem from the color of the capsule or tablet (e.g., "yellow jackets," "blue devils," and "reds").

Normally, barbiturate users take these drugs by mouth. The average sedative dose is about 10 to 70 milligrams. When taken in this fashion, the drug enters the blood through the walls of the small intestine. Some barbiturates, such as phenobarbital, are absorbed more slowly than others and are therefore classified as long-acting barbiturates. Undoubtedly, it is the slow action of phenobarbital that accounts for its low incidence of abuse. Apparently, barbiturate abusers prefer the faster-acting ones—i.e., secobarbital, pentobarbital, and amobarbital.

When taken in prescribed amounts, barbiturates are relatively safe, but in instances of extensive and prolonged use, physical dependence can develop. However, this only happens when the total daily intake of the drug significantly exceeds the normal therapeutic level prescribed by a physician. This means that patients can, for example, take barbiturates daily for sedative purposes or as an aid to sleep without developing physical dependence. However, for individuals who deliberately resort to maintaining high levels of barbiturate use, cessation will produce a withdrawal syndrome more severe than that caused by any other drug. This may result in insomnia, muscle spasms, delirium, and convulsions. Consequently, withdrawal must be conducted under close medical supervision if the likelihood of death is to be minimized.

Since the early 1970s, a new nonbarbiturate depressant, methaqualone (Quaalude), has appeared on the illicit scene. Methaqualone is a powerful sedative and muscle relaxant that possesses many of the depressant properties of barbiturates. Its initial popularity before 1973 probably stemmed from the fact that the drug was not controlled by U.S. federal law or by most of the states. However, since this time the drug has been placed under strict control, causing the incidence of its abuse to decline.

TRANQUILIZERS

In the past 25 years there has been a dramatic growth in the use of tranquilizers. Although tranquilizers can be considered depressants, they do differ from barbiturates in the extent of their actions on the central nervous system. Generally, these drugs produce a relaxing tranquility without impairment of high-thinking facilities or the inducement of sleep. "Major tranquilizers" like reserpine and chlorpromzine have been successfully used to reduce the anxieties and tensions of mental patients.

There is a group of so-called "mild tranquilizers" commonly prescribed to deal with the everyday tensions of many healthy people. These drugs include: meprobamate (Miltown), chlordiazepoxide (Librium), and diazepam (Valium). There is medical evidence to show that these drugs produce psychological and physical dependency with repeated and high levels of usage. For this reason the widespread prescribing of tranquilizers as a means of overcoming the pressures and tensions of life has worried many who fear the creation of a legalized drug culture.

"GLUE SNIFFING"

Since the early 1960s the practice of sniffing materials containing volatile solvents (airplane glue or model cement, for example) has grown in popularity. Within recent years another dimension has been added to the problem with the increasing number of incidents involving the sniffing of aerosol gas propellants such as freon. All materials used in sniffing contain volatile or gaseous substances that are primarily central nervous system depressants.

Although toluene seems to be the most popular solvent to sniff, there are others that can produce comparable physiological effects. These chemicals include naphtha, methyl ethyl ketone, gasoline, and trichloroethylene.

The usual immediate effects of sniffing are a feeling of exhilaration and euphoria combined with slurred speech, impaired judgment, and double vision. Finally, the user may experience drowsiness and stupor, with these depressant effects slowly wearing off as the user returns to a normal state. Most experts believe that users become physiologically dependent on the effects achieved by sniffing. There is, however, little evidence to suggest that the practice of solvent inhalation is addictive. But sniffers do expose themselves to the danger of liver, heart, and brain damage from the chemicals they have inhaled. Even worse, sniffing of some solvents, particularly halogenated hydrocarbons, is accompanied by a significant risk of death.

STIMULANTS

AMPHETAMINES

Amphetamines are a group of synthetic drugs that stimulate the central nervous system. They are commonly referred to in the terminology of the drug culture as "uppers" or "speed." Ordinary therapeutic doses of 5 to 20 milligrams per day, taken orally, provide a feeling of well-being and increased alertness that is followed by a decrease in fatigue and a loss of appetite. However, these apparent benefits of the drug are accompanied by restlessness and instability or apprehension, and once the drug effects wear off, depression may set in.

In the United States, the most serious form of amphetamine abuse stems from the intravenous injection of amphetamine or its chemical derivative methamphetamine. The desire for a more intense amphetamine experience is the primary motive for this route of administration. The initial sensation of a "flash" or "rush," followed by an intense feeling of pleasure, constitutes the principal appeal of the intravenous route for the "speed freak." During a "speed binge," the individual may inject 500 to 1000 mg of amphetamines every 2 to 3 hours. Users have reported experiencing a euphoria that produces hyperactivity, with a feeling of clarity of vision as well as hallucinations. As the effect of the amphetamines wears off, the individual lapses into a period of exhaustion and may sleep continuously for one or two days. Following this, the user often experiences a prolonged period of severe depression lasting from days to weeks.

The repeated use of amphetamines does lead to a strong psychological dependency, which encourages its continued administration. At this time there is some disagreement among medical specialists as to whether the repeated use of amphetamines does create physical dependence. Several investigators are of the opinion that the prolonged sleep, chronic fatigue, and sensation of hunger that follow the repeated administration of amphetamines constitute withdrawal sickness.

Amphetamines are marketed in a confusing array of proprietary formulations and under different trade names. They may be called "bennies" and "dexies," street names for Benzedrine and Dexedrine, two trademark forms of amphetamine. Methamphetamine is also sold under numerous trade names that include Mededrine and Dexosyn. In light of the reduced production quotas that have been imposed on amphetamine manufacturers by U.S. government regulations, an increasing percentage of the amphetamines sold on the illicit market is being synthesized in clandestine drug laboratories.

Drugs having pharmacological properties similar to those of amphetamines, but which are chemically unrelated, are also being increasingly abused. These include phenmetrazine and phendimetrazine, two drugs commonly prescribed for weight control.

COCAINE

Between 1884 and 1887, Sigmund Freud created something of a sensation in European medical circles by describing his experiments with a new drug. What he reported was a substance of seemingly limitless potential as a source of "exhilaration and lasting euphoria" that permitted "intensive mental or physical work [to be] performed without fatigue. . . . It is as though the need for food and sleep was completely banished."

The object of Freud's enthusiasm was cocaine, a drug stimulant extracted from the leaves of *Erythroxylon coca*, a plant grown in the Andes Mountains of South America and tropical Asia (see Figure 9-6). At one time cocaine had wide medical application as a local painkiller or anesthetic. However, this function has now been largely replaced by other drugs, namely, procaine and lidocaine. Cocaine is also a powerful stimulant to the central nervous system, and its effects resemble those caused by the amphetamines; namely, increased alertness and vigor accompanied by the suppression of hunger, fatigue, and boredom. Most commonly, cocaine is sniffed or "snorted" and is absorbed into the body through the mucous membranes of the nose.

One form of cocaine gaining widespread popularity in the drug culture is known as "crack." The process used to make crack is simple. Ordinary

Figure 9-6. Coca leaves and illicit forms of cocaine. *Courtesy* Drug Enforcement Administration, Washington, D.C.

cocaine is mixed with baking soda and water into a solution that is then heated in a pot. This material is then dried and broken into tiny chunks that dealers sell as crack rocks. Crack is free-base cocaine and is sufficiently volatile to be smoked, usually in glass pipes. Smoking crack produces a quick high that is much more intense than ordinary cocaine, which must be snorted. Within minutes the flash high of crack is followed by a crashing low that leaves the user craving for another hit.

In the United States, cocaine abuse is on the rise. Cocaine generates confidence and produces increased alertness giving a false illusion that one is doing well at an assigned task. Many people are apparently using cocaine to improve their ability to work and to keep going when tired. Another reason for the popularity of the drug is its reputation for being harmless. Actually, this reputation is untrue. While there is no evidence of physical dependency accompanying cocaine's repeated use, abstention from cocaine after prolonged use does bring on severe bouts of mental depression which produce a very strong compulsion to resume the drug's use. In fact, laboratory experiments with animals have demonstrated beyond dispute that cocaine produces the strongest psychological compulsions for continued use of all the commonly abused drugs.

The United States spends millions of dollars annually in attempting to control the cultivation of the coca leaf in various South American countries and to prevent cocaine trafficking into the United States. Three-quarters of the cocaine smuggled into the United States is refined at clandestine laboratories located in Columbia. The profits are astronomical. A kilo of cocaine purchased for $5000 in Bolivia may sell at wholesale in Columbia for $50,000 and at retail in the United States for $300,000.

DRUG-ABUSE LAWS

Although the previous sections have attempted to classify drugs according to their physiological effects on the body, for practical purposes of law enforcement, the legal community requires a thorough knowledge of drug classification and definitions as they are delineated by drug laws. As may often happen, the medical and legal definitions or classifications of a drug bear little resemblance to one another. The provisions of drug laws are of particular interest to the criminalist, for they may impose specific analytical requirements on a drug analysis. For example, the severity of a penalty associated with the manufacture, distribution, possession, and use of a drug may depend on the weight of the drug or its concentration in a mixture. In such cases, the chemist's report must contain all information that is needed to properly charge a suspect under the provisions of the existing law.

The provisions of any drug-control law are an outgrowth of national and local law enforcement requirements and customs, as well as the result of moral and political philosophies. These factors have combined to produce a wide spectrum of national and local drug-control laws. Although their detailed discussion is beyond the intended scope of this book, a brief description of the U.S. federal law known as the Controlled Substances Act of 1970 will serve to illustrate a legal drug-classification system that has been created to prevent and control drug abuse. The fact that many states have modeled their own drug-control laws after this act represents an important step in establishing uniform drug-control laws throughout the United States.

CONTROLLED SUBSTANCES ACT OF 1970

The federal law establishes five schedules of classification (to be outlined below) for controlled dangerous substances on the basis of a drug's potential for abuse, potential for physical and psychological dependence, and medical value. This classification system is extremely flexible in that the U.S. Attorney General has the authority to add, delete, or reschedule a drug as more information becomes available. In addition, controlled dangerous substances listed in schedules I and II are subject to manufacturing quotas set by the Attorney General. For example, some 8 billion doses of amphetamines were manufactured in the United States in 1971. In 1972, production quotas were established reducing amphetamine production approximately 80 percent below 1971 levels.

The criminal penalties for the unauthorized manufacture, sale, or possession of controlled dangerous substances are related to the schedules as well. The most severe penalties are associated with drugs listed in schedules I and II. For example, for narcotics included in schedules I and II, a first offense is punishable by up to 15 years in prison and up to a $25,000 fine. Table 9-2 summarizes the control mechanisms and penalties for each schedule of the Controlled Substances Act.

Table 9-2.

CONTROL MECHANISMS OF THE CONTROLLED SUBSTANCES ACT

Schedule	Registration	Record Keeping	Manufacturing Quotas	Distribution Restrictions	Dispensing Limits
I	Required	Separate	Yes	Order forms	Research use only
II	Required	Separate	Yes	Order forms	Rx: written; no refills
III	Required	Readily retrievable	No *but* Some drugs limited by Schedule II quotas	Records required	Rx: written or oral; with medical authorization, refills up to 5 times in 6 months
IV	Required	Readily retrievable	No *but* Some drugs limited by Schedule II quotas	Records required	Rx: written or oral; with medical authorization, refills up to 5 times in 6 months
V	Required	Readily retrievable	No *but* Some drugs limited by Schedule II quotas	Records required	Over-the-counter (Rx drugs limited to MD's order)

Source: *Drug Enforcement Administration.*

Table 9-2. (continued)

Import-Export		Security	Manufacturer/ Distributor Reports to Drug Enforcement Administration	Criminal Penalties for Trafficking (First Offense)	
Narcotic	Nonnarcotic			Narcotic	Non- Narcotic
Permit	Permit	Vault/safe	Yes	15 years/ $25,000	5 years/ $15,000
Permit	Permit	Vault/safe	Yes	15 years/ $25,000	5 years/ $15,000
Permit	Declaration	Secure storage area	Yes Narcotic	5 years/ $15,000	5 years/ $15,000
			No Nonnarcotic		
Permit	Declaration	Secure storage area	Manufacturer only Narcotic	3 years/ $10,000	3 years/ $10,000
			No Nonnarcotic		
Permit to import	Declaration	Secure storage area	Manufacturer only Narcotic	1 year/ $5000	1 year/ $5000
Declaration to export			No Nonnarcotic		

Schedule I. Schedule I drugs are deemed to have a high potential for abuse; have no currently accepted medical use in the United States; and/or lack accepted safety for use in treatment under medical supervision. Drugs controlled under this schedule include heroin, marijuana, methaqualone, and LSD.

Schedule II. Schedule II drugs have a high potential for abuse; a currently accepted medical use or a medical use with severe restrictions; and a potential for severe psychological or physical dependence. Schedule II drugs include opium and its derivatives not listed in schedule I, cocaine, methadone, most amphetamine preparations, and most barbiturate preparations containing amobarbital, secobarbital, and pentobarbital. In 1978, phencyclidine was moved from schedule III to II.

Schedule III. Schedule III drugs have a potential for abuse less than those in schedules I and II; have a currently accepted medical use in the United States; and have a potential for low or moderate physical dependence or high psychological dependence. Schedule III controls, among other substances, all barbiturate preparations (except phenobarbital) not covered under schedule II and certain codeine preparations.

Schedule IV. Schedule IV drugs have a low potential for abuse relative to schedule III drugs; have a current medical use in the United States; and their abuse may lead to limited dependence relative to schedule III drugs. Drugs controlled in this schedule include propoxphene, phenobarbital, and tranquilizers such as meprobamate (Miltown), diazepam (Valium), and chlordiazepoxide (Librium).

Schedule V. Schedule V drugs must show low abuse potential; have medical use in the United States; and have less potential for producing dependence than schedule IV drugs. Schedule V controls certain opiate drug mixtures that contain nonnarcotic medicinal ingredients.

Under the Controlled Substances Act, a compound must be specifically classified in one of the five schedules if its use is to be considered illegal. This requirement has given rise to the existence of so-called designer drugs as a means of circumventing this law. Designer drugs are substances which are chemically related to some controlled drugs and are pharmacologically very potent. These substances are manufactured by skilled individuals in clandestine laboratories with the knowledge that their products will not be covered by the Controlled Substances Act. For instance, the compound fentanyl is a powerful narcotic that is commercially marketed for medical use and is also listed as a controlled dangerous substance. This drug is about 100 times as potent as morphine. Currently, there are a number of substances chemically related to fentanyl that have been synthesized by underground chemists and sold on the street. The first such substance encountered was sold under the street name of "China White." These drugs have been responsible for more than 100 overdose deaths in California. As designer drugs, such as China White, are identified and linked to drug abuse, they have been placed in appropriate schedules.

DRUG IDENTIFICATION

One only has to look into the evidence vaults of crime laboratories to appreciate the assortment of drug specimens that confront the criminalist. The presence of a huge array of powders, tablets, capsules, vegetable matter, liquids, pipes, cigarettes, cookers, and syringes is testimony to the vitality and sophistication of the illicit drug market. If outward appearance is not evidence enough of the difficult analytical chore facing the forensic chemist, consider the complexity of the drug preparations themselves. Usually these contain active drug ingredients of unknown origin and identity as well as additives—e.g., sugar, starch, and quinine—that dilute their potency and stretch their value on the illicit marketplace. Do not forget that illicit dealers are not hampered by governmental regulations that ensure the quality and consistency of a product.

When a forensic chemist picks up a drug specimen for analysis, anything can be expected to be found, and all contingencies must be prepared for. The analysis must leave no room for error, for its results will have a direct bearing on the process of determining the guilt or innocence of a defendant. There is no middle ground in drug identification—either the specimen is a specific drug or it is not—and once a positive conclusion is drawn, the chemist must be prepared to support and defend the validity of the results in a court of law.

The challenge or difficulty of forensic drug identification comes in selecting analytical procedures that will ensure a specific identification of a drug. Presented with a substance of unknown origin and composition, the forensic chemist must develop a plan of action that will ultimately yield the drug's identity. This plan, or scheme of analysis, is divided into two phases. First, faced with the prospect that the unknown substance may be any one of a thousand or more commonly encountered drugs, the analyst must employ screening tests to reduce these possibilities to a small and manageable number. This objective is often accomplished by subjecting the material to a series of color tests that will produce characteristic colors for the more commonly encountered illicit drugs. Even if these tests should produce negative results, their value lies in having excluded drugs from further consideration.

Once the number of possibilities has been substantially reduced, the second phase of the analysis must be devoted to pinpointing and confirming the drug's identity. In an era in which crime laboratories are receiving voluminous quantities of drug evidence, it would certainly be impractical to subject a drug to all the chemical and instrumental tests that are at the disposal of the modern criminalist. Indeed, it is more realistic to look on these techniques as constituting a large analytical arsenal. It is up to the chemist, aided by training and experience, to choose tests that will most conveniently furnish the identity of a particular drug.

In some cases, the analytical scheme will consist of a series of nonspecific or presumptive tests. Each test in itself is insufficient to prove the drug's identity; however, the proper analytical scheme will encompass a combination of test results that are characteristic of one and only one chemical substance—the drug under investigation. Furthermore, experimental evidence must exist to confirm that the probability of any other substance responding in an identical manner to the scheme selected is so small as to be beyond any reasonable scientific certainty.

There are several tests that forensic chemists normally rely on to comprise a routine drug-identification scheme. These are color tests, microcrystalline tests, chromatography, spectrophotometry, and mass spectrometry.

COLOR TESTS

Many drugs yield characteristic colors when brought into contact with specific chemical reagents. Not only do these tests provide a useful indicator of a drug's presence, but they are also utilized by investigators in the field to examine materials suspected of containing a drug.[2] However, it must be emphasized that color tests are useful for screening purposes only and are never taken as conclusive identification of unknown drugs.

Five primary color test reagents are listed and described below:

1. Marquis (2% formaldehyde in sulfuric acid). The reagent turns purple in the presence of heroin and morphine and most opium derivatives. Marquis will also become orange-brown when mixed with amphetamines and methamphetamine.

2. Dillie-Koppanyi (1% cobalt acetate in methanol is first added to the suspect material followed by 5% isopropylamine in methanol). This is a valuable screening test for barbiturates in whose presence the reagent turns violet-blue in color.

3. Duquenois-Levine (solution A is a mixture of 2% vanillin and 1% acetaldehyde in ethyl alcohol; solution B is concentrated hydrochloric acid; solution C is chloroform). This is a valuable color test for marijuana, performed by adding solutions A, B, and C, respectively, to the suspect vegetation. A positive result is shown by a purple color in the chloroform layer.

---

[2] Field test color kits for drugs can be purchased from various commercial manufacturers.

4. Van Urk (1% solution of p-dimethylaminobenzaldehyde in 10% concentrated hydrochloric acid and ethyl alcohol). Reagent turns blue-purple in the presence of LSD. However, owing to the extremely small quantities of LSD in illicit preparations, this test is difficult to conduct under field conditions.

5. Scott Test (solution A is 2% cobalt thiocyanate dissolved in water and glycerine [1:1]; solution B is concentrated hydrochloric acid; solution C is chloroform). This is a color test for cocaine. A powder containing cocaine will turn solution A blue. Upon addition of B, the blue color is transformed to a clear pink color. Upon addition of C, if cocaine is present, the blue color reappears in the chloroform layer.

MICROCRYSTALLINE TESTS

A technique considerably more specific than color tests is the microcrystalline test. Here, a drop of a chemical reagent is added to a small quantity of the drug on a microscopic slide. After a short time, a chemical reaction ensues, producing a crystalline precipitate. It is the size and shape of the crystals, under microscope examination, that are highly characteristic of the drug. Crystal tests for heroin are illustrated in Figure 9-7(a) and (b).

Over the years analysts have developed hundreds of crystal tests to characterize the most commonly abused drugs. These tests are rapid and often do not require the isolation of a drug from its diluents, however, because diluents can sometimes alter or modify the shape of the crystal, the examiner must develop experience in interpreting the results of the test.

It is important to note that most color and crystal tests are largely empirical—that is, scientists do not fully understand why they produce the results that they do. From the forensic chemist's point of view, this is not important. The fact is that when the tests are properly chosen and are used in proper combination, their results constitute an analytical scheme that is characteristic for one and only one drug.

CHROMATOGRAPHY

The techniques of thin-layer and gas chromatography are especially well suited to the needs of the drug analyst because they separate drugs from their diluents while providing for their tentative identification. The basic principles of these techniques have already been described in Chapter 5.

Because chromatography requires a comparison of either R_f or retention-time values between questioned and known drugs, the analyst must have some clue as to the identity of the illicit material before utilizing these techniques. Hence, in a typical drug analysis, chromatography accompanies and complements color and crystal tests.

(a)

(b)

Figure 9-7. (a) A photomicrograph of heroin crystals in the presence of 10% sodium acetate. (b) A photomicrograph of heroin crystals in the presence of mercuric iodine.

SPECTROPHOTOMETRY

The selective absorption of light by drugs in the UV and IR regions of the electromagnetic spectrum provides a valuable technique for characterizing drugs. The ultraviolet spectrum is not conclusive for the positive identification of a drug because other materials may very well produce an indistinguishable spectrum. Nevertheless, UV spectrophotometry is often a useful technique for establishing the *probable* identity of a drug. For example, if an unknown yields a UV spectrum that resembles amphetamine (see Figure 9-8), thousands of substances are immediately eliminated from consideration, and efforts can now begin to identify the material from a relatively small number of possibilities. A comprehensive collection of UV drug spectra will give the analyst a ready index that can rapidly be searched in order to tentatively identify a drug, or failing that, to at least exclude certain drugs from consideration.

Infrared spectrophotometry is one of the few analytical techniques available to the chemist that can specifically identify a substance. The pattern of an infrared spectrum is unique for each compound and can thus be thought of as being analogous to a "fingerprint" of the compound. The combination of preliminary screening tests with a final verification by infrared

Figure 9-8. Ultraviolet spectrum of amphetamine.

spectrophotometry offers an ideal approach to drug identification. Unfortunately, the technique does present some problems to the criminalist because the substance to be identified must be as pure as possible. This requirement often necessitates employing lengthy purification steps to prepare the sample for IR analysis. The IR spectra of heroin and secobarbital were shown in Figure 5-15.

MASS SPECTROMETRY

The technique of chromatography is particularly suited for analyzing drugs of abuse since it can readily separate a drug from other substances which may be present in the drug preparation. Chromatography does, however, suffer from the drawback of not being able to provide the analyst with a specific identification of the material under investigation. This deficiency has been overcome by linking the gas chromatograph to a mass spectrometer (see discussion on pp. 130–132) to yield a very powerful combination known as *gas chromatography-mass spectrometry* (GC-MS). As a sample emerges from the gas chromatograph, it immediately enters the mass spectrometer. Here, the sample is exposed to high-energy electrons which cause the sample molecules to fragment or break apart. With few exceptions, no two substances fragment in the same fashion; hence, this fragmentation pattern serves as a "fingerprint" of a chemical substance. The fragmentation pattern of heroin is shown in Figure 5-16.

With data obtained from a GC-MS determination, a forensic analyst can with one instrument separate the components of a complex drug mixture and then unequivocally identify each substance present in the mixture.

THE IDENTIFICATION OF MARIJUANA

Enforcement of laws prohibiting the sale and use of marijuana presently accounts for a high percentage of drug arrests in the United States. Any trial or hearing involving a seizure of marijuana requires an identification of the material before the issue of guilt or innocence can be decided.

Unlike most other drugs received by the crime laboratory, marijuana (*Cannabis sativa L.*) possesses botanical features that impart it with identifiable characteristics. Because the vast majority of marijuana specimens consist of small leaf fragments, their identification must be partially based on botanical features observed under the microscope by a trained expert. This approach is further augmented with a chemical test that will independently confirm the findings of the botanical examination.

The identification of marijuana by microscopic methods depends largely on observing short hairs having the shape of "bear claws" on the upper side of the leaf (see SEM photo in Figure 7-11). These hairs are known as *cysto-*

lithic hairs. Further verification of the identity of marijuana is confirmed by the presence of longer nonglandular hairs on the opposite side of the leaf.

The Duquenois-Levine color test, described on page 244, has been found to be a highly, but not totally specific, test for marijuana. However, when used in combination with a botanical examination, the results constitute a specific identification of marijuana. In addition, situations may arise in which the analyst is unable to obtain a microscopic identification of the marijuana leaf, as in the case of hashish or hashish oil. Here, the color test has to be supplemented by another examination, preferably thin-layer chromatography. This method involves separating chemical constituents found in the suspect resin on a thin-layer plate. The separated components are compared on the same plate to those obtained from a known marijuana extract, as shown in Figure 5-8. In this manner, a positive TLC comparison, when used in conjunction with the Duquenois-Levine color test, constitutes a specific identification for marijuana.

THE COLLECTION AND PRESERVATION OF DRUG EVIDENCE

The preparation of drug evidence for submission to the crime laboratory is normally a relatively simple task, accomplished with minimal precautions in the field. The field investigator has the responsibility of ensuring that the evidence is properly packaged and labeled for delivery to the laboratory. Considering the countless forms and varieties of drug evidence seized, it is not practical to prescribe any single packaging procedure for fulfilling these requirements. Generally, common sense is the best guide in such situations, keeping in mind that the package must prevent the loss of the contents and/or cross-contamination between specimens. Often the original container in which the drug was seized will suffice to meet these requirements. Specimens suspected of containing volatile solvents, such as those involved in glue-sniffing cases, must be packaged in an airtight container to prevent evaporation of the solvent.

All packages must be marked with information that is sufficient to ensure identification by the officer in future legal proceedings and to establish the chain of custody.

To aid the drug analyst, it would be helpful if the investigator could supply any background information that may relate to a drug's identity. In some instances, analysis time is markedly reduced when this information is at the disposal of the chemist. For the same reason, the results of drug-screening tests used in the field must also be transmitted to the laboratory. However, although these tests indicate the presence of a drug and may help the officer establish probable cause to search and arrest a suspect, they do not offer conclusive evidence of a drug's identity.

REVIEW QUESTIONS

1. Underlying emotional factors are the primary motives leading to the repeated use of a drug. (True, False)
2. Drugs such as alcohol, heroin, amphetamines, barbiturates, and cocaine can lead to a (high, low) degree of psychological dependence with repeated use.
3. The development of (psychological, physical) dependence on a drug is shown by withdrawal symptoms such as convulsions when the user stops taking the drug.
4. Abuse of barbiturates can lead to physical dependency. (True, False)
5. The repeated use of LSD will lead to physical dependency. (True, False)
6. Physical dependency develops only when the drug user adheres to a _____ schedule of drug intake.
7. Narcotic drugs are _____ that exert a _____ action on the central nervous system.
8. _____ is a gummy, milky juice exuded through a cut made in the unripe pod of the opium poppy.
9. The primary constituent of opium is _____.
10. _____ is a chemical derivative of morphine made by reacting morphine with acetic anhydride.
11. Methadone is classified as a narcotic drug even though it is not derived from opium or morphine. (True, False)
12. Drugs that cause marked alterations in normal thought processes, perceptions, and mood are called _____.
13. _____ is the sticky resin extracted from the marijuana plant.
14. The active ingredient of marijuana largely responsible for its hallucinogenic properties is _____.
15. The potency of a marijuana preparation depends on the proportion of the various plant parts in the mixture. (True, False)
16. A marijuana preparation having the highest THC content is _____.
17. LSD is a chemical derivative of _____. This chemical is obtained from the ergot fungus that grows on certain grasses and grains.
18. The drug phencyclidine is often manufactured for the illicit market in _____ laboratories.
19. Alcohol (stimulates, depresses) the central nervous system.
20. _____ are called "downers" because they depress the actions of the central nervous system.
21. Phenobarbital is an example of a (short-, long-) acting barbiturate.
22. _____ is a powerful sedative and muscle relaxant that possesses many of the depressant properties of barbiturates.

23. _____ are drugs used for the relief of anxiety and tension without inducing sleep.

24. Glue sniffing stimulates the central nervous system. (True, False)

25. _____ are a group of synthetic drugs that stimulate the central nervous system.

26. The most severe form of amphetamine abuse stems from its (oral, intravenous) administration.

27. An increasing percentage of amphetamines available on the illicit market originate from _____ drug laboratories.

28. _____ is extracted from the leaf of the coca plant.

29. Traditionally cocaine is _____ into the nostrils.

30. The 1970 federal drug control law is known as _____.

31. Federal law establishes _____ schedules of classification for the control of dangerous drugs.

32. Drugs that have no accepted medical use are placed in schedule _____.

33. Librium and Valium are listed in schedule _____.

34. Color tests are used to identify drugs conclusively. (True, False)

35. The _____ color test turns purple in the presence of heroin.

36. The _____ color test turns orange-brown in the presence of amphetamines.

37. The Duquenois-Levine test is a valuable color test for _____.

38. The _____ test is a widely used color test for cocaine.

39. _____ tests tentatively identify drugs by the size and shape of crystals formed when the drug is mixed with specific reagents.

40. _____ provides a means of separating drugs from their diluents while making a tentative identification.

41. The pattern of an _____ absorption spectrum is unique for each drug and thus is a specific test for identification.

42. The microscopic identification of marijuana largely depends on observing short hairs on the leaf known as _____ hairs.

43. All packages containing drugs must be marked for identification by the police officer before being sent to the laboratory in order to maintain the _____.

FURTHER REFERENCES

Dal Cason, T. A., R. Fox, and R. S. Frank, "Investigations of Clandestine Drug Manufacturing Laboratories," *Analytical Chemistry*, 52 (1980), 804A.

Fulton, Charles C., *Modern Microcrystal Tests for Drugs*. New York: Wiley-Interscience, 1969.

Hofmann, Fredrick G., *A Handbook on Drug and Alcohol Abuse*, 2nd ed. New York: Oxford University Press, 1983.

Humphreys, I. J., "The Work of the Drugs Intelligence Laboratory, Home Office Forensic Science Service," *Bulletin on Narcotics*, 36 (1984), 33.

Klein, M., A. V. Kruegel, and S. P. Sobol, eds., *Instrumental Applications in Forensic Drug Chemistry*. Washington, D.C.: U.S. Government Printing Office, 1979.

Lowry, W. T., and James C. Garriott, *Forensic Toxicology: Controlled Substances and Dangerous Drugs*. New York: Plenum Press, 1979.

Manura, J. J., J-M Chao, and R. Saferstein, "The Forensic Identification of Heroin," *Journal of Forensic Sciences*, 23 (1978), 44.

Moffat, A. E., et al., eds. *Clarke's Isolation and Identification of Drugs*, 2nd ed. London: Pharmaceutical Press, 1986.

Siegel, J. A., "Forensic Identification of Controlled Substances," in *Forensic Science Handbook*, Vol. 2, R. Saferstein, ed. Englewood Cliffs, N.J.: Prentice-Hall, Inc., 1987.

Thornton, J. I., and G. R. Nakamura, "The Identification of Marijuana," *Journal of the Forensic Science Society*, 12 (1972), 461.

AUDIOVISUAL PRESENTATIONS

Cocaine Abuse (80 35-mm slides and audio tape). Police Science Services, Niles, Ill.

Heroin (80 35-mm slides and audio tape). Police Science Services, Niles, Ill.

PCP and the Hallucinogens (80 35-mm slides and audio tape). Police Science Services, Niles, Ill.

The Drug Scene (80 35-mm slides and audio tape). Police Science Services, Niles, Ill.

10

Forensic Toxicology

It is no secret that, in spite of the concerted effort that law enforcement agencies are making to prevent the distribution and sale of illicit drugs, thousands die every year from the intentional or unintentional administration of drugs, and many more innocent lives are lost as a result of the erratic and frequently uncontrollable behavior of individuals who are under the influence of drugs. Thus, one should not automatically attribute these occurrences to the wide proliferation of illicit drug markets. For example, in the United States alone, drug manufacturers produce enough barbiturates each year to provide every man, woman, and child with about 40 pills. In a recent five-year period in New York City, there were 8500 cases of barbiturate poisoning and 1100 of the victims died but only half of these 1100 were called suicide.

All the statistical and medical evidence presently available shows ethyl alcohol, a legal over-the-counter drug, to be the most heavily abused drug in Western countries. In the United States, nearly 25,000 automobile deaths each year are alcohol-related, with a rate of injury requiring hospital treatment exceeding two million persons per year. This death toll of human beings on the road, as well as the untold damage to life, limb, and property, is testimony in itself to the dangerous consequences of alcohol abuse.

At a time when the uncontrolled use of drugs has become a worldwide problem affecting all segments of society, the role of the toxicologist has taken on new and added significance. Toxicologists are charged with the responsibility for detecting and identifying the presence of drugs and poisons in body fluids, tissues, and organs. Their services are not just required in such legal institutions as crime laboratories and medical examiners' offices; they also reach into hospital laboratories—where the possibility of identifying a drug overdose may represent the difference between life and death, and into various health facilities responsible for monitoring the intake of drugs and other toxic substances. Primary examples include blood tests performed on children exposed to leaded paints, or the analysis of the urine of addicts enrolled in methadone maintenance programs.

The role of the forensic toxicologist is limited to matters that pertain to violations of criminal law. However, the assignment of the responsibility for performing toxicological services in a criminal justice system does vary considerably throughout the United States. In those systems that have a crime laboratory independent of the medical examiner, this responsibility may reside with one or the other, or may be shared by both. Some systems, however, take advantage of the expertise residing in governmental health department laboratories and assign to them this role. Nevertheless, it is a fact that whatever facility is ultimately assigned this work, its caseload will reflect the prevailing popularity of drugs that are abused in the community. In most cases, this means that the forensic toxicologist must expect to be confronted with numerous requests relating to the determination of the presence of alcohol in the body.

TOXICOLOGY OF ALCOHOL

THE FATE OF ALCOHOL IN THE BODY

The subject of the analysis of alcohol immediately confronts us with the primary objective of forensic toxicology—the detection and isolation of drugs in the body for the express purpose of determining their influence on human behavior. In the case of alcohol, however, the problem is further complicated by practical considerations. The predominant role of the automobile in our society has mandated the imposition of laws designed to protect the public from the drinking driver. In practice, this has meant that toxicologists have had to devise rapid and specific procedures for measuring the degree of alcohol intoxication. The methods utilized must be suitably designed to test hundreds of thousands of motorists annually without causing them undue physical harm or unreasonable inconveniences, while at the same time providing reliable diagnoses that can be supported and defended within the framework of the legal system.

Alcohol, or ethyl alcohol, is a colorless liquid normally diluted with water and consumed as a beverage. Logically, the most obvious measure of intoxication would be the amount of liquor a person has consumed. Unfortunately, most arrests are made after the fact, when such information is not available to legal authorities; furthermore, even if this data could be collected, numerous related factors, such as body weight and the rate of alcohol's absorption into the body, are so extremely variable that it would be impossible to prescribe uniform standards that would yield reliable alcohol intoxication levels.

Like any other depressant, alcohol has its principal effect on the central nervous system, particularly the brain. The extent of the depression is proportional to the concentration of alcohol within the nerve cells. The nerve functions most susceptible to the action of alcohol are found in the surface areas of the forebrain. Later, as the subject absorbs alcohol to a greater extent, the functions of the central and rear portions of the brain are affected. The nerve functions that are most resistant, and that are the last to fail, are those centered in the brain's medulla, which regulates such vital functions as respiration and heart activity.

Theoretically, if one wanted a true determination of the quantity of alcohol that was impairing normal body functions, it would be best to remove a portion of brain tissue and perform a direct analysis on it for alcohol content. For obvious reasons this cannot be done on living subjects. Consequently, toxicologists have concentrated their efforts on the blood, for it is the blood that provides the medium for circulating alcohol throughout the body, carrying it to all tissues, including the brain. Fortunately, experimental evidence supports this approach and shows blood-alcohol concentration to be directly proportional to the concentration of alcohol in the brain. From the medico-legal point of view, blood-alcohol levels have become the accepted standard for relating alcohol intake to its effect on the body.

Alcohol appears in the blood within minutes after it has been taken by mouth, and slowly increases in concentration while it is being absorbed from the stomach and the small intestine into the bloodstream. When all the alcohol has been absorbed, a maximum alcohol level is reached in the blood, and the postabsorption period begins. Then the alcohol concentration slowly decreases until a zero level is again reached.

There are many factors that determine the rate at which alcohol is absorbed into the bloodstream. These include the total time taken to consume the drink, the alcohol content of the beverage, the amount consumed, and the quantity and type of food that may be present in the stomach at the time of drinking. With so many variables, it is difficult to predict just how long the absorption process will require. For example, beer is absorbed more slowly than is an equivalent concentration of alcohol in water. This is apparently because of the carbohydrates present in beer. Also, alcohol consumed on an empty stomach is absorbed faster than an equivalent amount of alcohol taken when there is food in the stomach. The longer the total time required for complete absorption to occur, the lower will be the peak alcohol concentration in the blood (see Figure 10-1). Depending on a combination of factors, maximum blood-alcohol concentration may not be reached until two or three hours have elapsed from the time of consumption. However, under

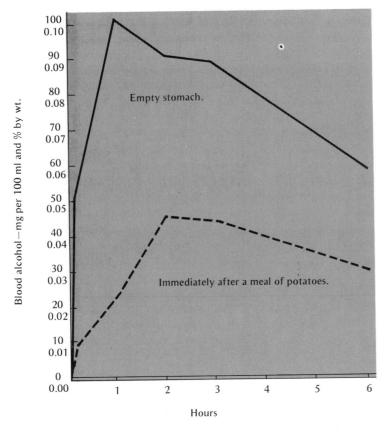

Figure 10-1. Blood alcohol concentrations after ingestion of 2 ounces of pure alcohol mixed in 8 ounces of water (equivalent to about 5 ounces of 80-proof vodka). *Source:* U.S. Dept. of Transportation, Washington, D.C.

normal social drinking conditions, it takes anywhere from 30 to 90 minutes from the time of the final drink until the absorption process is completed.

During the absorption phase, alcohol slowly enters the body's bloodstream and is carried to all parts of the body. When the absorption period is completed, the alcohol will become distributed uniformly throughout the watery portions of the body—that is to say, throughout about two-thirds of the body volume. Fat, bones, and hair are low in water content and therefore contain little alcohol, whereas alcohol concentration in the rest of the body is fairly uniform. Hence, if blood is not available, as may be the case in some postmortem situations, a medical examiner always has the option of selecting a water-rich organ or fluid—e.g., brain, cerebrospinal fluid, or vitreous humor—for determining the body's alcohol content to a reasonable degree of accuracy.

As the alcohol is circulated by the bloodstream, the body proceeds at once to begin the task of eliminating its presence. Elimination is accomplished through two mechanisms—oxidation and excretion. Nearly all the alcohol (90 to 95 percent) consumed is eventually oxidized to carbon dioxide and water. Oxidation takes place almost entirely in the liver. Here, in the presence of the enzyme alcohol dehydrogenase, the alcohol is converted into acetaldehyde and then to acetic acid. The acetic acid is subsequently oxidized in practically all parts of the body to carbon dioxide and water.

The remaining portion of alcohol is excreted unchanged in the breath, urine, and perspiration. Most significantly, extensive experimental evidence has verified that the amount of alcohol exhaled in the breath is in direct proportion to the concentration of alcohol in the blood. This observation has had a tremendous impact on the technology and procedures used for blood-alcohol testing. The development of instruments to reliably measure breath for its alcohol content has made possible the testing of millions of persons in a rapid, safe, and convenient manner.

The fate of alcohol in the body is therefore relatively simple—namely, absorption into the bloodstream, distribution throughout the body's water, and finally, elimination by oxidation and excretion. The elimination or "burn-off" rate of alcohol varies in different individuals; 0.015 percent w/v per hour seems to be an average value once the absorption process is complete.[1] However, it must be emphasized that this figure is an average that may vary by as much as 30 percent between individuals.

ALCOHOL IN THE CIRCULATORY SYSTEM

The extent to which an individual may be under the influence of alcohol is usually determined by measuring the quantity of alcohol present in the blood system. Normally, this is accomplished in one of two ways: (1) by direct chemical analysis of the blood for its alcohol content; and (2) by measurement of the alcohol content of the breath and a subsequent relating of this value to blood-alcohol concentration. In either case, the significance and meaning of the results can better be understood when the movement of alcohol through the circulatory system is studied.

Man, like all vertebrates, has a closed circulatory system, which consists basically of a heart and numerous arteries, capillaries, and veins. An artery is a blood vessel carrying blood away from the heart, and a **vein** is a vessel carrying blood back toward the heart. **Capillaries** are tiny blood vessels that

---

[1] In the United States, laws that define blood-alcohol levels almost exclusively use the unit percent weight per volume—% w/v. Hence, 0.015% w/v is equivalent to 0.015 grams of alcohol per 100 milliliters of blood, or 15 milligrams of alcohol per 100 milliliters of blood.

interconnect the arteries with the veins. It is across the thin walls of the capillaries that the exchange of materials between the blood and the other tissues
takes place. A schematic diagram of the circulatory system is shown in Figure 10-2.

Let us now proceed to trace the movement of alcohol through the
human circulatory system. After alcohol is ingested, it moves down the
esophagus into the stomach. About 20 percent of the alcohol is absorbed
through the stomach walls into the portal vein of the blood system. The
remaining alcohol passes into the blood through the walls of the small intestine. Once in the blood, the alcohol is carried to the liver, where the process
of its destruction starts as the blood (carrying the alcohol) moves up to the
heart. The blood enters the upper right chamber of the heart, called the right
atrium (or auricle), and is forced into the lower right chamber of the heart,
known as the right ventricle. Having returned to the heart from its circulation through the tissues, the blood at this time contains very little oxygen

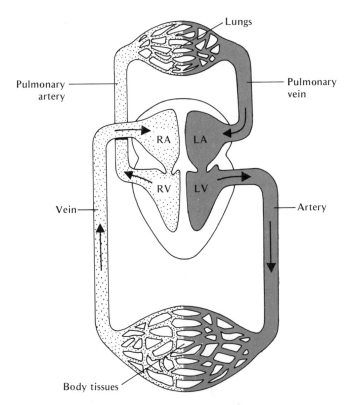

Figure 10-2. Simplified diagram of the human circulatory system. Dark
vessels contain oxygenated blood; light vessels contain deoxygenated
blood.

and much carbon dioxide. Consequently, the blood must be pumped up to the lungs, through the pulmonary artery, to be replenished with oxygen.

It is in the lungs that the respiratory system bridges with the circulatory system so that oxygen can enter the blood and carbon dioxide can leave it. As shown in Figure 10-3(a), the pulmonary artery branches into capillaries lying in close proximity to tiny pear-shaped sacs called **alveoli**. There are about 250 million alveoli in the lungs, all located at the ends of the bronchial tubes. The bronchial tubes themselves connect into the windpipe (trachea), which leads up to the mouth and nose; see Figure 10-3(b). It is at the surface of the alveolar sacs that blood flowing through the capillaries comes in contact with fresh oxygenated air in the sacs. A rapid exchange now proceeds to take place between the fresh air in the sacs and the spent air in the blood. Oxygen passes through the walls of the alveoli into the blood while carbon dioxide is discharged from the blood into the air; see Figure 10-3(a). If, while this exchange is taking place, alcohol or any other volatile substance happens to be in the blood, it too will pass into the alveoli. During the act of breathing, the carbon dioxide and alcohol are expelled through the nose and mouth, and the alveoli sacs are replenished with fresh oxygenated air breathed into the lungs, thus allowing the process to begin all over again.

The distribution of alcohol between the blood and alveolar air is very much analogous to the example of a gas dissolved in an enclosed beaker of water that was described on page 110. Here again, one can use Henry's Law to explain how the alcohol will divide itself between the air and blood. Henry's Law may now be restated as follows: When a volatile chemical (alcohol) is dissolved in a liquid (blood) and is brought to equilibrium with air (alveolar breath), there is a fixed ratio between the concentration of the volatile compound (alcohol) in air (alveolar breath) and its concentration in the liquid (blood), and this ratio is constant for a given temperature.

The temperature at which the breath leaves the mouth is normally 34°C. At this temperature, experimental evidence has shown that the ratio of alcohol in the blood to alcohol in alveoli air is approximately 2100 to 1. In other words, one milliliter of blood will contain nearly the same amount of alcohol as 2100 milliliters of alveolar breath. Henry's Law thus becomes a basis for relating breath to blood-alcohol concentration.

Now let's return to the circulating blood. After emerging from the lungs, the oxygenated blood is rushed back to the upper left chamber of the heart (left atrium) by the pulmonary vein. When the left atrium contracts, it forces the blood through a valve into the left ventricle, which is the lower left chamber of the heart. The left ventricle then pumps the freshly oxygenated blood into the arteries, which carry the blood to all parts of the body. Each of these arteries, in turn, branches into smaller arteries, which eventually connect with the numerous tiny capillaries embedded in the tissues. Here the alcohol moves out of the blood and into the tissues. The blood then runs

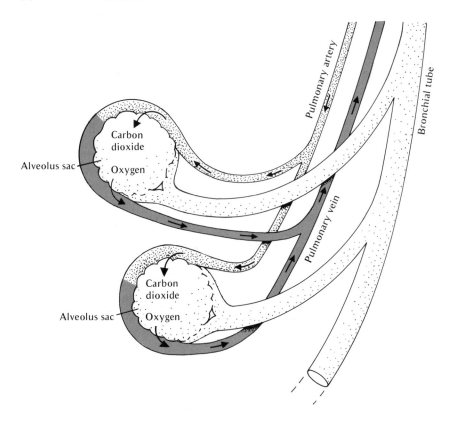

Figure 10-3(a). Gas exchange in the lungs. Blood flows from the pulmonary artery into vessels that lie close to the walls of the alveoli sacs. Here the blood gives up its carbon dioxide and absorbs oxygen. The oxygenated blood leaves the lungs via the pulmonary vein, and returns to the heart.

from the capillaries into tiny veins that fuse to form larger and larger veins. These veins eventually lead back to the heart to complete the circuit.

During the period of absorption, the concentration of alcohol in the arterial blood will be considerably higher as compared to the concentration of alcohol in the venous blood. One typical study revealed a subject's arterial blood-alcohol level to be 41 percent higher than the venous level 30 minutes after the last drink.[2] This difference is thought to exist because of the rapid diffusion of alcohol into the body tissues from venous blood during the early phases of absorption. Because the administration of a blood test requires drawing venous blood from the arm, this test is clearly to the advantage of a subject who may still be in the absorption stage. However, once

<hr />

[2] R. B. Forney et al., *Quarterly Journal of Studies on Alcohol*, 25 (1964), 205.

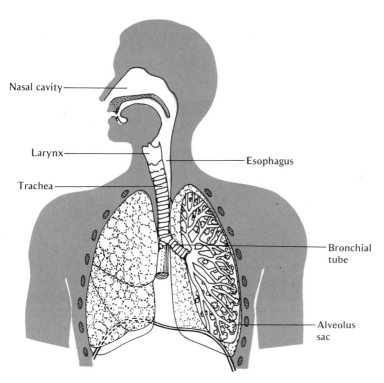

Nasal cavity

Larynx

Trachea

Esophagus

Bronchial
tube

Alveolus
sac

Figure 10-3(b). The respiratory system. The trachea connects the nose and mouth to the bronchial tubes. The bronchial tubes divide into numerous branches that terminate in the alveoli sacs in the lungs.

absorption is complete, the alcohol will become equally distributed throughout the blood system.

A breath test reflects the alcohol concentration in the pulmonary artery. Breath-test results obtained during the absorption phase may be higher than results obtained from a simultaneous direct analysis of venous blood. However, the former are more reflective of the concentration of alcohol reaching the brain and therefore more accurately reflect the effects of alcohol on the subject. Again, once absorption is complete, the difference between a blood and breath test should be minimal.

THE BREATHALYZER

From a practical point of view, the idea of drawing blood from a vein to test motorists suspected of being under the influence of alcohol simply does not offer itself as a convenient method for monitoring alcoholic drivers. The need to have the suspect transported to a location where a medically qualified person can draw blood would be a costly and time-consuming operation, considering the hundreds of tests that the average police department must conduct every year. Thus, breath analysis serves a very useful purpose in providing an easily obtainable specimen along with a rapid and accurate result.

One breath-testing instrument that has become widely employed for testing individuals suspected of being under the influence of alcohol is known as the Breathalyzer. The Breathalyzer was first developed in 1954 by R. F. Borkenstein, who at that time was a captain in the Indiana State Police. Although it has since undergone several modifications, the basic theory and design of the instrument have not changed. The Breathalyzer and an accompanying schematic diagram of its parts are illustrated in Figure 10-4(a) and (b).

Simply, the Breathalyzer is a device for collecting and measuring the alcohol content of alveolar breath. When the valve is in the TAKE position, the subject is required to blow into a mouthpiece that leads into a metal cylinder. As the subject is blowing, the pressure of the exhaled breath raises a piston to a height that exposes two vent holes near the top of a heated cylinder. When the last breath has been expired, the piston settles down to a predetermined position covering the vent holes and trapping the last portion of air (alveolar breath) in the cylinder. The amount of breath collected in this manner is 52.5 ml or 1/40th of 2100 ml.[3] We have already seen that the amount of alcohol contained within 2100 milliliters of alveolar breath approximates that within 1 milliliter of blood. Hence, in essence, the Breathalyzer is designed to measure alcohol concentration present in 1/40th of a milliliter of blood.

Figure 10-4(a). The Breathalyzer. *Courtesy* Smith & Wesson Electronics Co., Pittsburgh, Pennsylvania.

---

[3]Actually, the collection cylinder is designed to hold 56.5 ml of breath. This is because having left the mouth at 34°C, the breath will expand when heated to 50°C in the cylinder. Furthermore, added breath is needed to compensate for the air that remains in the delivery tube leading to the test ampoule.

Figure 10-4(b). Schematic diagram of a Breathalyzer. *Courtesy* Smith & Wesson Electronics Co., Pittsburg, Pennsylvania.

When the valve is placed in the ANALYZE position, the piston drops, causing the trapped sample of alveolar air to pass into a glass ampoule that contains 3 ml of 0.025 percent potassium dichromate and 0.025 percent silver nitrate in sulfuric acid and water. Any alcohol present in the breath immediately dissolves in the dichromate solution and is oxidized to acetic acid. In the oxidation process, potassium dichromate is also destroyed. It is the extent of this destruction that is measured by the Breathalyzer and is related to the quantity of alcohol passed into the ampoule.

Basically, the Breathalyzer is a spectrophotometer (see Chapter 5) that has been specially designed to measure the absorption of light passing through the potassium dichromate solution at a single wavelength. To better understand its operation, let's examine what is happening in the ampoule when alcohol is converted to acetic acid. Whenever a chemical reaction takes place between two or more substances, chemists use a chemical equation as a shorthand method to describe the changes taking place. The equation serves two purposes. It identifies the participants, and it describes the quantitative aspects of the reaction.

The following equation depicts the chemical reaction taking place in the ampoule:

$$2K_2Cr_2O_7 \; + \; 3C_2H_5OH \; + \; 8H_2SO_4 \quad \rightarrow$$

potassium dichromate   ethyl alcohol   sulfuric acid   yields

$$2Cr_2(SO_4)_3 \; + \; 2K_2SO_4 \; + \; 3CH_3COOH \; + \; 11H_2O$$

chromium sulfate   potassium sulfate   acetic acid   water

From this chemical equation we can see that there is always a fixed relationship between the number of potassium dichromate molecules reacting with the alcohol. Two molecules of potassium dichromate always combine with three molecules of ethyl alcohol. Hence, by determining the amount of potassium dichromate consumed, one has an indirect way of determining the quantity of alcohol that was originally present. Silver nitrate is also present in the Breathalyzer ampoule; however, this substance acts only as a catalyst to speed up the rate of reaction between potassium and ethyl alcohol. As a catalyst, silver nitrate undergoes no net change itself during the reaction.

Potassium dichromate is yellow in color and is known to absorb visible light in the wavelength region of 420 nanometers. In accordance with Beer's Law (see page 125), $A = kc$, the quantity of light absorbed by potassium dichromate is directly proportional to its concentration. As the reaction proceeds, the concentration and hence the light absorbance of potassium dichromate will diminish in proportion to the amount of alcohol consumed. The Breathalyzer indirectly determines the quantity of alcohol consumed by measuring the absorption of light by potassium dichromate before and after its reaction to alcohol.

Because the Breathalyzer determines alcohol concentration by measuring a change in light absorption, its operation entails two measurements. First, referring to the schematic diagram in Figure 10-4(b), the light source is positioned somewhere between a test ampoule and a sealed standard ampoule, both having a similar chemical composition, so that the intensity of the light passing through each is the same. At this time, there will be an equal electrical signal coming from each of the photocells located behind the ampoules as shown by a "zero" reading on the null meter. The light source is mechanically connected to a pointer that is located above a scale calibrated to read directly in blood-alcohol percentage. The pointer is now manually set to read "zero." The filters incorporated into the design of the Breathalyzer will allow only a narrow band of wavelengths in the region of 420 nanometers to pass through the ampoules and reach the photocells.

The captured alveolar air is now bubbled into the test ampoule in the manner previously described, and the operator must wait 90 seconds for the chemical reaction to be complete. If alcohol was present in the breath, its oxidation to acetic acid will be accompanied by a corresponding decline in the potassium dichromate concentration, and this in turn will be reflected by a decrease in light absorption in the test ampoule. To compensate for this decrease, the operator must move the light source away from the test ampoule toward the standard ampoule in order to return the null meter to a "zero" reading. When the light source is moved to its new position, the pointer moves a distance that reflects the blood-alcohol percentage as read off the scale.

It is well recognized that almost the only volatile substances encountered in significant concentrations in the blood or breath of subjects operating a motor vehicle are acetone, acetaldehyde, methanol, isopropyl alcohol, and paraldehyde. Acetone, which might be present on the breath of an untreated diabetic, does not give a test result under the reaction conditions of the Breathalyzer. Isopropyl alcohol and paraldehyde have a distinct odor that can be recognized on the breath. However, it must be emphasized that all of these interfering substances are highly toxic, and their presence in the blood in concentrations sufficient to give an apparent blood-alcohol reading of 0.04 to .05 percent w/v would be associated with severe poisoning or death.

Since its development in the 1950s, the Breathalyzer has been one of the most popular breath-testing devices in the law enforcement community. However, recent technology has made possible the incorporation of new operational and design concepts into breath-testing instruments. Emphasis is currently being placed on automating the breath testing procedure to minimize the chance of operator error. Additionally, trends clearly point to the eventual widespread use of breath testers free of any chemical reagents. In particular, breath testers which operate on the principle of infrared light absorption are becoming increasingly popular within the law enforcement community.

An evidential testing instrument which incorporates the principle of infrared light absorption is shown in Figure 10-5. In principle these instruments operate no differently than the spectrophotometers described on pp. 125–126. If alcohol is present in the subject's breath, it will be captured in the instrument's breath chamber. As shown in Figure 10-6, a beam of infrared light is aimed through the chamber. A filter is used to select a wavelength of infrared light at which alcohol will absorb. As the infrared light passes through the chamber, it will interact with the alcohol and cause the light to decrease in intensity. The decrease in light intensity is measured by a photo-

Figure 10-5. An infrared breath-testing instrument—the Intoxilyzer 5000. *Courtesy* Federal Signal Corp., Park Forest South, Illinois.

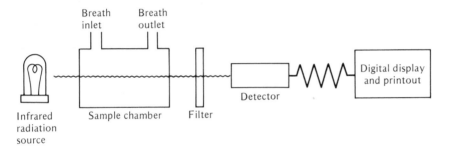

Figure 10-6. A schematic diagram of an infrared breath-testing instrument.

electric detector which gives a signal proportional to the concentration of alcohol present in the captured breath sample. This information is processed by an electronic microprocessor, and the percent blood-alcohol concentration is displayed on a digital readout. Also, the blood-alcohol level can be printed on a card to produce a permanent record of the test result. Some infrared breath testers aim a second infrared wavelength beam into the same chamber in order to check for the presence of acetone in the breath.

Another emerging trend in breath testing is the utilization of portable hand-held, roadside testers. One such instrument is shown in Figure 10-7. This device, about the size of a pack of cigarettes, weighs 5 ounces and uses a fuel cell to measure the alcohol content of a breath sample. The fuel cell absorbs the alcohol from the breath sample, oxidizes it, and produces an electrical current proportional to the breath-alcohol content. This instrument can provide up to 3,000 tests before the fuel cell needs replacement. Breath test results obtained with devices such as those shown in Figure 10-7 must be considered preliminary and nonevidential in nature. They should

Figure 10-7. The Alco-Sensor II. *Courtesy of Intoximeters, Inc. St. Louis, Mo.*

only serve to establish probable cause for requiring an individual to submit to a more thorough breath or blood test.

THE ANALYSIS OF BLOOD FOR ALCOHOL

Before the widespread use of the Breathalyzer, toxicologists had to rely extensively on a direct chemical analysis of the blood for quantitating alcohol levels. Today, many of these procedures are still used in toxicology laboratories. Almost all of them take advantage of alcohol's volatility and first require the separation of the alcohol from the blood by distillation. Alcohol's concentration in the distillate can be determined when a measured volume of potassium dichromate solution of known concentration is slowly added until all the alcohol is completely consumed. In this process, known as titration, the potassium dichromate is added from a graduated buret, as shown in Figure 10-8. A colored indicator is used to detect the point at which all of the alcohol has been oxidized to acetic acid. A change in the color of the indicator signals when the analyst should stop the addition of potassium dichromate.

Gas chromatography offers the toxicologist the most widely used approach for determining alcohol levels in blood. When proper gas chromatographic conditions are used, alcohol can be separated from other volatiles

Figure 10-8. A typical titration set-up.

that may be present in blood. By comparing the resultant alcohol peak area to ones obtained with known blood-alcohol standards, the investigator can calculate the alcohol level with a high degree of accuracy (see Figure 10-9).

A more recent procedure developed for alcohol analysis involves the oxidation of alcohol in the presence of the enzyme alcohol dehydrogenase and a coenzyme diphosphopyridine nucleotide (DPN). As the oxidation proceeds, DPN is converted into another chemical species, DPN-H_2. The extent of this conversion is measured spectrophotometrically and is related to alcohol concentration.

COLLECTION AND PRESERVATION OF BLOOD

Blood must always be drawn under medically accepted conditions by a qualified individual. It is important that before the suspect's skin is penetrated with a sterile needle or lancet, a nonalcoholic disinfectant be applied. This

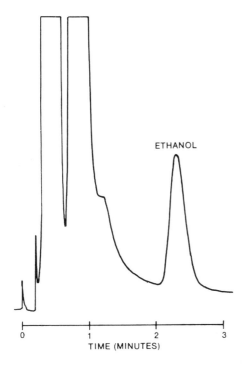

ETHANOL

0   1   2   3

TIME (MINUTES)

Figure 10-9. Gas chromatogram showing ethyl alcohol (ethanol) in whole blood. *Courtesy* Varian Instruments, California.

procedure will negate any argument that an alcoholic disinfectant may have inadvertently contributed to a falsely high blood-alcohol result. Nonalcoholic disinfectants such as aqueous benzalkonium chloride (Zepiran), aqueous mercuric chloride, or povidone-iodine (Betadine) are recommended for this purpose.

Once blood is removed from an individual, its preservation will be best ensured when it has been sealed in an airtight container after an anticoagulant and a preservative have been added. The blood should be stored in a refrigerator until delivery to the toxicology laboratory. The addition of an anticoagulant, such as EDTA or potassium oxalate, will prevent clotting; and a preservative, such as sodium fluoride, will inhibit the growth of microorganisms capable of destroying alcohol.

A recent study performed to determine the stability of alcohol in blood, removed from living individuals, found that the most significant factors affecting alcohol's stability in blood are storage temperature, the presence of a preservative, and the time of storage.[4] It is worth noting that not a single blood specimen examined showed an increase in alcohol level with time. Failure to keep the blood refrigerated or to add sodium fluoride resulted in a

---

[4] G. A. Brown et al., "The Stability of Ethanol in Stored Blood," *Analytica Chimica Acta*, 66 (1973), 271.

substantial decline in alcohol concentration. Longer storage times also reduced blood-alcohol levels. Hence, failure to adhere to all or any of the proper preservation requirements for blood will work toward the benefit of the suspect and to the detriment of society.

The collection of post-mortem blood samples for alcohol determination requires added precautions as compared to living subjects. Ethyl alcohol may be generated in a *deceased individual* as a result of bacterial action. Therefore, it is best to collect a number of blood samples from different body sites. For example, blood may be removed from the heart and from the femoral (leg) and cubital (arm) veins. Each sample should be placed in a clean airtight container containing an anticoagulant and sodium fluoride preservative and should be refrigerated. It is expected that blood-alcohol levels attributed solely to alcohol consumption would result in nearly similar results for all blood samples collected from the same person.

ALCOHOL AND THE LAW

Constitutionally, every state in the United States is charged with the responsibility of establishing and administering statutes regulating the operation of motor vehicles. Although it might be expected that such an arrangement would encourage diverse laws defining permissible blood-alcohol levels, this has not been the case. Both the American Medical Association and the National Safety Council have been able to exert considerable influence in convincing the states to establish uniform and reasonable blood-alcohol standards.

Between 1939 and 1964, 39 states and the District of Columbia enacted legislation that followed the recommendations of the American Medical Association and the National Safety Council in specifying that a person having a blood-alcohol concentration in excess of 0.15 percent w/v was to be considered under the influence of alcohol.[5] However, continued experimental studies have since shown that there is a clear correlation between drinking and driving impairment for blood-alcohol levels much below 0.15 percent w/v. As a result of these studies, in 1960 the American Medical Association and in 1965 the National Safety Council recommended lowering the presumptive level at which an individual was considered to be under the influence of alcohol to 0.10 percent w/v. All the states, as well as the District of Columbia, and most possessions of the United States have complied with this recommendation. In fact, most states have now established *per se* laws, meaning that any individual meeting or exceeding a defined blood-alcohol level (usually 0.10 percent) shall be deemed to be intoxicated. No other proof of alcohol impairment is necessary. As shown in Figure 10-10, one is about 4 times more likely to become involved in an automobile accident at the .08

---

[5] 0.15% w/v is equivalent to 0.15 grams of alcohol per 100 milliliters of blood, or 150 milligrams per 100 milliliters.

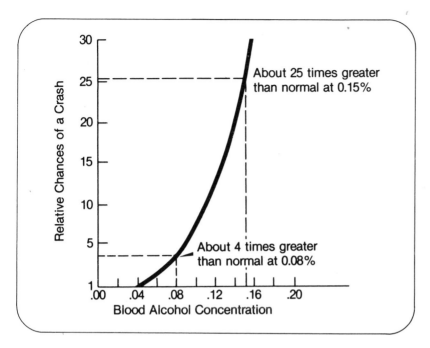

Figure 10-10. Diagram of increased driving risk in relation to blood alcohol concentration. *Source:* U.S. Dept. of Transportation, Washington, D.C.

percent level as compared to a sober individual. At the 0.15 percent level, the chances are 25 times greater for involvement in an automobile accident as compared to a sober driver. The reader may *estimate* the relationship of blood-alcohol levels to body weight and the quantity of 80-proof liquor consumed by referring to Figure 10-11.

The trend toward lowering the impairment level continues; in 1972, the Committee on Alcohol and Drugs of the National Safety Council suggested that a blood concentration of 0.08 percent w/v indicates impairment in driving performance. Already, two states—Idaho and Utah—have adopted such a standard.

Several Western countries have also set .08 percent w/v as the blood level above which it is an offense to drive a motor vehicle. These countries include Great Britain, Canada, Australia, and Switzerland. In addition, a few countries have even lower levels: Norway and Sweden designate 0.05 percent w/v, and Czechoslovakia has an allowable limit of 0.03 percent w/v.

In order to prevent a person's refusal to take a test for alcohol intoxication on the constitutional grounds of self-incrimination, the National Highway Traffic Safety Administration recommended an "implied consent" law. By 1973, all the states had complied with this recommendation. In accordance

HOW TO TELL WHAT YOUR BLOOD ALCOHOL LEVEL IS AFTER DRINKING

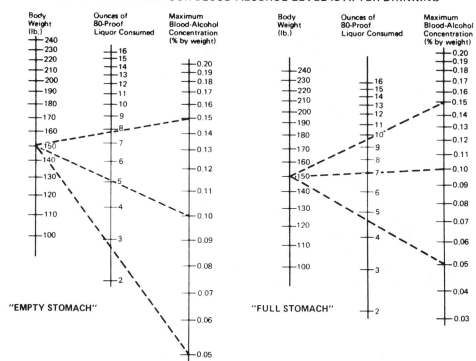

Figure 10-11. In order to use the above diagram, lay a straightedge across your weight and number of ounces of liquor you've consumed on an empty or full stomach. The point where the edge hits the right-hand column is your maximum blood-alcohol level. The rate of elimination of alcohol from the bloodstream is approximately 0.015% per hour. Therefore, to calculate your actual blood-alcohol level, subtract 0.015 from the number indicated on the right-hand column for each hour from the start of drinking.

with this statute, the operation of a motor vehicle on a public highway automatically carries with it the stipulation that the driver will have the choice of either submitting to a test for alcohol intoxication if requested, or be subject to loss of the license for some designated period—usually six months to one year.

The leading case relating to the constitutionality of collecting a blood specimen for alcohol testing, as well as for obtaining other types of physical evidence from a suspect without consent, is *Schmerber* v. *California*.[6] While being treated at a Los Angeles hospital for injuries sustained in an automobile collision, Schmerber was arrested on a charge of having driven under the influence of alcohol. A blood sample was subsequently obtained from

---

[6] 384 U.S. 757 (1966).

Schmerber by a physician at the direction of the police over the objection of the defendant. On appeal to the U.S. Supreme Court, the defendant argued that his privilege against self-incrimination had been violated by the introduction of the results of the blood test at his trial. The Court ruled against the defendant, reasoning that the Fifth Amendment only prohibits compelling a suspect to give "testimonial" evidence that may prove to be self-incriminating; furnishing "physical" evidence, such as fingerprints, photographs, measurements, and blood samples, the Court ruled, was protection not afforded by the Fifth Amendment.

The Court also addressed the question of whether Schmerber was subjected to an unreasonable search and seizure by the taking of a blood specimen without a search warrant. The Court upheld the blood removal, reasoning in this case that the police were confronted with an emergency situation. By the time police officials would have obtained the warrant, the blood levels would have declined significantly as a result of natural body elimination processes. In effect, the evidence would have been destroyed. The Court also emphasized that the blood specimen was taken in a medically accepted manner and without unreasonable force.

It must be emphasized that this opinion in no way condones the warrantless taking of blood for alcohol or drug testing under all circumstances. The reasonableness of actions a police officer may take to compel an individual to yield evidence can only be judged on a case-by-case basis.

THE ROLE OF THE TOXICOLOGIST

Once the forensic toxicologist ventures beyond the analysis of alcohol, he immediately confronts an encyclopedic maze of drugs and poisons. Only a cursory discussion of the problem and handicaps imposed on the toxicologist is enough to develop a sense of appreciation for the accomplishments and ingenuity of the scientists who occupy this branch of forensic science. The toxicologist is originally presented with body fluids and/or organs and is normally requested to examine them for the presence of drugs and poisons. If he or she is fortunate, which is not often, some clue as to the type of toxic substance present may develop from the victim's symptoms, a post-mortem pathological examination, an examination of the victim's personal effects, or the nearby presence of empty drug containers or house chemicals. Without such supportive information, the toxicologist is forced into using general screening procedures with the hope of narrowing thousands of possibilities to one.

If this task in itself does not seem monumental, consider that the toxicologist is not dealing with drugs at the concentration levels found in powders and pills. By the time a drug specimen reaches the toxicology laboratory, it has been dissipated and distributed throughout the body. Where the drug analyst may have gram or milligram quantities of material to work with, the toxicologist must be satisfied with nanogram or at best microgram amounts, and these are only acquired after careful extraction from body fluids and organs.

Furthermore, the body is an active chemistry laboratory, and no one can appreciate this observation more than a toxicologist. Few substances enter and completely leave the body in the same chemical state. The drug that is injected is not always the substance extracted from the body tissues. Therefore a thorough understanding of how the body alters or metabolizes the chemical structure of a drug is essential in ultimately detecting the presence of a drug. It would, for example, be a futile and frustrating effort on the part of any toxicologist to undertake an exhaustive search for heroin in the human body. This drug is almost immediately metabolized to morphine on entering the bloodstream. Even with this information, the search may still prove impossible unless the examiner is also aware of the fact that only a small percentage of morphine is excreted unchanged in urine. For the most part, morphine becomes chemically bonded to body carbohydrates before its elimination in urine. Thus, the successful detection of morphine requires that its extraction be planned in accordance with a knowledge of its chemical fate in the body.

Last, when and if the toxicologist has surmounted all these obstacles and has finally detected, identified, and quantitated a drug or poison, he must be prepared to assess the substance's toxicity. Unfortunately, there is very little published information relating to the toxic levels of most drugs. Even when such data is available, its interpretation must be predicated on the assumption that the victim's physiological behavior is in agreement with that experienced by the subjects of previous studies. In some cases, such an assumption may not be entirely valid without knowing the subject's case history. No experienced toxicologist would be terribly surprised to find an individual walking around with a toxic level of a drug that would have killed most others.

Toxicology is made infinitely easier once it is recognized that the toxicologist's capabilities are directly dependent on the input received from the attending physician, medical examiner, and police investigator. It is a tribute to forensic toxicologists, who must often labor under conditions that do not afford such cooperation, that they can achieve the high level of proficiency that they do.

Generally, with a deceased person, the medical examiner is in a position to make the necessary decisions regarding what biological specimens must be shipped to the toxicology laboratory for analysis. However, the living person suspected of being under the influence of a drug presents a completely different problem, and there are few options available. When possible, both blood and urine are to be taken from any suspected drug user. The entire urine void is to be collected and submitted for toxicological analysis. Preferably, two consecutive voids should be collected in separate specimen containers. When a licensed physician or registered nurse is available, a sample of blood should also be collected. The amount of blood taken is dependent on the type of examination to be conducted. Comprehensive toxicological tests for drugs and poisons can conveniently be carried out on a minimum of 10 cc of blood. A determination solely for the presence of alcohol will require much less—approximately 5 cc of blood. However, it must be emphasized that many therapeutic drugs, such as tranquilizers and barbiturates, when taken in combination with a small, nonintoxicating amount of alcohol, will produce behavioral patterns resembling alcohol intoxication. For this reason, it is particularly important that the toxicologist be given an adequate amount of blood so he will have the option of performing a comprehensive analysis for drugs in cases of low alcohol concentrations.

TECHNIQUES USED IN TOXICOLOGY

For the toxicologist, the upsurge in drug use and abuse has meant that the overwhelming majority of fatal and nonfatal toxic agents are drugs. Not surprisingly, it is a relatively small number of drugs, namely, those discussed in Chapter 9, that comprise nearly all the toxic agents encountered. Of these, alcohol and the barbiturates normally account for 90 percent or more of the drugs encountered in a typical toxicology laboratory.

Like the drug analyst, the toxicologist must devise an analytical scheme that will successfully detect, isolate, and specifically identify a toxic substance. In doing so, the first chore will be to selectively remove and isolate drugs and other toxic agents from the biological materials submitted as evidence. Because drugs do constitute a large portion of the toxic materials found, a good deal of effort will necessarily have to be devoted to their extraction and detection. The procedures used are numerous, and their description is too detailed for inclusion in an introductory text such as this is intended to be. We can best understand the underlying principle of drug extraction by observing that a very large number of drugs fall into the categories of acids and bases.

Although there are a number of definitions for these two classes, a reasonably simple one states that an acid is a compound that sheds a hydrogen ion (or a hydrogen minus its electron) with reasonable ease. Conversely, a base is a molecule that can pick up a hydrogen ion shed by an acid. The idea of acidity and basicity can be expressed in terms of a simple numerical value that relates to the concentration of the hydrogen ion (H^+) in a liquid medium such as water. Chemists use what is called the *pH scale* to do this. This scale runs from 0 to 14.

$$pH = \underline{0\ 1\ 2\ 3\ 4\ 5\ 6\ 7\ 8\ 9\ 10\ 11\ 12\ 13\ 14}$$

$$\leftarrow \text{Increasing} \longrightarrow \text{Neutral} \longrightarrow \text{Increasing} \rightarrow$$
$$\text{acidity} \qquad\qquad\qquad \text{basicity}$$

Normally, water is neither acid or basic—in other words, it is neutral, and has a pH of 7. However, when an acidic substance—e.g., sulfuric acid or hydrochloric acid—is added to the water, it adds excess hydrogen ions, and the pH value becomes less than 7. The lower the number, the more acidic the water. Similarly, when a basic substance—e.g., sodium hydroxide or ammonium hydroxide—is added to water, it removes hydrogen ions, thus making water basic. The more basic the water, the higher its pH value.

By controlling the pH of a water solution into which blood or tissues are dissolved, the toxicologist can conveniently control the type of drug that will be recovered. For example, acid drugs are easily extracted from an acidified water solution (pH less than 7) with organic solvents such as chloroform. Similarly, basic drugs are readily removed from a basic water solution (pH greater than 7) with organic solvents. This relatively simple approach gives the toxicologist a general technique for extracting and categorizing drugs. Some of the more commonly encountered drugs may be classified as follows:

Acid Drugs	Basic Drugs
Barbiturates	Phencyclidine
Acetylsalicylic acid (Aspirin)	Methadone
	Amphetamines
	Cocaine

Once the specimen has been extracted and separated into acidic and basic fractions, the toxicologist can proceed to identify the drugs present in a manner similar to that described in Chapter 9 (see Figure 10-12). The techniques of color tests, microcrystalline tests, chromatography, and spectrophotometry are all at the disposal of the toxicologist to be used in appropriate combination to complete the identification process. In addition, many toxicology laboratories have added the mass spectrometer (see Chapter 5) to their arsenal of instruments. The high sensitivity and specificity of this technique make it highly suitable for identifying small concentrations of drugs. The combination gas chromatograph/mass spectrometer/computer promises the toxicologist a one-step identification procedure of unequalled sensitivity and specificity (see page 130).

A recent development called immunoassay is proving to be a useful analytical procedure in toxicology laboratories. The principles of immunoassay are very different from any of the techniques we have so far discussed. Suffice it to say at this point that immunoassay is based on specific drug antibody reactions. The primary advantage of immunoassay is its ability to detect small concentrations of drugs in body fluids and organs. In fact, this technique offers the best approach for detecting the low drug levels normally associated with the smoking of marijuana. We will learn more about this concept in Chapter 12.

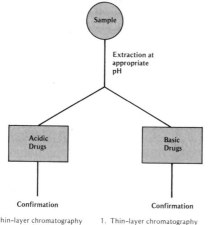

Confirmation

1. Thin-layer chromatography
2. Gas chromatography
3. Ultraviolet spectrophotometry
4. Mass spectrometry
5. Immunoassay

Confirmation

1. Thin-layer chromatography
2. Gas chromatography
3. Ultraviolet spectrophotometry
4. Mass spectrometry
5. Immunoassay

Figure 10-12. Biological fluids and tissues are extracted for acidic and basic drugs by controlling the pH of a water solution in which they are dissolved. Once this is accomplished, the toxicologist will analyze for drugs by utilizing a variety of test procedures.

These days the forensic toxicologist only occasionally encounters a group of poisons known as "heavy metals." These include arsenic, bismuth, antimony, mercury, and thallium. To screen for many of these metals, the investigator may dissolve the suspect body fluid or tissue in a hydrochloric acid solution and insert a copper strip into the solution (the Reinsch test). The appearance of a silvery or dark coating on the copper is indicative of the presence of a heavy metal. Such a finding must be confirmed by the use of analytical techniques suitable for inorganic analysis, namely, atomic absorption spectrophotometry, emission spectroscopy, or X-ray diffraction.

Carbon monoxide still represents one of the most common poisons encountered in a forensic laboratory. When carbon monoxide enters the human body, it is primarily absorbed by the red blood cells, where it combines with hemoglobin to form carboxyhemoglobin. An average red blood cell contains about 280 million molecules of hemoglobin. It is with hemoglobin that oxygen normally combines allowing the blood to transport the oxygen throughout the body. However, if a high percentage of the hemoglobin combines with carbon monoxide, not enough is left to carry sufficient oxygen to the tissues, and death by asphyxiation shortly follows.

There are two basic methods for measuring the concentration of carbon monoxide in the blood. Spectrophotometric methods can examine the visible spectrum of blood to determine the relative amount of carboxyhemoglobin to oxyhemoglobin or total hemoglobin; or a volume of blood can be treated with a reagent to liberate the carbon monoxide, which is then measured by gas chromatography.

The amount of carbon monoxide in blood is generally expressed as "percent saturation." This actually represents the extent to which the available hemoglobin has been converted to carboxyhemoglobin. The transition from normal or occupational levels of carbon monoxide to toxic levels is not sharply defined. It depends, among other things, on the age, health, and general fitness of each individual. In a healthy middle-aged individual, a carbon monoxide blood saturation greater than 50 to 60 percent is considered fatal. However, in combination with alcohol or other depressants, fatal levels may be significantly lower. For instance, a carbon monoxide saturation of 35 to 40 percent may prove fatal in the presence of a blood-alcohol concentration of 0.20 percent w/v. Interestingly, chain smokers may have a carbon monoxide level of 8 to 10 percent from the carbon monoxide in cigarette smoke.

Inhalation of automobile fumes is a relatively common way chosen by people to commit suicide. A garden or vacuum cleaner hose is often used to connect the tailpipe with the vehicle's interior, or the engine is allowed to run in a closed garage. A level of carbon monoxide sufficient to cause death accumulates in 5 to 10 minutes in a closed single-car garage.

The level of carbon monoxide in the blood of a victim found dead at the scene of a fire is of significance in ascertaining whether or not foul play has occurred. The presence of high levels of carbon monoxide in the blood is proof that the victim breathed the combustion products of the fire and was therefore alive when the fire began. Many attempts at covering up a murder by setting fire to a victim's house or car have been uncovered in this manner.

THE SIGNIFICANCE OF TOXICOLOGICAL FINDINGS

Once the drug is found and identified, the toxicologist is called upon to assess its influence on the behavior of the individual under examination. The task of interpreting the results of a toxicology find is one of the more difficult chores facing the toxicologist. We have already seen that many of the world's countries have created laws designating a specific blood-alcohol level at which an individual is presumed to be under the influence of alcohol. These levels were established as a result of numerous studies carried out over a period of years to measure the effects of alcohol levels on driving performance. However, no such legal guidelines are available to the toxicologist who must offer an opinion as to how a drug other than alcohol affects an individual's performance or physical state.

For many drugs, blood concentration levels can readily be determined and can be used to *estimate* the pharmacological effects of the drug on the individual. For a deceased person, drug levels present in various body organs and tissues can be ascertained to provide additional information about an individual's state at the time of death. However, before conclusions can be drawn about drug-induced behavior other factors must also be taken into consideration. These include the age, physical condition, and tolerance of the drug user. With the prolonged use of a drug, an individual may become less responsive to a drug's effects and will be able to tolerate drug blood concentrations that would normally be fatal to the casual drug user. Therefore, knowledge of an individual's history of drug use is very important in evaluating drug concentrations found by the toxicologist. Another consideration may be additive or synergistic effects provided by the interaction of two or more drugs. The combination of two or more drugs may produce a highly intoxicated or comatose state even though none of the drugs alone is present at high or toxic levels. The combination of alcohol with barbiturates or narcotics is a common example of a potentially lethal drug combination.

The concentration of a drug present in urine is a poor indicator of how extensively an individual's behavior or state is influenced by the drug. Urine is formed outside the body's circulatory system, and consequently drug levels can build up in it over a relatively long period of time. In fact, some drugs are found in the urine one to three days after thay have been taken and long after their effects on the user have disappeared. Nevertheless, the value of this information should not be discounted. Urine drug levels, like blood levels, are best used by law enforcement authorities and the courts to corroborate other investigative and medical findings pertaining to an individual's condition. Hence, for the individual who is arrested for suspicion of being under the influence of a drug, a toxicologist's determinations will supplement the observations of the arresting officer, including the results of balance and coordination tests performed on the suspect at the time of apprehension. For a deceased person, the ultimate responsibility for establishing a cause of death rests with the medical examiner or coroner. However, before a conclusive determination is made, the examining physician is dependent on the skills of the forensic toxicologist to demonstrate the presence of absence of a drug or poison in the tissues or body fluids of the deceased. It is only through the combined efforts of the toxicologist and the medical examiner (or coroner) that society can be assured that death investigations will achieve high professional and legal standards.

REVIEW QUESTIONS

1. The most heavily abused drug in the Western world is _____.
2. Toxicologists are only employed by crime laboratories. (True, False)
3. The amount of alcohol present in the blood (is, is not) directly proportional to the concentration of alcohol in the brain.
4. Blood levels have become the accepted standard for relating alcohol intake to its effect on the body. (True, False)
5. Alcohol consumed on an empty stomach is absorbed (faster, slower) than an equivalent amount of alcohol taken when there is food in the stomach.

6. Under normal drinking conditions, alcohol concentration in the blood peaks in _____ to _____ minutes.

7. In the postabsorption period, alcohol is distributed uniformly between the _____ portions of the body.

8. Elimination of alcohol from the body is accomplished by _____ and _____.

9. Ninety to 95 percent of the alcohol is _____ to carbon dioxide.

10. The oxidation of alcohol takes place almost entirely in the _____.

11. The amount of alcohol exhaled in the _____ is directly proportional to the concentration of the alcohol in the blood.

12. Alcohol is eliminated from the blood at an average rate of _____ percent w/v.

13. Alcohol is absorbed into the blood from the _____ and _____.

14. An _____ carries blood away from the heart; a _____ carries blood back to the heart.

15. The _____ artery carries deoxygenated blood from the heart to the lungs.

16. Alcohol passes from the blood capillaries into the _____ sacs located in the lungs.

17. One milliliter of blood will contain the same amount of alcohol as approximately _____ milliliters of alveolar breath.

18. During the period when alcohol is being absorbed into the blood, the alcohol concentration in venous blood will be (higher, lower) than that in arterial blood.

19. In a Breathalyzer ampoule, the ethyl alcohol reacts with _____ in a fixed ratio.

20. The Breathalyzer measures the (absorption, emission) of light by potassium dichromate before and after its reaction with alcohol.

21. Silver nitrate is present in a Breathalyzer ampoule as a _____ to speed up the rate of reaction.

22. Alcohol can be separated from other volatiles present in blood and can be quantitated by the technique of _____.

23. Breath testers that operate on the principle of _____ light absorption of alcohol are becoming increasingly popular with the law enforcement community.

24. Portable hand-held, roadside breath testers for alcohol provide evidential test results. (True, False)

25. When drawing blood for alcohol testing, the suspect's skin must first be wiped with a _____ disinfectant.

26. Failure to add a preservative, such as sodium fluoride, to blood may lead to a(n) (decline, increase) in alcohol concentration.
27. Most states have established _____ percent w/v as the impairment limit for blood-alcohol concentration.
28. In the case of _____, the Supreme Court ruled that the taking of nontestimonial evidence, such as a blood sample, was not in violation of a suspect's Fifth Amendment privileges.
29. Heroin is changed upon entering the body into _____.
30. The body fluids _____ and _____ are both desirable for the toxicological examination of a living person suspected of being under the influence of a drug.
31. A large number of drugs can be classified chemically as _____ and _____.
32. Water having a pH value (less, greater) than 7 is basic.
33. Barbiturates are classified as _____ drugs.
34. Drugs are extracted from body fluids and tissues by carefully controlling the _____ of the medium in which the sample has been dissolved.
35. The technique of _____ is based on specific drug antibody reactions.
36. The gas _____ will combine with hemoglobin in the blood to form carboxyhemoglobin, thus interfering with the transportation of oxygen in the blood.
37. The amount of carbon monoxide present in blood is usually expressed as _____.
38. Blood levels of drugs can alone be used to draw definitive conclusions about the effects of a drug on an individual. (True, False)
39. The interaction of alcohol and barbiturates in the body can produce a _____ effect.
40. The level of a drug present in the urine is by itself a (good, poor) indicator of how extensively an individual is affected by a drug.
41. Urine and blood drug levels are best used by law enforcement authorities and the courts to _____ other investigative and medical findings pertaining to an individual's condition.

FURTHER REFERENCES

Caplan, Y. H., "The Determination of Alcohol in Blood and Breath," in *Forensic Science Handbook*, R. Saferstein, ed. Englewood Cliffs, N.J.: Prentice-Hall, Inc., 1982.

Cravey, R. H., and R. C. Baselt, eds., *Introduction to Forensic Toxicology.* Davis, Calif.: Biomedical Publications, 1981.

Cravey, Robert H., and Naresh C. Jain, "Current Status of Blood Alcohol Methods," *Journal of Chromatographic Science*, 12 (1974), 209.

Curry, A. S., *Poison Detection in Human Organs*, 3rd ed. Springfield, Ill.: Charles C. Thomas, Publisher, 1976.

Freimuth, Henry C., "Forensic Aspects of Alcohol," in *Medicological Investigation of Death*, 2nd ed., Werner U. Spitz and Russell S. Fisher, eds. Springfield, Ill.: Charles C. Thomas, Publisher, 1980.

Jain, Naresh C., and Robert H. Cravey, "Analysis of Alcohol. I. A Review of Chemical and Infrared Methods," *Journal of Chromatographic Science*, 10 (1972), 257.

——— , "Analysis of Alcohol. II. A Review of Gas Chromatographic Methods," *Journal of Chromatographic Science*, 10 (1972), 263.

Mason, M. F., and K. M. Dubowski, "Alcohol, Traffic, and Chemical Testing in the United States: A Résume and Some Remaining Problems," *Clinical Chemistry*, 20 (1974), 126.

Moffat, A. E., et al., eds. *Clarke's Isolation and Identification of Drugs*, 2nd ed. London: Pharmaceutical Press, 1986.

National Safety Council, *Alcohol and the Impaired Driver*. Chicago: National Safety Council, 1976.

11

Forensic Aspects of Arson and Explosive Investigations

Arson and explosions often present the criminal investigator with complex and difficult circumstances to investigate. Normally, these incidents are committed at the convenience of a perpetrator who has thoroughly planned the criminal act and has left the crime scene long before any official investigation is launched. Furthermore, proof of the commission of the offense is rendered more difficult to obtain because of the extensive destruction that frequently dominates the crime scene. The contribution of the criminalist is only one aspect of a comprehensive and difficult investigative process that must establish a motive, the modus operandi, and a suspect.

In practice, the criminalist's function is a rather limited one; usually he is expected only to detect and identify relevant chemical materials collected at the scene, and to reconstruct and identify ignitors or detonating mechanisms. Although a chemist can identify trace amounts of gasoline or kerosene in debris, there is no scientific test that will determine whether or not an arsonist has used a pile of rubbish or paper to start a fire. Furthermore, a fire can have many accidental causes, including faulty wiring, overheated electric motors, improperly cleaned and regulated heating systems, and cigarette smoking—and these usually leave no chemical traces. Thus, the final determination as to the cause of a fire or explosion must take numerous factors into consideration and requires an extensive on-site investigation. The ultimate determination must be made by an investigator whose training and knowledge have been augmented by the practical experiences of fire and explosive investigation.

283

THE CHEMISTRY OF FIRE

Man's early search to explain the physical concepts underlying the behavior of matter always bestowed a central and fundamental role on fire. To ancient Greek philosophers, fire was one of the four basic elements from which all matter was derived. The alchemist thought of fire as an instrument of transformation to be used for changing one element into another. One ancient recipe expresses its mystical power as follows:

> Now the substance of cinnabar is such that the more it is heated, the more exquisite are its sublimations. Cinnabar will become mercury, and passing through a series of other sublimations, it is again turned into cinnabar, and thus it enables man to enjoy eternal life.

Today, man knows of fire not as an element of matter, but as a transformation process during which oxygen is united with some other substance to produce noticeable quantities of heat and light (a flame). Therefore, any insight into why and how a fire is initiated and sustained must begin with the knowledge of the fundamental chemical reaction of fire—oxidation.

A simple description of oxidation is one that has oxygen combining with other substances to produce new products. Thus, we may write the chemical equation for the burning of methane gas, a major component of natural gas, as follows:

$$CH_4 + 2O_2 \rightarrow CO_2 + 2H_2O$$

methane   oxygen yields carbon   water
            dioxide

However, not all oxidation proceeds in the manner that one associates with fire. For example, oxygen combines with many metals to form oxides. Thus, iron forms a red-brown iron oxide, the familiar rust; as shown below:

$$4\,Fe + 3O_2 \rightarrow 2Fe_2O_3$$

iron   oxygen yields iron oxide

Yet chemical equations do not give us the complete insight into the oxidation process. Other factors must be taken into consideration if we are to understand all the implications of oxidation, or, for that matter, any other chemical reaction. We know that when methane unites with oxygen, it burns; but the mere mixing of methane and oxygen will not produce a fire, nor will, for example, gasoline burn when it is simply exposed to air. However, light a match in the presence of any one of these fuel-air mixtures (assuming proper proportions) and you have an instant fire. What are the reasons behind these differences? Why do some oxidations proceed with the outward appearances that we associate with a fire, while others do not? Why do we need a match to initiate some oxidations while others proceed at room temperature? The explanation lies in a fundamental but abstract concept—energy.

Energy can be defined as the capacity for doing work. Energy takes many forms such as heat energy, electrical energy, mechanical energy, nuclear energy, light energy, or chemical energy. For example, when methane is burned, the stored chemical energy in methane is converted to energy in the form of heat and light. This heat may be used to boil water or to provide high-pressure steam to turn a turbine. This is an example of converting chemical energy to heat energy to mechanical energy. The turbine can then be used to generate electricity, involving a transformation from mechanical to electrical energy. Electrical energy may then be used to turn a motor. In other words, energy can enable work to be done; heat is energy.

The quantity of heat evolved from a particular chemical reaction arises out of the breaking and formation of chemical bonds. For instance, methane is a molecule composed of one atom of carbon bonded with four hydrogen atoms:

$$H-\underset{\underset{H}{|}}{\overset{\overset{H}{|}}{C}}-H$$

Oxygen is a molecule that is formed by bonding two atoms of the element oxygen:

$$O=O$$

In chemical changes, atoms are not lost but are merely redistributed during the chemical reaction; thus, the products of methane's oxidation will be carbon dioxide:

$$O=C=O$$

and water:

$$H-O-H$$

This rearrangement, however, means that the bonds holding the atoms together must be broken and new bonds formed. We now have arrived at a fundamental observation in our dissection of a chemical reaction—that molecules must absorb energy to break apart their chemical bonds, and that they will liberate energy when their bonds are reformed. The amount of energy needed to break a bond and the quantity of energy liberated when a bond is formed are characteristic of the type of chemical bond involved. Hence, a chemical reaction involves a change in energy content; energy is going in and energy is given off. The quantities of energies involved are different for each reaction and are determined by the participants of the chemical reaction.

All oxidation reactions, including the combustion of methane, are examples of reactions in which more energy is liberated than what is required to break the various bonds. This excess energy is liberated as heat and often as light and is known as the **heat of combustion**. Such reactions are said to be **exothermic**. Table 11-1 summarizes the heats of combustion of a few of the more important fuels from the standpoint of fire investigation.

Although we will not be concerned with them, there are reactions that require more energy than what they will eventually liberate. These reactions are known as **endothermic** reactions.

It is apparent from the above considerations that all reactions require an energy input to start them. We can perhaps think of this requirement as an invisible energy barrier that has been erected between the reactants and the products of a reaction (see Figure 11-1). The higher this barrier, the more energy will be required to initiate the reaction. Where does this initial energy come from? There are many sources of energy; however, for the purpose of this discussion it will only be necessary to look at one—heat.

The energy barrier that exists in the conversion of iron to rust is a relatively small one, and it can be surmounted with the help of heat energy present in the surrounding environment at normal outdoor temperatures. Not so for methane or gasoline—here the energy barriers are quite high, and a high temperature must be applied to start the oxidation of these fuels. Hence, before any fire can result, the temperature of these fuels must be

Table 11-1.

HEATS OF COMBUSTION OF FUELS

Fuel	Heat of Combustion*
Crude oil	19,650 BTU/gal
Diesel fuel	19,550 BTU/lb
Gasoline	19,250 BTU/lb
Methane	995 BTU/cu ft
Natural gas	128-1868 BTU/cu ft
Octane	121,300 BTU/gal
Wood	7500 BTU/gal
Coal—Bituminous	11,000-14,000 BTU/lb
Anthracite	13,351 BTU/lb

Source: *John D. DeHaan, Kirk's Fire Investigation, 2nd ed. (New York: John Wiley & Sons, 1983).*
BTU (British Thermal Unit) is defined as the quantity of heat required to raise the temperature of 1 pound of water 1°F at or near its point of maximum density.

$CH_4 + 2O_2$ $CO_2 + 2H_2O$

Figure 11-1. An energy barrier must be hurdled before reactants such as methane and oxygen can combine with one another to form the products of carbon dioxide and water.

raised to a value that will allow the heat energy input to exceed the energy barrier. Table 11-2 shows that this temperature, known as the ignition temperature, is quite high for common fuels. Once the combustion starts, a sufficient amount of heat is liberated to keep the reaction going by itself. In essence, the fire becomes a chain reaction, absorbing a portion of its own liberated heat in order to generate even more heat. The fire will continue to burn until either the supply of oxygen or the fuel is exhausted.

Normally, an ordinary lighted match offers itself as a convenient ignitor of fuels. However, the fire investigator must also consider other potential sources of ignition—e.g., electrical discharges, sparks, and chemicals—while reconstructing the initiation of a fire. All of these sources have temperatures in excess of what is needed to meet the ignition temperature requirement of most fuels.

Although the liberation of energy explains many important features of oxidation, it does not offer a complete explanation for all the characteristics of the reaction. Obviously, although all oxidations liberate energy, they are not all accompanied by the presence of a flame; witness the oxidation of iron to rust. There is, therefore, one other important consideration that must be taken into account before our understanding of oxidation and fire is com-

Table 11-2.

IGNITION TEMPERATURES OF SOME COMMON FUELS

Fuel	Ignition Temperature °F
Acetone	1000
Benzene	1045
Fuel oil #2	495
Gasoline	495
Kerosene (fuel oil #1)	445
n-Octaine	428
Petroleum ether	550
Turpentine	488

Source: *John D. DeHaan,* Kirk's Fire Investigation, *2nd. ed. (New York: John Wiley & Sons, 1983).*

plete. This additional factor is the rate or speed at which the reaction takes place.

Simply, we can picture a chemical reaction, such as oxidation, taking place when molecules combine or collide with one another. Essentially, the faster the molecules move, the greater will be the number of collisions taking place between them and the faster will be the rate of reaction. There are many factors that influence the rate at which these collisions take place. In our description of fire and oxidation we need only be concerned with two: the physical state of the fuel and temperature.

A fuel will only achieve a reaction rate with oxygen sufficient to produce a flame when it is in the gaseous state, for it is only in this state that molecules can collide frequently enough to support a flaming fire. This remains true even though the fuel that may be feeding the flame is a solid, e.g., wood, paper, cloth, plastic, or a liquid such as gasoline or kerosene. How then does a liquid or solid maintain a gaseous reaction? In the case of a liquid fuel, the temperature must be high enough to vaporize the fuel. The vapor that forms burns when it mixes with oxygen and combusts as a flame. The **flash point** is the *lowest* temperature at which a liquid gives off sufficient vapor to form a mixture with air that will support combustion. Once the flash point is reached, the fuel can be ignited by some outside source of temperature to start a fire. The ignition temperature is always considerably higher than the flash point. For example, gasoline has a flash point of −50°F; however, it takes an ignition temperature of 495°F to start a gasoline fire. With a solid fuel, the process of generating vapor is more complex. Wood, or any other solid fuel, will only burn when it is exposed to heat that is hot enough to decompose the solid into gaseous products. This chemical breakdown of solid material is known as **pyrolysis**. It is the numerous gaseous products of pyrolysis that combine with oxygen to produce a fire. Here again fire can be described as a chain reaction. A match or other source of heat initiates the pyrolysis of the solid fuel, the gaseous products react with oxygen in the air to produce heat and light, and this heat in turn is used to pyrolyze more solid fuel into volatile gases.

As we have seen from our discussion about a gaseous fuel, air (oxygen) and sufficient heat are the basic ingredients of a flaming fire. There is also one other consideration—the gas fuel-air mix. Gaseous fuel and air will only burn if their composition lies within certain limits. If the fuel concentration is too low (lean) or too great (rich), combustion will not occur. The concentration range between the upper and lower limits is called the **flammable range**. For example, the flammable range for gasoline is 1.3 to 6.0 percent.

Although a flaming fire will only be supported by a gaseous fuel, there are instances in which a fuel can burn without the presence of a flame. Witness the burning cigarette or the red glow of hot charcoals. These are examples of a phenomenon known as **glowing combustion** or **smouldering**. Here combustion is taking place on the surface of a solid fuel in the absence of heat sufficiently high enough to pyrolyze the fuel. Interestingly, this phenomenon generally ensues long after the flames have gone out. Wood, for example, tends to burn with a flame until all of its pyrolyzable components have been expended; however, wood's carbonaceous residue will continue to smoulder long after the flame has extinguished itself.

We may now consider the conversion of iron to rust to be an example of an extremely slow oxidation process, a situation that exists because of the inability of the iron atoms to achieve a gaseous state. For this reason, the combination of oxygen with iron to produce rust is restricted to the surface area of the metal exposed to air, a limitation that severely reduces the rate of reaction. On the other hand, the reaction of methane and oxygen is an example of oxidation in which all the reactants are in the gaseous state. Hence, this reaction proceeds at a rapid rate as reflected by the production of noticeable quantities of heat and light (a flame).

Most typically, the rate of a chemical reaction increases when the temperature is raised. The magnitude of the increase in rate with temperature varies from one reaction to another and also from one temperature range to another. For most reactions, a $10°C$ ($18°F$) rise in temperature doubles or triples the reaction rate. This observation explains in part why burning is so rapid. As the fire spreads, it raises the temperature of the fuel-air mixture, thus increasing the rate of reaction; this in turn generates more heat, again increasing the rate of reaction. It is only when the fuel or oxygen is depleted that this vicious cycle will come to a halt.

One rather interesting phenomenon that is often invoked by arson suspects as being the cause of a fire is **spontaneous combustion**. Actually, the conditions under which spontaneous combustion can develop are rather limited and in fact rarely account for the cause of a fire. Spontaneous combustion is the result of a natural heat-producing process in poorly ventilated containers or areas. For example, hay stored in barns offers itself as an excellent growing medium for bacteria whose activities will generate heat. If the hay is not properly ventilated, the heat will build to a level that will support other types of heat-producing chemical reactions in the hay. Eventually, as the heat rises, the ignition temperature of hay is reached, spontaneously setting off a fire.

Another known example of spontaneous combustion involves the ignition of improperly ventilated containers containing rags soaked with certain types of highly unsaturated oils, such as linseed oil. It is conceivable that heat will build up to the point of ignition as a result of a slow heat-producing chemical oxidation between the air and the oil. Of course, storage conditions will have to encourage the accumulation of the heat over a prolonged period of time. However, spontaneous combustion will not occur with hydrocarbon lubricating oils, and it is not expected to occur with most of the fats and oils that are found in a household.

Until now we have only referred to oxidation reactions that rely on air as the sole source of oxygen. However, we need not restrict ourselves to this type of situation. For example, explosives are substances that undergo a rapid exothermic oxidation reaction with the production of large quantities of gases. It is this sudden buildup of gas pressure that constitutes the nature of an explosion. Detonation occurs so rapidly that oxygen in the air cannot participate in the reaction; thus, many explosives must have their own source of oxygen. Chemicals that supply oxygen are known as **oxidizing agents**. One such agent is found in black powder, a low explosive, which is composed of a mixture of the following chemical ingredients:

75% potassium nitrate (KNO_3)
15% charcoal (C)
10% sulfur (S)

In this combination, oxygen containing potassium nitrate acts as an oxidizing agent for the charcoal and sulfur fuels. As heat is applied to black powder, oxygen is liberated from potassium nitrate and simultaneously combines with charcoal and sulfur to produce heat and gases (symbolized by ↑), as represented in the following chemical equation:

$$3C + S + 2KNO_3 \rightarrow 3CO_2 \uparrow + N_2 \uparrow + K_2S + \text{heat}$$

| carbon | sulfur | potassium nitrate | yields | carbon dioxide | nitrogen | potassium sulfide | |

Some explosives have their oxygen and fuel components combined within one molecule. For example, nitroglycerin, the major constituent of dynamite, has a chemical structure that combines carbon, hydrogen, nitrogen, and oxygen:

$$
\begin{array}{ccccc}
 & H & H & H & \\
 & | & | & | & \\
H- & C- & C- & C- & H \\
 & | & | & | & \\
 & O & O & O & \\
 & | & | & | & \\
 & NO_2 & NO_2 & NO_2 &
\end{array}
$$

When nitroglycerin detonates, large quantities of energy are released as the molecule decomposes, and the oxygen recombines to produce large volumes of carbon dioxide, nitrogen, and water.

In summary, three requirements must be satisfied if combustion is to be initiated and sustained:

1. A fuel must be present.

2. Oxygen must be available in sufficient quantity to combine with the fuel.

3. Heat must be applied to initiate the combustion, and sufficient heat must be generated to sustain the reaction.

SEARCHING THE FIRE SCENE

It is important that the arson investigator begin examining the fire scene for signs of arson as soon as the fire has been extinguished. Time is constantly working against the arson investigator. Experience has shown that most arsons are started with petroleum-based accelerants such as gasoline or kerosene. If any petroleum residues remain after the fire is extinguished, they will evaporate within a matter of hours and certainly within a few days. Furthermore, safety and health conditions may necessitate that clean-up and salvage operations begin as quickly as possible. Once this occurs, it will be impossible to conduct a meaningful investigation of the fire scene.

The necessity to begin an *immediate* investigation of the circumstances surrounding a fire even takes precedence over the requirement to obtain a search warrant to enter and search a premise. The Supreme Court, in explaining its position on this issue, stated in part:

> Fire officials are charged not only with extinguishing fires, but with finding their causes. Prompt determination of the fire's origin may be necessary to prevent its recurrence, as through the detection of continuing dangers such as faulty wiring or a defective furnace. Immediate investigation may also be necessary to preserve evidence from intentional or accidental destruction. And, of course, the sooner the officials complete their duties, the less will be their subsequent interference with the privacy and the recovery efforts of the victims. For these reasons, officials need no warrant to remain in a building for a reasonable time to investigate the cause of a blaze after it has been extinguished. And if the warrantless entry to put out the fire and determine its cause is constitutional, the warrantless seizure of evidence while inspecting the premises for these purposes also is constitutional. . . .
>
> In determining what constitutes a reasonable time to investigate, appropriate recognition must be given to the exigencies that confront officials serving under these conditions, as well as to individuals' reasonable expectations of privacy.[1]

A search of the fire scene must focus on finding the fire's origin, for it is this area that will prove most productive in any search for an accelerant or ignition device. In a search to determine the specific point of origin of a fire, the investigator may uncover some telltale signs of arson. For instance, there may be evidence of separate and unconnected fires or the use of "streamers"

---

[1] *Michigan* v. *Tyler*, 56 L.Ed.2d 486 (1978).

to spread the fire from one area to another. For example, the arsonist may have spread a trail of gasoline or paper to cause the fire to move rapidly from one room to another. Additionally, the presence of containers capable of holding an accelerant or the finding of an ignition device ranging in sophistication from a candle to a time-delay device certainly will arouse suspicions of an arson-caused fire. Simultaneously with these efforts, investigators should look for signs of breaking and entering and theft, and they should begin interviewing any eyewitnesses to the fire.

There are no fast and simple rules for identifying a fire's origin. Normally, a fire has a tendency to move in an upward direction, and thus the probable origin will most likely be located closest to the lowest point that shows the most intense characteristics of burning. However, there are many factors that can contribute to the deviation of a fire from normal behavior. Prevailing drafts and winds; secondary fires due to collapsing floors and roofs; the physical arrangement of the burning structure; stairways, elevator shafts; holes in the floor, wall, or roof; and the effects of the fire fighter in suppressing the fire are all factors that the knowledgeable fire investigator must consider before determining conclusive findings.

Once located, the point of origin should be protected as necessary to permit careful investigation. As at any crime scene, nothing should be touched or moved before notes, sketches, and photographs are taken. An examination must also be made for possible accidental causes, as well as for evidence of arson. The most common materials used by an arsonist to assure the rapid spread and intensity of a fire are gasoline and kerosene, or, for that matter, any volatile flammable liquid. Fortunately, only under the most ideal of conditions will combustible liquids be entirely consumed during a fire. When the liquid is poured over a large area, it is highly likely that a portion of it will seep into a porous surface, such as cracks in the floor, upholstery, rags, plaster, wallboards, or carpet, where enough of it remains unchanged so that it can be detected in the crime laboratory. In addition, when a fire has been extinguished with water, the rate of evaporation of volatile fluids may have been slowed down because water cools and covers materials through which the combustible liquid may have soaked. Fortunately the presence of water does not interfere with laboratory methods utilized to detect and characterize flammable liquid residues.

The fire investigator's search for traces of flammable liquid residues may be aided by the use of a highly sensitive portable vapor detector or "sniffer" (Figure 11-2). This device can rapidly screen suspect materials for the presence of volatile residues by sucking in the air surrounding the questioned sample. The air is passed over a heated filament; if a combustible vapor is present, it oxidizes and immediately increases the temperature of the filament. The rise in filament temperature is then registered as a deflection on the detector's meter. Of course, such a device is not a conclusive test for a flammable vapor, but it does provide the investigator with an excellent screening device for checking suspect samples at the fire scene.

Figure 11-2. Portable hydrocarbon detector. *Courtesy* New Jersey State Police.

COLLECTION AND PRESERVATION
OF ARSON EVIDENCE

As a matter of routine, two to three quarts of ash and soot debris must be collected at the point of origin of a fire when arson is suspected. The collection should include all porous materials and all other substances thought likely to contain flammable residues. These include such things as wood flooring, rugs, upholstery, and rags. Specimens are to be immediately packaged in an airtight container so no loss can occur through evaporation. New, clean paint cans are good containers as they are low-cost, airtight, and unbreakable and are available in a variety of sizes. Wide-mouthed glass jars are also useful for packaging suspect specimens, provided that they contain airtight lids. If need be, large bulky samples will have to be cut to size at the scene so that they will fit into available containers. Plastic bags are not suitable for packaging specimens because they react with hydrocarbons and will permit volatile hydrocarbon vapors to be depleted.

It is important that the collection of all materials suspected of containing volatile liquids be accompanied by a thorough sampling of similar but uncontaminated control specimens from another area of the fire scene. For example, if an investigator collects carpeting at the point of origin, he must sample the same carpet from another part of the room where he is reasonably sure that no flammable substance was placed. In the laboratory, the criminalist will check the control to be sure that it is free of any flammables. This procedure will reduce the possibility and subsequent argument that the carpet was exposed to a flammable liquid such as a cleaning solution during the normal course of its maintenance. In addition, laboratory tests on the unburned control material may have to be performed in order to help analyze the breakdown products arising from the burned material's exposure to intense heat during the fire.

Needless to say, fluids found in open bottles or cans must be collected and sealed. Even when such containers appear to be empty, the investigator is wise to seal and preserve them in case they contain trace amounts of liquids or vapors. At the same time, a thorough search of the scene should be undertaken for ignitors. The most common ignitor is the match. Normally, the match is completely consumed during a fire and is impossible to locate. However, there have been cases in which, by force of habit, matches have been extinguished and tossed aside only to be recovered later by the investigator. This evidence may prove valuable if the criminalist can successfully fit the match to a book found in the possession of a suspect, as shown in Figure 11-3 (a) and (b). There are, in addition, many other types of devices that an arsonist can construct to start a fire. These might include a burning cigarette, firearms, ammunition, a mechanical match striker, electrical sparking devices, and a "Molotov cocktail." Relatively complex mechanical devices are much more likely to survive the fire for later discovery. The broken glass and wick of the Molotov cocktail, if recovered, must be preserved as well.

(a)

(b)

Figure 11-3. Three matches (spec. 3, 4, 5) discarded at the scene of an arson are each shown to fit into a match book (spec. 1) found in the suspect's possession. Such evidence provides a strong link between the crime scene and suspect. *Courtesy* New Jersey State Police.

One important piece of evidence which is not to be overlooked by arson investigators is the clothing of the suspect perpetrator. If this individual is arrested within a few hours of initiating the fire, residual quantities of the accelerant may still be present in the clothing. As we will see in the next section, the forensic laboratory can detect extremely small quantities of accelerant materials, making the examination of a suspect's clothing a feasible investigative approach. Each item of clothing should be placed in a separate airtight container, preferably a new, clean paint can.

THE ANALYSIS OF FLAMMABLE RESIDUES

Criminalists are nearly unanimous in judging the gas chromatograph to be the most sensitive and reliable instrument for detecting and characterizing flammable residues. The vast majority of arsons are initiated by petroleum distillates such as gasoline and kerosene; these liquids are actually composed of a complex mixture of hydrocarbons. Basically, the gas chromatograph separates the hydrocarbon components and produces a chromatographic pattern characteristic of a particular petroleum product.

The easiest way to recover accelerant residues from fire-scene debris is to heat the airtight container in which the sample is sent to the laboratory. When the container is heated, any volatile residue present in the debris will be driven off and will be trapped in the container's enclosed air space. The vapor or "headspace" is removed with a syringe, as shown in Figure 11-4. When the vapor is injected into the gas chromatograph, it is separated into

Figure 11-4. Removal of vapor from an enclosed container prior to gas chromatographic analysis. *Courtesy* New Jersey State Police.

its components, and each peak is recorded on the chromatogram. The identity of the volatile residue is determined when the pattern of the resultant chromatogram is compared to patterns produced by known petroleum products. For example, in Figure 11-5 a gas chromatographic analysis of debris recovered from a fire site shows a chromatogram similar to a known gasoline standard, thus proving the presence of gasoline. In the absence of any recognizable pattern the individual peaks can be identified when the investigator compares their retention times to known hydrocarbon standards (e.g., hexane, benzene, toluene, and xylenes).

One major disadvantage of the "headspace" technique described above is that the size of the syringe limits the volume of vapor which can be removed from the container and injected into the gas chromatograph. In order to overcome this deficiency, many crime laboratories have begun to augment the "headspace" technique with a method called vapor concentration. One setup for accomplishing this analysis is shown in Figure 11-6. Here the container holding the debris collected at the fire scene is heated to about 100°C while nitrogen gas flows through the container. At this temperature a significant quantity of accelerant will vaporize into the container's airspace. As the nitrogen gas flows through the airspace, it will force any accelerant present to pass through a tube containing a chemical adsorbent which is usually charcoal or Tenax. Either one of these adsorbents will retain or trap accelerant vapors. In this manner, the forensic analyst can flush out the vapor content of the can. The accelerant trapped on the chemical adsorbent is either driven off by heat directly into a gas chromatograph or extracted by a small volume of solvent (carbon disulfide) for injection into the gas chromatograph.

The major advantage of using vapor concentration in conjunction with gas chromatography is its extreme sensitivity. Gasoline volumes as low as 0.025 microliter (0.000000025 liter) can be detected and identified in this manner, far surpassing all other techniques known to the forensic scientist.

Although the gas chromatograph can readily distinguish gasoline from other flammable liquids such as kerosene, turpentine, and naphtha, it offers no solution for the identification of gasoline by brand name. In an era of fluctuating gasoline markets, exchange agreements among the various oil companies makes such an identification uncertain at best anyway. However, a procedure that has proven quite useful for associating a *liquid* gasoline sample to a particular brand stems from the knowledge that some brands of gasoline are distinguishable from one another by the colored dye additives that manufacturers put into them. These dyes are readily separated into characteristic patterns on a thin-layer chromatographic plate. However, the failure of some oil companies to consistently add the same dyes does limit the utility of this procedure. Also, it is highly possible for two or more manufacturers of gasoline to use the same dye in similar grade gasolines.

Even with these limitations, the above technique has proven a useful investigative tool for tentatively identifying a source of gasoline, or at least

Figure 11-5. (Top) Gas chromatograph of vapor from a genuine gasoline sample. (Bottom) Gas chromatograph of vapor from debris recovered at fire site. Note the similarity of the known gasoline to vapor removed from the debris. *Courtesy* New Jersey State Police.

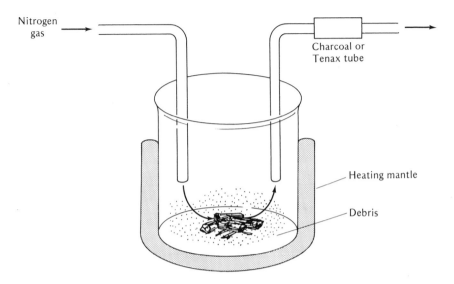

Figure 11-6. Apparatus for accelerant recovery by vapor concentration. The vapor in the enclosed container is swept onto a chemical adsorbent where it's trapped for later analysis.

for eliminating a suspected source. For example, an investigator may request the crime laboratory to undertake such an analysis in order to pinpoint a gasoline to a particular gas station. Here, it is important that the criminalist be supplied with known gasoline samples from all local and suspect stations for comparison to the unknown. These specimens must be collected as quickly as possible in order to minimize the possibility that the dye composition at the pumps will be altered by fresh gasoline deliveries.

Unfortunately, the dye composition of gasoline is of no value when one is dealing with gasoline residues absorbed into other materials. At the present time, no reliable procedure has been devised to compare such gasoline residues as to their suspected sources.

TYPES OF EXPLOSIVES

The ready accessibility of potentially explosive laboratory chemicals, dynamite, and in some countries, an assortment of military explosives, has provided the criminal element of society with a very lethal weapon. Although worldwide politically motivated bombings have received considerable publicity, it is a fact that in the United States the vast majority of bombing incidents are perpetrated by isolated individuals rather than by organized terrorists. Unfortunately for society, explosives have become attractive weapons to be used by the criminal bent on revenge, the destruction of commercial operations, or just plain mischief.

Most bombing incidents that confront police agencies today involve the use of homemade explosives and incendiary devices. The design of such weapons is limited only by the imagination and ingenuity of the bomber. Like arson investigation, bomb investigation requires the close cooperation of a group of highly specialized individuals trained and experienced in bomb disposal, bomb-site investigation, forensic analysis, and criminal investigation. To the criminalist falls the responsibility of detecting and identifying explosive chemicals recovered from the crime scene as well as identifying the detonating mechanisms. It is this special responsibility that will concern us for the remainder of this chapter.

Like fire, an explosion is the product of combustion accompanied by the creation of gases and heat. However, the distinguishing characteristic of an explosion is the rapid rate at which the reaction proceeds. It is the sudden buildup of expanding gas pressure at the origin of the explosion that produces the violent physical disruption of the surrounding environment. Consider, for example, the effect of confining an explosive charge to a relatively small enclosed container. Upon detonation, the explosive almost instantaneously produces large volumes of gases that begin to exert enormously high pressures on the interior walls of the container. In addition, the heat energy released by the explosion serves to expand the gases, causing them to push on the walls with an even greater force. If we could observe the effects of an exploding lead pipe in slow motion, we would first see the pipe's walls stretch and balloon under pressures as high as several hundred tons per square inch. Finally, the walls would fragment and fly outward in all directions. It is this flying debris or schrapnel that constitutes a great danger to life and limb in the immediate vicinity of this kind of an explosion.

Upon release from confinement, the gaseous products of the explosion suddenly expand and compress layers of surrounding air as they move outward from the origin of the explosion. This blast effect, or outward rush of gases, at a rate that may be as high as 7000 miles per hour, creates an artificial gale that can overthrow walls, collapse roofs, and disturb any object in its path. If a bomb is sufficiently powerful, the more serious damage will be inflicted by the blast effect rather than by fragmentation debris.

The speed at which explosives decompose varies greatly from one to another and permits their classification as high and low explosives. In the low explosive, this speed is called the **speed of deflagration (burning)**. In the high explosive, it is called the **speed of detonation**. Low explosives, such as black and smokeless powders, decompose relatively slowly at rates that vary up to 1000 meters per second. Because of their slow burning rates, they produce a propelling or throwing action that makes them suitable as propellants for ammunition or skyrockets. However, the danger of this group of explosives must not be underestimated, for when any one of them is confined to a relatively small container, it can explode with a force as lethal as any known explosive. **High explosives include dynamite, TNT, PETN, and RDX.**

They detonate almost instantaneously at rates from 1000 to 8500 meters per second, producing a smashing or shattering effect on their target.

LOW EXPLOSIVES

The most widely used explosives in the low explosive group are black powder and smokeless powder. The popularity of these two explosives is enhanced by their accessibility to the public. Both are available in any gun store, and black powder can easily be made from ingredients purchased at any chemical supply house as well. Black powder is a relatively stable mixture of potassium or sodium nitrate, charcoal, and sulfur. Unconfined, it merely burns; it is, in fact, used as a medium for carrying a flame to an explosive charge. A safety fuse usually consists of black powder wrapped in a fabric or plastic casing. When ignited, a sufficient length of fuse will burn at a rate slow enough to allow an individual adequate time to leave the site of the pending explosion. Black powder, like any other low explosive, only becomes explosive and lethal when it is confined.

Actually, the only ingredients required for a low explosive are fuel and a good oxidizing agent. Thus, the oxidizing agent potassium chlorate, for example, when it is mixed with sugar, produces a popular and accessible explosive mix. When it is confined to a small container—e.g., a pipe—and ignited by the flame of a safety fuse, this mixture can explode with a force equivalent to a stick of 40 percent dynamite. Some other commonly encountered ingredients that may be combined with chlorate to produce an explosive are carbon, sulfur, starch, phosphorous, and magnesium filings. Chlorate mixtures may also be ignited by the heat generated from a chemical reaction. For instance, sufficient heat can be generated to initiate combustion when concentrated sulfuric acid comes in contact with a sugar-chlorate mix.

The safest and most powerful low explosive is smokeless powder. This explosive usually consists of nitrated cotton or nitrocellulose (single-base powder) or nitroglycerin mixed with nitrocellulose (double-base powder). The powder is manufactured in a variety of grain sizes and shapes depending on the desired application.

Another form of low explosive is created when a considerable quantity of natural gas escapes into a confined area and mixes with a sufficient amount of air. If ignited, this mixture will result in simultaneous combustion, with the sudden production of large volumes of gases and heat. In a building, walls are forced outward by the expanding gases, causing the roof to fall into the interiors, and objects are thrown outward and scattered in erratic directions with no semblance of pattern.

Mixtures of air and a gaseous fuel will only explode or burn within a limited concentration range. For example, the concentration limits for methane in air ranges from 5.3 to 13.9 percent. In the presence of too much air, the fuel will become too diluted and will not respond to efforts to ignite it; on the other hand, if the fuel becomes too concentrated, ignition will be prevented because there is not enough oxygen to support the combustion. Mixtures at or near the upper concentration limit ("rich" mixtures) will explode; however, some gas will remain unconsumed because there is not enough oxygen to complete the combustion. As air rushes back into the origin of the explosion, it combines with the residual hot gas and a fire is produced that is characterized by a "whoosh" sound. Often this fire may prove to be more destructive than the explosion that preceded it. Mixtures near the lower end of the limit ("lean" mixtures) generally cause an explosion without accompanying damage due to fire.

HIGH EXPLOSIVES

The sensitivity of a high explosive provides a convenient basis for its classification into two groups. The first group, initiating explosives, are ultrasensitive to heat, shock, or friction, and under normal conditions will detonate violently instead of burning. For this reason, they are used to detonate other explosives through a chain reaction and are often referred to as *primers*. Initiating explosives provide the major ingredient of a blasting cap and include lead azide, lead styphnate, and mercury fulminate. Because of their extreme sensitivity, these explosives are rarely used as the main charge of a homemade bomb.

The second group, noninitiating explosives, are relatively insensitive to heat, shock, or friction and will normally burn rather than detonate if they are ignited in small quantities in the open air. This group comprises the majority of high explosives used for commercial and military blasting. Some common examples of noninitiating explosives are: dynamite, TNT (trinitrotoluene), PETN (pentaerythritol tetranitrate), RDX (cyclotrimethylenetrinitramine), and tetryl (2,4,6-trinitrophenylmethylnitramine).

It is an irony of history that the prize most symbolic of man's search for peace—the Nobel Peace Prize—should bear the name of the developer of one of man's most lethal discoveries—dynamite. In 1867, the Swedish chemist Alfred Nobel, searching for a method to desensitize nitroglycerin, found that when kieselguhr, a variety of diatomaceous earth, absorbed a large portion of nitrogylcerin, it became far less sensitive but still retained its explosive force. Nobel later decided to use pulp as an absorbent because kieselguhr was a heat-absorbing material. Thus, pulp dynamite was the beginning of what is now known as the straight dynamite series, the gradations of which are specified according to the percentage of nitroglycerin used. These dynamites are used when a quick shattering action is desired. Present-day straight dynamites also include sodium nitrate, which serves to furnish oxygen for complete combustion, along with a small percentage of a stabilizer— e.g., calcium carbonate. The strength rating of a straight dynamite is designated by the weight percentage of nitroglycerin in the formula; a 40-percent straight dynamite contains 40 percent, a 60-percent grade contains 60 percent, and so forth. However, the concept that the actual blasting power developed by different strengths is in direct proportion to the percent markings is erroneous. Actually, a 60-percent straight dynamite, rather than being three times as strong as a 20 percent, is only one and one-half times as strong.

Today, there are hundreds of dynamite formulations commercially available that can perform a variety of blasting tasks. In some types of dynamites the proportion of nitrogylcerin is reduced by substituting other strength-imparting ingredients, such as ammonium nitrate. Ammonium nitrate intensifies the explosive action of dynamite by furnishing oxygen, but the resulting blast is accompanied by less of a shattering action as compared to straight dynamites. This type of dynamite has a definite advantage in quarry operations and on construction projects in which the material to be blasted is of medium hardness.

Gelatin dynamites are formulated by the dissolving of nitrocellulose in the nitroglycerin to form a rubberlike gel. Gelatin dynamites are characterized by their water-resistant nature and are employed for all types of blasting under wet conditions.

In recent years the availability of nitroglycerin-based dynamite has markedly declined. Manufacturers are abandoning the use of nitroglycerin in favor of explosives containing less expensive and more stable ingredients, such as ammonium nitrate, nitrostarch, and monomethylamine nitrate (MMAN). Water gel explosives, such as those formulated with MMAN and ammonium nitrate, are characterized by their water-resistant nature and are employed for all types of blasting under wet conditions.

No discussion of high explosives would be complete without a mention of military high explosives. In many countries outside the United States, the accessibility of high explosives to terrorist organizations makes them very common constituents of homemade bombs. RDX is the most popular and powerful of the military explosives. This explosive is often encountered in the form of a pliable plastic of doughlike consistency known as *composition C–4* (a U.S. military designation).

TNT was produced and used on an enormous scale during World War II and may be considered the most important military bursting charge explosive. Alone or in combination with other explosives, it has found wide application in shells, bombs, grenades, demolition explosives, and propellent compositions. Interestingly, military "dynamite" contains no nitroglycerin but is actually composed of a mixture of RDX and TNT. Like other military explosives, TNT is rarely encountered in bombings in the United States.

PETN is used by the military in TNT mixtures for small-caliber projectiles and grenades. Commercially, the chemical is used as the explosive core in detonating fuse or primacord. Instead of the slower-burning safety fuse, a detonating fuse is often used to interconnect a series of explosive charges so that they will detonate simultaneously.

Unlike low explosives, bombs made of high explosives must be detonated by an initiating explosion. In most cases, detonators are blasting caps composed of copper or aluminum cases filled with lead azide as an initiating charge and PETN or RDX as a detonating charge. Blasting caps can be initiated by means of a burning safety fuse or by an electrical current (see Figure 11-7).

Homemade bombs camouflaged in packages, suitcases, etc., are for the most part usually initiated with an electrical blasting cap wired to a battery.

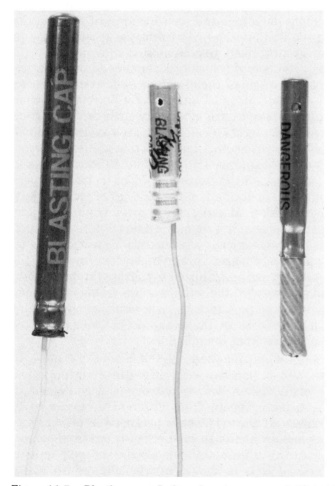

Figure 11-7.   Blasting caps. Left and center caps are initiated by an electrical current; the right cap is initiated by a safety fuse.

An unlimited number of switching-mechanism designs have been devised for setting off these devices; favored are clocks and mercury switches. There are certain situations in which individual bombers prefer to employ outside electrical sources. For instance, most automobile bombs are detonated when the ignition switch of a car is turned on.

COLLECTION AND ANALYSIS OF EXPLOSIVES

The single most important step in the detection and analysis of explosive residues is the collection of appropriate samples from the explosion scene. Invariably, there remains at the site of the explosion undetonated residues of the explosive. The ultimate detection and identification of these in the laboratory will depend on the bomb-scene investigator's skill and ability to recognize and sample the areas most likely to contain such materials.

The most obvious characteristic of a high or a contained low explosion is the presence of a crater at the origin of the blast. Once the crater has been located, all loose soil and other debris must immediately be removed from the interior of the hole and be preserved for laboratory analysis. Other good sources of explosive residues are objects located near the origin of detonation. Wood, insulation, rubber, or other soft materials that are readily penetrated often collect traces of the explosive. However, nonporous objects in close proximity to the blast must not be overlooked. For instance, experience has shown that residues can be located on the surfaces of metal objects found near the site of an explosion. Material blown away from the blast's origin should also be recovered because it, too, may retain explosive residues.

The entire area must be systematically searched with great care to recover any trace of a detonating mechanism or any other item foreign to the explosion site. Wire-mesh screens are best utilized for sifting through debris. In pipe-bomb explosions, particles of the explosive are frequently found adhering to the pipe cap or to the pipe threads, as a result of either being impacted into the metal by the force of the explosion or being deposited in the threads during the construction of the bomb.

All materials collected for examination by the laboratory must be placed in sealed containers and be labeled with all pertinent information. Soil and other soft loose materials are best stored in metal containers or plastic bags. Debris and articles collected from different areas are to be packaged in separate containers. If the evidence is packaged in plastic bags, do not place these bags in close proximity to each other. It has been demonstrated that some explosives can diffuse through plastic and contaminate nearby containers. Sharp-edged objects should not be allowed to pierce the sides of a plastic bag. It is best to place these types of items in metal containers.

When the bomb-scene debris and other material arrive in the laboratory, everything is first examined microscopically so that particles of unconsumed explosive can be detected. Portions of the recovered debris and detonating mechanism, if found, are carefully viewed under a low-power stereoscopic microscope in a painstaking effort to locate particles of the explosive. Black and smokeless powder are relatively easy to locate in debris because of their characteristic shape and colors (see Figure 11-8). However, dynamite and other high explosives present the microscopist with a much more difficult task and often have to be detected by other means.

Following microscopic examination, the recovered debris is thoroughly rinsed with acetone. The high solubility of most explosives in acetone will assure their quick removal from the debris. Once collected, the acetone extract is concentrated and analyzed utilizing color spot tests, thin-layer chromatography, and high-performance liquid chromatography (see p. 116–117). The presence of an explosive will be indicated by a well-defined spot on a TLC plate with an R_f value corresponding to a known explosive—e.g., nitroglycerin, RDX, or PETN. The high sensitivity of high-performance liquid chromatography (HPLC) also makes it very useful for the analysis of trace evidence of explosives. The HPLC operates at room temperature and hence will not cause explosives, many of which are temperature-sensitive, to decompose during their analysis. When a water-gel explosive containing ammonium nitrate and MMAN or a low explosive is suspected, the debris should be rinsed with water so that water-soluble substances (e.g., MMAN, nitrates, and chlorates) will be extracted.

Figure 11-8. Samples of smokeless powders. *Courtesy* Bureau of Alcohol, Tobacco, and Firearms, U.S. Treasury Dept., Washington, D.C.

Table 11-3.

COLOR SPOT TESTS FOR COMMON EXPLOSIVES

| | Reagent | | |
Substance	*Griess*[a]	*Diphenylamine*[b]	*Alcoholic KOH*[c]
Chlorate	No color	Blue	No color
Nitrate	Pink to Red	Blue	No color
Nitrocellulose	Pink	Blue-black	No color
Nitroglycerin	Pink to red	Blue	No color
PETN	Pink to red	Blue	No color
RDX	Pink to red	Blue	No color
TNT	No color	No color	Red
Tetryl	Pink to red	Blue	Red-violet

[a]Griess Reagent:
Solution 1—Dissolve 1 g sulfanilic acid in 100 ml of 30% acetic acid.
Solution 2—Dissolve 0.5 g N-(1-napthyl) ethylenediamine in 100 ml of methyl alcohol.
Add solutions 1 and 2 and a few milligrams of zinc dust to the suspect extract.
[b]Diphenylamine Reagent:
Dissolve 1 g diphenylamine in 100 ml concentrated sulfuric acid.
[c]Alcoholic KOH Reagent:
Dissolve 10 g of potassium hydroxide in 100 ml of absolute alcohol.

Table 11-3 lists a number of simple color tests the examiner can perform on the acetone and water extracts in order to screen for the presence of organic and inorganic explosives, respectively.

When sufficient quantities of explosives are recoverable, confirmatory tests may be performed by either infrared spectrophotometry or X-ray diffraction. The former produces a unique "fingerprint" pattern for an organic explosive, as shown by the IR spectrum of RDX in Figure 11-9. The latter provides a unique diffraction pattern for inorganic substances, as exemplified by the diffraction pattern for potassium nitrate and potassium chlorate shows in Figure 6-11 (a) and (b) (page 152).

An explosive "taggant" program has been proposed by the U.S. Treasury Department to further enhance a bomb-scene investigator's chances of recovering useful evidence at a post-explosion scene. Under this proposal, tiny color-coded chips, the size of sand grains, would be added to commercial explosives during their manufacture. Some of these chips would be expected to survive an explosion and be capable of recovery at explosion scenes. To aid in their recovery, the chips are made both fluorescent and magnetic-sensitive. Hence, taggants can be searched for at the explosion site with the use of magnetic tools and ultraviolet light.

The taggant chip is arranged in a color sequence that indicates where the explosive was made and when it was produced (Figure 11-10). With this

Figure 11-9. Infrared spectrum of RDX.

307

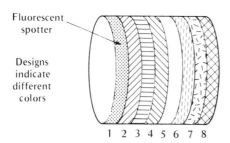

Fluorescent spotter

Designs indicate different colors

1 2 3 4 5 6 7 8

Figure 11-10. Cross section of a taggant. The color sequence of the recovered taggant is observed with the aid of a low-power microscope. The colors are then matched to a color code to yield vital information about the explosive's plant of manufacture, production lot, and purchasers of the explosive material.

knowledge, upon recovery the explosive can be traced through its distribution chain to its final legal possessor. The taggant colors are readily observed and are read with the aid of a low-power microscope.

At present, there are no plans to institute a taggant program in the United States. While some European countries are considering the adoption of explosives taggants, it is extremely doubtful that taggants will be found in any significant number of bombing incidents in the foreseeable future.

REVIEW QUESTIONS

1. The absence of chemical residues always rules out the possibility of arson. (True, False)
2. The combination of oxygen with other substances to produce new chemical products is called _____.
3. All oxidation reactions produce noticeable quantities of heat and light. (True, False)
4. _____ is the capacity for doing work.
5. Burning methane for the purpose of heating water to produce steam in order to drive a turbine is an example of converting _____ energy to _____ energy.
6. The quantity of heat evolved from a chemical reaction arises out of the _____ and _____ of chemical bonds.
7. Molecules must (absorb, liberate) energy to break their bonds and will (absorb, liberate) energy when their bonds are reformed.
8. All oxidation reactions (absorb, liberate) heat.
9. Reactions that liberate heat are said to be _____.
10. Excess heat energy liberated by an oxidation reaction is called the _____.
11. A chemical reaction in which heat is absorbed from the surroundings is said to be _____.
12. All reactions require an energy input to start them. (True, False)

13. The minimum temperature at which a fuel will burn is known as the _____ temperature.
14. A fuel will only achieve a sufficient reaction rate with oxygen to produce a flame when it is in the (gaseous, liquid) state.
15. The lowest temperature at which a liquid fuel will produce enough vapor to burn is the _____.
16. _____ is the chemical breakdown of a solid material to gaseous products.
17. _____ is a phenomenon in which a fuel will burn without the presence of a flame.
18. The rate of a chemical reaction (increases, decreases) as the temperature rises.
19. _____ describes a fire caused by a natural heat-producing process.
20. Oxidizing agents supply _____ to a chemical reaction.
21. Three ingredients of black powder are _____, _____, and _____.
22. An immediate search of a fire scene can commence without obtaining a search warrant. (True, False)
23. A search of the fire scene must focus on finding the fire's _____.
24. The probable origin of a fire will most likely be located closest to the lowest point that shows the most intense characteristics of burning. (True, False)
25. The collection of debris at the origin of a fire should include all (porous, nonporous) materials.
26. _____ containers must be used to package all materials suspected of containing hydrocarbon residues.
27. The most sensitive and reliable instrument for detecting and characterizing flammable residues is the (gas chromatograph, infrared spectrophotometer).
28. The criminalist (can, cannot) identify gasoline residues by brand name.
29. Gasoline dyes are best separated by the technique of _____.
30. Combustion accompanied by the creation of large volumes of gases describes an _____.
31. Explosives that decompose at relatively slow rates are classified as _____ explosives.
32. _____ explosives detonate almost instantaneously to produce a smashing or shattering effect.
33. The most widely used low explosives are _____ and _____.
34. A low explosive only becomes explosive and lethal when it is _____.
35. Air and a gaseous fuel will burn when mixed at any concentration range. (True, False)

36. High explosives can be classified either as _____ or _____ explosives.
37. The blasting power of different dynamite strengths (is, is not) in direct proportion to the weight percentage of nitroglycerin.
38. The most widely used explosive in the military is _____.
39. The explosive core in detonating cord is _____.
40. A high explosive is normally detonated by an _____ explosive contained within a blasting cap.
41. An obvious characteristic of a high explosive is the presence of a _____ at the origin of the blast.
42. The single most important step in the detection of explosive residues is the _____ of appropriate samples from the explosion scene.
43. Unconsumed explosive residues may be detected in the laboratory through a careful _____ examination of the debris.
44. Debris recovered from the site of an explosion is routinely rinsed with _____ in an attempt to recover high explosive residues.
45. Once collected, the acetone extract is initially analyzed by _____, _____, and _____.
46. The technique of _____ produces a unique absorption spectrum for an organic explosive.
47. The technique of _____ provides a unique diffraction pattern for the identification of the inorganic constituents of explosives.

FURTHER REFERENCES

Camp, Michael J., "Analytical Techniques in Arson Investigation," *Analytical Chemistry*, 52 (1980), 422A.

DeHaan, John D., *Kirk's Fire Investigation*, 2nd ed. New York: John Wiley & Sons, 1983.

Meyer, Eugene, *Chemistry of Hazardous Materials*. Englewood Cliffs, N.J.: Prentice-Hall, Inc., 1977.

Midkiff, C. R., "Arson and Explosive Investigation," in *Forensic Science Handbook*, R. Saferstein, ed. Englewood Cliffs, N.J.: Prentice-Hall, Inc., 1982.

Roblee, C. L., and A. J. McKechnic, *The Investigation of Fires*. Englewood Cliffs, N.J.: Prentice-Hall, Inc., 1981.

Saferstein, R., and S. A. Park, "Application of Dynamic Headspace Analysis to Laboratory and Field Arson Investigations," *Journal of Forensic Sciences*, 27 (1982), 484.

Stoffel, J. F., *Explosives and Homemade Bombs*, 2nd ed. Springfield, Ill.: Charles C. Thomas, Publisher, 1972.

Washington, W. D., and C. R. Midkiff, "Explosive Residues in Bombing Scene Investigations. New Technology Applied to Their Detection and Identification," in *Forensic Science*, 2nd ed., G. Davies, ed. Washington, D.C.: American Chemical Society, 1986.

Yinon, J., and S. Zitrin, *The Analysis of Explosives.* Oxford, England: Pergamon Press, 1981.

AUDIOVISUAL PRESENTATION

Arson Investigation (80 35-mm slides and audio tape). Gulf Publishing Co., Houston, Texas.

12

Forensic Serology

In 1901, Karl Landsteiner announced one of the most significant discoveries of this century—the typing of blood—a finding that 29 years later was to earn for him a Nobel Prize. For years before the new century, physicians had attempted to transfuse blood from one individual to another. Their efforts often ended in failure because the transfused blood had a tendency to coagulate in the body of the recipient, causing instantaneous death. It was Landsteiner who first recognized that all human blood was not the same; instead, he found blood to be distinguishable by its group or type. Out of Landsteiner's work came the classification system that we presently call the A-B-O system. Now for the first time physicians had the key for properly matching the blood of a donor to a correct recipient. One blood type cannot be mixed with a different blood type without disastrous consequences. This discovery of course had important implications for blood transfusion and the millions of lives it has since saved. Meanwhile, Landsteiner's findings had opened up a completely new field of research in the biological sciences. Now others were to pursue the identification of other characteristics that could further differentiate blood. By 1937, the Rh factor in blood was demonstrated, and shortly thereafter, numerous blood factors or groups were discovered. At present, more than 100 different blood factors have been shown to exist. However, of all the known blood factors, those belonging to the A-B-O system are still by far the most important for properly matching a donor and recipient for a transfusion.

The intriguing aspect of all these findings, as far as forensic science is concerned, is that in theory no two individuals, except for identical twins, can be expected to have the same combination of blood factors. In other words, blood factors are controlled genetically and have the potential of being a highly distinctive feature for personal identification. What makes this observation so relevant is the high frequency of occurrence of blood-stains at crime scenes, especially crimes of the most serious nature—i.e., homicides, assaults, and rapes. Consider, for example, the situation in which a transfer of blood takes place between the victim and assailant during a struggle; that is, the victim's blood is transferred to the suspect's garment or vice versa. If, as has been suggested, the criminalist can individualize human blood by identifying all of its known factors, the result could be evidence of the strongest kind for linking the suspect to the crime scene.

Unfortunately, we must separate theory from reality. The goal of truly individualizing human blood is still many years away. The problem of iden-tifying most blood factors in whole blood is in itself a difficult task; however, in the crime laboratory the task is further complicated by the fact that prac-tically all blood evidence is received in the form of dried stains. As blood dries, some of its characteristic blood factors are destroyed; and as the stain continues to age, the destruction slowly extends to most of the other factors. Even a task as relatively simple as determining the A-B-O classification of blood becomes much more difficult when applied to dried bloodstains.

During the past decade, chiefly owing to research efforts of the Metro-politan Police Laboratory in London, the individualization of dried blood has become one of the most exciting and promising research areas in foren-sic science. As forensic serologists pursue the detection and identification of various blood characteristics, their ability to associate a bloodstain to a particular individual with a known degree of probability has increased dramatically. The fact is that the individualization of bloodstains now has become a distinct possibility—but one that can only be achieved through the willingness of crime laboratories to commit time, brainpower, and money to unravel the mysteries of blood.

THE NATURE OF BLOOD

ANTIGENS AND ANTIBODIES

The word *blood* actually refers to a highly complex mixture of cells, en-zymes, proteins, and inorganic substances. The fluid portion of blood is called plasma. Plasma is composed principally of water and accounts for 55 percent of blood content. Suspended in the plasma are solid materials consisting chiefly of cells—i.e., red blood cells (erythrocytes), white blood cells (leukocytes), and platelets. The solid portion of blood accounts for 45 percent of its content. Blood clots when a protein in the plasma known as *fibrin* traps and enmeshes the red blood cells. If one were to remove the clotted material, a pale yellowish liquid known as serum would be left.

Obviously, considering the complexity of blood, any discussion of its function and chemistry would have to be an extensive one, extending beyond the scope of this text. It is certainly far more relevant at this point to concentrate our discussion on those blood components that are directly pertinent to the forensic aspects of blood identification—the red blood cells and the blood serum.

Functionally, red blood cells transport oxygen from the lungs to the body tissues and in turn remove carbon dioxide from tissues by transporting it back to the lungs, where it is exhaled. However, for reasons unrelated to the red blood cell's transporting mission, there resides on the surface of each cell millions of characteristic chemical structures called antigens. It is these antigens that impart blood-type characteristics to the red blood cells. Blood antigens are grouped into systems depending on their relationship to each other. More than fifteen blood antigen systems have been identified to date; of these, the A-B-O, M-N, and Rh systems are the most important.

If an individual is type A, this simply indicates that each red blood cell has A antigens located on its surface; similarly, all type B persons have B antigens; and the red blood cells of type AB contain both A and B antigens. Type O persons will have neither A nor B antigens on their cells. Hence, it is the presence or absence of the A and B antigens on the red blood cells that determines a person's blood type in the A-B-O system.

Another important blood antigen has been designated as the Rh factor, or D antigen. Those people having the D antigen are said to be *Rh positive*; those not having this antigen are *Rh negative*. In routine blood banking, it is the presence or absence of the three antigens, A, B, and D that must be determined in testing for the compatibility of the donor and recipient.

Serum is important because it contains certain proteins known as antibodies. The fundamental principle of blood typing is that for every antigen, there exists a specific antibody. Each antibody symbol contains the prefix *anti*, followed by the name of the antigen for which it is specific. Hence, anti-A is specific only for A antigen, anti-B for B antigen, and anti-D for D antigen. The serum-containing antibody is referred to as the antiserum, meaning a serum that reacts against something (antigens).

An antibody will only react with its specific antigen and no other. Thus, if serum containing anti-B is added to red blood cells carrying the antigen B, the two will immediately combine, causing the antibody to attach itself to the cell. Antibodies are normally bivalent—that is, they have two reactive sites. This means that each antibody can simultaneously be attached to antigens located on two different red blood cells. This creates a vast network of cross-linked cells usually seen as clumping or agglutination (see Figure 12-1).

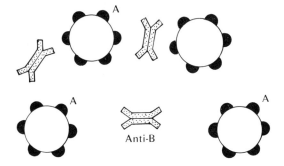

Red blood cells containing A antigens
will not combine with B antibodies

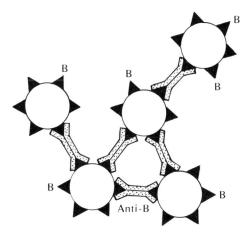

Red blood cells containing B antigens
are agglutinated or clumped together
in the presence of B antibodies   Figure 12-1.

Lets look a little more closely at this phenomenon. In normal blood, shown in Figure 12-2 (a), antigens on red blood cells and antibodies can coexist without destroying each other because the antibodies present are not specific toward any of the antigens. However, suppose a foreign serum added to the blood introduces a new antibody. The occurrence of a specific antigen-antibody reaction will immediately cause the red blood cells to link together, or agglutinate, as shown in Figure 12-2 (b).

Evidently, nature has taken this situation into account, for when we examine the serum of type A blood, we find anti-B and no anti-A. Similarly, type B blood contains only anti-A, type O blood has both anti-A and anti-B,

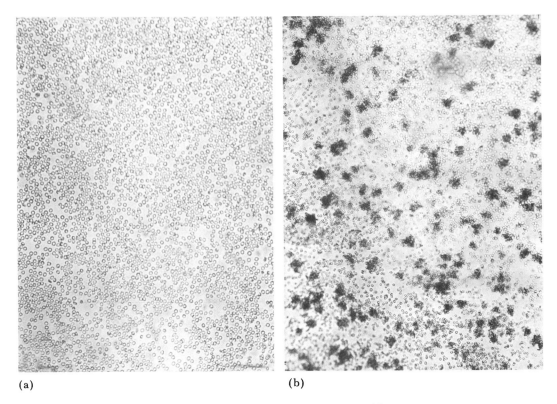

(a)   (b)

Figure 12-2. (a) Microscopic view of normal red blood cells (225X). (b) Microscopic view of agglutinated red blood cells (225X). *Courtesy* Linda Jankowski.

and type AB blood contains neither anti-A nor anti-B. The antigen and antibody components of normal blood are summarized below:

Blood Type	Antigens on Red Blood Cells	Antibodies in Serum
A	A	Anti-B
B	B	Anti-A
AB	AB	Neither anti-A nor anti-B
O	Neither A nor B	Both anti-A and anti-B

The reasons for the fatal consequences of mixing incompatible blood during a transfusion should now be quite obvious. For example, the transfusion of type A blood into a type B patient will cause the natural anti-A in the blood of the type B patient to react promptly with the incoming A antigens, resulting in agglutination. In addition, the incoming anti-B of the donor will react with the B antigens of the patient.

IMMUNOASSAY TECHNIQUES

The concept of a specific antigen-antibody reaction is one that is finding application in other areas unrelated to the blood typing of individuals. Most significantly, this approach has been extended to the detection of drugs in blood and urine. Antibodies that are capable of reacting with drugs do not naturally exist; however, they can be produced in animals such as rabbits by first combining the drug with a protein and injecting this combination into the animal. This drug-protein complex now acts as an antigen stimulating the animal to produce antibodies (see Figure 12-3). The recovered blood serum of the animal will now contain antibodies that are specific or nearly specific toward the drug.

There are at present a number of immunological assay techniques commercially available for detecting drugs through an antigen-antibody reaction. One such technique, enzyme-multiplied immunoassay technique (EMIT), is gaining widespread popularity among toxicologists because of its speed and high sensitivity for detecting drugs in blood and urine. A typical EMIT analysis begins by adding to a subject's blood or urine antibodies that will bind to the drug being measured. For example, if someone's urine is being checked for the presence of methadone, one would add methadone antibodies to the urine. Any methadone drug present in the urine will immediately combine with these antibodies. Then enzyme-labeled methadone drug is added to the urine. Methadone antibodies which did not interact with the methadone drug will now combine with the enzyme-labeled methadone. The quantity of enzyme-labeled methadone left uncombined is then measured and this value is related to the concentration of methadone drug originally present in the urine.

One of the most frequent uses of the EMIT technique in forensic laboratories has been for screening urines of suspected marijuana smokers. In marijuana, THC is considered the primary pharmacologically active agent (see page 229). In order to facilitate its elimination, the body converts THC to a series of substances or metabolites which are more readily excreted. The

Drug   Protein carrier   Drug Antibodies

Figure 12-3.

major THC metabolite found in urine is a substance called *THC-9-carboxylic acid*. It is against this metabolite that antibodies are prepared for testing by the EMIT technique. Normally, the urine of marijuana smokers will contain THC-9-carboxylic acid in a very small quantity (less than one-millionth of a gram); however, this is a level that is readily detected by the EMIT procedure.

The greatest problem associated with marijuana's detection in urine is interpretation. While smoking marijuana will result in the detection of THC metabolite, it is very difficult to determine when the individual actually used marijuana. In individuals who smoke marijuana frequently, detection is possible within 2–5 days after the last use of the drug. However, some individuals may yield positive results up to 10 days after the last use of marijuana.

Though EMIT is presently the most popular immunoassay technique in forensic laboratories, there are other immunoassay procedures commercially available. For example, radioimmunoassay (RIA) uses drugs which are labeled with radioactive tags. Whether an analyst is using an enzyme tag as in EMIT or a radioactive tag as in RIA, one must be cautioned that immunoassay techniques are not totally specific for any drug. Substances having a chemical structure similar to the drug in question may cross-react with the antibody to give a false positive reaction. Hence, positive immunoassay tests must always be confirmed by another reliable analytical procedure. The issue of specificity, along with other questions relating to the reliability of RIA, was raised during the murder trial of Dr. Jascalevich, which is described in detail on pages 20–28.

BLOOD TYPING

The term serology is used to describe a broad scope of laboratory tests that utilize specific antigen and serum antibody reactions. The most widespread application of serology is the typing of whole blood for its A-B-O identity. In determining the A-B-O blood type, only two antiserums are needed—anti-A and anti-B. For routine blood typing, both of these antiserums are commercially available.

Table 12-1 summarizes how the identity of each of the four blood groups is established when the blood is tested with anti-A and anti-B serum. Blood of type A will be agglutinated by anti-A serum; blood of type B will be agglutinated by anti-B serum; AB blood will be agglutinated by both anti-A and anti-B; and blood of type O will not be agglutinated by either the anti-A or anti-B serum.

The identification of natural antibodies present in blood offers another route to the determination of blood type. Testing blood for the presence of anti-A and anti-B requires using red blood cells that have known antigens. Again, these cells are commercially available. Hence, when A cells are added to a blood specimen, agglutination will only occur in the presence of anti-B. All four A-B-O types can be identified in this manner by testing blood with known A and B cells as summarized in Table 12-2.

Table 12-1.

IDENTIFICATION OF BLOOD WITH KNOWN ANTISERUM

Anti-A Serum + Whole Blood	Anti-B Serum + Whole Blood	Antigen Present	Blood Type
+	−	A	A
−	+	B	B
+	+	A and B	AB
−	−	Neither A nor B	O

Note:
+ *shows agglutination.*
− *shows absence of agglutination.*

Table 12-2.

IDENTIFICATION OF BLOOD WITH KNOWN CELLS

A Cells + Blood	B Cells + Blood	Antibody Present	Blood Type
+	−	Anti-A	B
−	+	Anti-B	A
+	+	Both anti-A and anti-B	O
−	−	Neither anti-A nor anti-B	AB

Note:
+ *shows agglutination.*
− *shows absence of agglutination.*

The population distribution of blood types varies with location and race throughout the world. In the United States, a typical distribution is as follows:

O	A	B	AB
43%	42%	12%	3%

FORENSIC CHARACTERIZATION OF BLOODSTAINS

The criminalist must be prepared to answer the following questions when examining dried blood: (1) Is it blood? (2) From what species did the blood originate? (3) If the blood is of human origin, how closely can it be associated to a particular individual?

The determination of blood is best made by means of a preliminary color test. For many years the most commonly used test for this purpose was the benzidine color test; however, because benzidine has been identified as a known carcinogen, its use has generally been discontinued, and the chemical phenolphthalein is usually substituted in its place.[1] Both the benzidine and phenolphthalein color tests are based on the observation that blood hemoglobin possesses peroxidaselike activity. Peroxidases are enzymes that accelerate the oxidation of several classes of organic compounds by peroxides. When a bloodstain, phenolphthalein reagent, and hydrogen peroxide are all mixed together, the blood's hemoglobin will cause the formation of a deep pink color.

The phenolphthalein test is not a specific test for blood; there are some vegetable materials, for instance, that also turn phenolphthalein pink. These substances include potatoes and horseradish. However, it is unlikely that such materials will be encountered in criminal situations, and thus from a practical point of view, a positive phenolphthalein test is highly indicative of blood.

Another important identification test for blood is the luminol test.[2] Unlike the benzidine and phenolphthalein tests, the reaction of luminol with blood results in the production of light rather than color. By spraying luminol reagent onto a suspect item, large areas can be quickly screened for the presence of bloodstains. The sprayed objects must be located in a darkened area while being viewed for the emission of light (luminescence). Because the luminol test is exceedingly sensitive, it has been used successfully for locating minute traces of bloodstains at crime scenes and for visualizing bloodstain patterns that would not have been seen under normal lighting conditions (Figure 12-4).

The identification of blood can be made more specific if microcrystalline tests are performed on the material. There are several tests available; the two most popular ones are the Takayama and Teichmann tests. Both of these depend on the addition of specific chemicals to the blood so that characteristic crystals with hemoglobin derivatives will be formed. The criminalist must be cautioned that crystal tests are far less sensitive than color tests for blood's identification and are more susceptible to interferences from contaminants that may be present in the stain.

Once the stain has been characterized as blood, the serologist will have to determine whether the stain is of human or animal origin. For this purpose, the standard test used is the precipitin test. Precipitin tests are based on the fact that when animals (usually rabbits) are injected with human blood, antibodies are formed that react with the invading human blood to

[1] R. S. Higaki and W. M. S. Philp, "A Study of the Sensitivity, Stability and Specificity of Phenolphthalein as an Indicator Test for Blood," *The Canadian Society of Forensic Science Journal*, 9 (1976), 97.
[2] The luminol reagent is prepared by mixing 0.1 g 3-amino-phthalhydrazide and 5.0 g sodium carbonate in 100 ml of distilled water. Before use, 0.7 g of sodium perborate is added to the solution.

(a)

(b)

Figure 12-4. (a) A section of a linoleum floor photographed under normal light. This floor was located in the residence of a missing person. (b) Same section of the floor shown above after spraying with liminol. A circular pattern was revealed. It was concluded that the circular blood pattern was left by the bottom of a bucket carried about during the cleaning up of the blood. A small clump of sponge, blood, and hair was found near where this photograph was taken. *Courtesy* North Carolina State Bureau of Investigation.

neutralize its presence. The investigator can recover these antibodies by bleeding the animal and isolating the blood serum. This serum will contain antibodies that specifically react with human antigens. For this reason, the serum is known as human antiserum. In the same manner, by injecting rabbits with the blood of other known animals, virtually any kind of animal antiserum can be produced. Currently, antiserums are commercially available for humans and for a variety of commonly encountered animals—e.g., dogs, cats, and deer.

A number of techniques have been devised for performing precipitin tests on bloodstains. The classical method is to layer an extract of the blood-stain on top of the human antiserum in a capillary tube. Human blood, or for that matter, any protein of human origin in the extract, will react specifically with antibodies present in the antiserum, as indicated by the formation of a cloudy ring or band at the interface of the two liquids (Figure 12-5).

Another method, called gel diffusion, takes advantage of the fact that antibodies and antigens will diffuse or move toward one another on an agar gel-coated plate. Here, the extracted bloodstain and the human antiserum are placed in separate holes opposite each other on the gel. If the blood is of human origin, a line of precipitation will form where the antigens and anti-bodies meet. Similarly, the antigens and antibodies can be induced to move toward one another under the influence of an electrical field. In the electrophoretic method (see page 120), the electrical potential is applied to the gel medium; a specific antigen antibody reaction will be denoted by a line

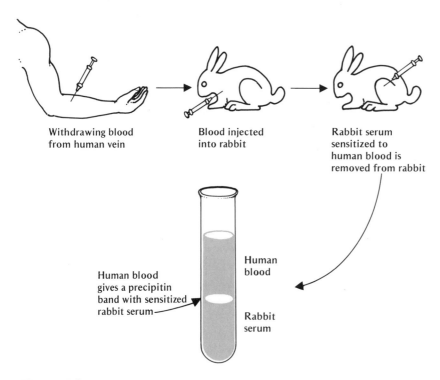

Withdrawing blood
from human vein

Blood injected
into rabbit

Rabbit serum
sensitized to
human blood is
removed from rabbit

Human blood
gives a precipitin
band with sensitized
rabbit serum

Human
blood

Rabbit
serum

Figure 12-5.

precipitation formed between the hole containing the blood extract and the hole containing the human antiserum (see Figure 12-6).

The precipitin test is very sensitive and requires only a small amount of blood for testing. Human bloodstains dried for as long as 10 to 15 years and longer may still give a positive precipitin reaction. Even extracts of tissue from mummies 4000 to 5000 years old have given positive reactions with this test. Furthermore, experience has shown that human bloodstains diluted by washing in water and left only with a faint color may still yield a positive precipitin reaction (see Figure 12-7).

Once it has been determined that the bloodstain is of human origin, an effort must be made to associate or disassociate the stain with a particular individual. In this situation, however, the forensic serologist is severely limited to only those blood factors that survive the drying and aging processes.

Antigen and antibody are added to their respective wells.

Antigen and antibody are being moved toward each other

Antigen and antibody have formed a visible precipitin line in the gel between the wells

Figure 12-7. Results of the precipitin test of dilutions of human serum up to 1 in 4096 against a human antiserum. A reaction is visible for blood up to 1 in 256. *Courtesy* Millipore Biomedica, Acton, Massachusetts.

Stains also vary considerably in purity and quantity, all of which make the analysis of dried blood much more complex than the analysis of whole blood. Until recently, existing procedures only permitted the typing of bloodstains by the A-B-O system; however, extensive research efforts have now made the characterization of other blood antigens, as well as some blood enzymes and proteins, feasible for routine dried-blood analysis.

In the earlier description of whole-blood typing, it was noted that the identification of A and B antigens was easily accomplished by directly reacting the blood with anti-A and anti-B serums. This identity of the antigens present was confirmed by visually observing the clumping or agglutination of the red blood cells. Unfortunately, one cannot use the same approach in dried-blood typing because red blood cells rupture on drying, leaving no cells in the stain to be agglutinated. However, although the cells may have disintegrated, the antigens present on their surfaces remain intact and are still identifiable by indirect means.

TYPING OF DRIED STAINS

The absorption-elution technique is the current method of choice for the indirect typing of bloodstains. As illustrated in Figure 12-8, the procedure consists of four steps:

Step 1: The antiserum is placed on the bloodstained material, allowing sufficient time for the antibodies to combine with their specific antigens.

Step 2: The unreacted serum is removed by being washed off the blood-stained material.

Step 3: Once an antibody combines with an antigen, it is possible to break the complex apart by a process known as **elution**. To do this, the stained material must be heated at 56°C. This allows the antibody-antigen bond to break, freeing both.

Step 4: When the eluted antibodies are combined with known red blood cells so that the presence or absence of agglutination can be observed, they can be identified. The identification of A-B-O type by the absorption-elution technique is summarized in Table 12-3.

This technique is sufficiently sensitive to type stains on a thread of fiber that is one-half inch in length. In addition, stains as old as eleven years have been typed by the absorption-elution procedure.

Further characterization of dried blood can be accomplished by the identification of other antigens located on the surface of the red blood cells. In addition to A-B-O, the M and N antigens and the Rh antigens have received attention from forensic laboratories in this respect. The presence of the M and N antigens in blood was first shown in 1927. Although these anti-

Step I

Treatment with antiserum.
Antibody binds to its
specific antigen.

Step II

Excess antibodies are
removed by washing.

Step III

Add known red
blood cells

Antibodies and antigens are
eluted or freed from one
another by heating the
stained material.

Step IV

Agglutination occurs if
antigens present on the
added blood cells were
originally on the stained
material as well.

Figure 12-8. The absorption-elution technique for typing dried blood-stains.

Table 12-3.

IDENTIFICATION OF BLOOD TYPES BY THE ABSORPTION-ELUTION TECHNIQUE

Bloodstains Tested with		Antigen Present on Stain	Blood Type
Anti-A + A Cells	Anti-B + B Cells		
+	−	A	A
−	+	B	B
+	+	Both A and B	AB
−	−	Neither A nor B	O

Note:
+ *shows agglutination*
− *shows absence of agglutination*

gens can survive in dried blood for nine months under ideal conditions, they have been found to be difficult to identify under realistic case conditions. Three blood groups belong to the M-N system: M, N, and MN. Their approximate frequency of occurrence in the white American population is 30 percent for M, 20 percent for N, and 50 percent for MN. Within the Rh system, five antigens, designated as C, D, E, c, and e may be detected in a bloodstain, although their full potential in bloodstain analysis is yet to be realized. The significance of Rh antigens has been made more apparent in disputed paternity cases in which whole-blood analysis is involved.

Secretors. The antigens of the A-B-O system are not confined exclusively to the red blood cells. Approximately 80 percent of individuals are classified as secretors—which means that their blood-type antigens are found in high concentration in most body fluids (e.g., saliva, semen, vaginal secretions, and gastric juice as well as in blood). In fact, saliva and semen have a higher concentration of A and B antigens than does blood. The value of this observation in criminal investigation is obvious. It is possible, for example, to type semen stains on the clothing of a victim of a sexual attack, or even the saliva deposited on the butt of a cigarette. Furthermore, it has been demonstrated that hair can be typed, although some criminalists have questioned the reliability of the technique. The A-B-O typing of solid tissue, such as muscle or skin, is also possible.

BLOOD ENZYMES AND PROTEINS

In addition to the antigenic systems discussed above, there are other substances found in the red blood cell that are becoming increasingly important for the individualization of bloodstains. These substances are called enzymes. Enzymes are proteins that have important functions in regulating many of the body's chemical reactions. Forensic serologists are particularly interested in enzymes that exist in different forms, or are polymorphic. These enzymes can actually be separated into protein components called iso-enzymes.

Let's look at one such enzyme, PGM, in order to understand its importance to the forensic serologist. The iso-enzymes of PGM (phosphoglucomutase) can be separated from one another by electrophoresis (see page 120–121). What is interesting and most important about this separation is the observation that all persons do not have the same PGM iso-enzymes. Actually, as shown in Figure 12-9, there are three common variations or types of PGM: PGM 1, PGM 2-1, and PGM 2. These variations are distributed unevenly throughout the population: PGM 1 is present in approximately 58 percent of the population; PGM 2-1 is in 36 percent; and PGM 2 in 6 percent. Thus, the identification of the PGM type in a dried bloodstain provides the forensic serologist with added statistical information with which to reduce the number of possible sources of the bloodstain.

Figure 12-9. Photograph and diagram of the separation of PGM iso-enzymes accomplished by electrophoresis. PGM can be grouped into one of three types: 1, 2-1, and 2 according to band patterns. Reproduced from *The Principles of Human Biochemical Genetics*, 2nd ed., by Harry Harris (New York: North-Holland Publishing Co., 1975), p. 61.

A number of years after the discovery of the three PGM variants described above, it was observed that these variants could actually be further subtyped by more refined electrophoretic techniques. Thus, instead of three PGM types, forensic scientists can now identify ten common PGM variants. This discovery has allowed forensic analysts to further narrow the possible source of a bloodstain. For example, where PGM 2-1 is present in 36 percent of the population, its subtypes PGM 2+1+, 2+1−, 2−1+, and 2−1− are found in approximately 25 percent, 5 percent, 4 percent, and 2 percent, respectively, of the population.

Apparently, there are numerous polymorphic enzymes in red blood cells that offer themselves as potential markers for determining blood origin. Also, a number of polymorphic proteins have been found to exist in blood serum. However, from a practical point of view, only those enzymes and proteins that are capable of surviving the drying and aging processes are of any value to the forensic serologist.

Because antigens, enzymes, and proteins occur independently of each other, the probability of a dried bloodstain having a particular combination of these factors is determined by the product of their distribution in the population. For example, if a bloodstain is found to be type A, then it can be concluded that such a stain could have originated from approximately 42 percent of the population. Now if it is also determined that this stain contains PGM 1, then its origin can be narrowed to 24 percent of the population (42% × 58% = 24%). Obviously, the more factors a serologist can find in a stain, the smaller will be its frequency of occurrence in a population. Hence, forensic researchers have made extensive efforts at uncovering blood factors which are identifiable in bloodstains (see Table 12-4).

Table 12-4.

BLOOD ENZYMES AND PROTEINS USED TO DISCRIMINATE BLOODSTAINS

Blood Factor	Abbreviation
Adensosine deaminase	ADA
Adenylate kinase	AK
Carbonic anhydrase II	CA II
Erythrocyte acid phosphatase	EAP
Esterase D	EsD
Glucose-6-Phosphate dehydrogenase	G6PD
Glyoxase I	GLO I
Group-specific component	Gc
Haptoglobin	Hp
Peptidase A	Pep A
Phosphoglucomutase	PGM
6-Phosphogluconate dehydrogenase	6PGD
Transferrin	Tf

Using only the commonest type of the A-B-O system and the commonest types of many of the polymorphic systems cited above, one would get:

Grouping System	Type	Frequency (approx.)
ABO	O	43%
ADA	1	90%
AK	1	91%
EAP	BA	43%
EsD	1	79%
GLO I	2-1	52%
Gc	1	50%
Hp	2-1	49%
PGM	1+1+	41%
6PGD	A	96%
Tf	CC	98%

The product of these frequencies shows that nearly 0.6 percent of the population will have this combination of blood types. Since the vast majority of people are expected to have less common types for at least some of these blood group systems, their frequency of occurrence will be far less than 0.6 percent. For instance, using the above grouping systems, the authors blood is found in only 0.04 percent of the population. Certainly, by expanding its ability to go beyond the A-B-O system, the crime laboratory has taken a significant step toward individualizing human blood, and in so doing has dramatically enhanced the value of bloodstain evidence.

In many criminal cases, the racial origin of a bloodstain located at a crime scene is not known. In this respect, the finding of certain polymorphic blood factors may provide a useful indicator of race. For example, detection of any of the following types: Pep A 2-1, Pep A 2, G6PD A, G6PD BA, Tf CD, CA II 2-1, and CA II 2 would indicate that the stain originated from a black donor. However, it must be cautioned that this approach cannot lead to definitive conclusions regarding race. Obviously, the offspring of racial intermarriages are very likely to contain some of these racial markers.

STAIN PATTERNS OF BLOOD

The crime-scene investigator must not overlook the fact that the location, distribution, and appearance of bloodstains and splatters may be useful for interpreting and reconstructing the events that must have occurred to have produced the bleeding. A thorough analysis of the significance of the position and shape of blood patterns with respect to their origin and trajectory is exceedingly complex and requires the services of an examiner who is experienced in such determinations. Most importantly, the interpretation of bloodstain patterns necessitates carefully planned control experiments utilizing surface materials comparable to those found at the crime scene.

An in-depth study of this subject has been published by Herbert L. MacDonell.[3] Many of Mr. MacDonell's observations and conclusions have important implications for any investigator who seeks to trace the direction, dropping distance, and angle of impact of a bloodstain. Some of them can be summarized as follows:

1. Surface texture is of paramount importance in the interpretation of bloodstain patterns, and correlations between standards and unknowns are valid only if identical surfaces are used. In general, the harder and

---

[3] Herbert L. MacDonell, *Bloodstain Pattern Interpretation* (Corning, N.Y.: Laboratory of Forensic Science, 1983).

(a)

(b)

Figure 12-10. (a) Bloodstain from a single drop of blood that struck a plastic wall tile after falling 42 inches. (b) Bloodstain from a single drop of blood that struck a heavy irregular textured wallpaper after falling 42 inches. Reprinted from Herbert L. MacDonell, *Flight Characteristics and Stain Patterns of Human Blood* (Washington, D.C.: U.S. Government Printing Office, 1971), pp. 36–37.

330

less porous the surface, the less splatter results. The effect of surface is shown in Figure 12-10 (a) and (b).

2. When a blood drop hits a hard smooth surface, it frequently breaks up on impact, casting off smaller droplets. These smaller droplets travel in the same direction as the original drop, ultimately terminating in a pattern that is tadpolelike, with the sharper or pointed ends always pointing back toward their origin. An example of this streaking is shown in Figure 12-11. This stain resulted from a drop of blood traveling at about 4 feet per second, right to left, and falling to the hard cardboard target at an angle of approximately 56 degrees.

3. It is possible to determine the impact angle of blood on a flat surface by measuring the degree of circular distortion of the stain. A drop of blood striking a surface at right angles gives rise to a nearly circular stain; as the angle decreases, the stain becomes elongated in shape. This progressive elongation is evident in Figure 12-12 (a) and (b).

Considerably more detailed information relating to blood patterns is available in MacDonell's treatise, which should certainly be consulted when such determinations are appropriate to an investigation.

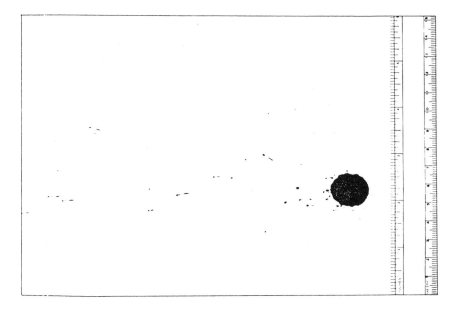

Figure 12-11. This stain came from a drop of blood traveling at about 4 feet per second, right to left. The pointed ends of the droplets are aimed toward their origin. The above figure is from Herbert L. MacDonell, *Flight Characteristics and Stain Patterns of Human Blood* (Washington, D.C.: U.S. Government Printing Office, 1971), p. 39.

(a)   (b)

Figure 12-12. (a) Pattern of a single drop of human blood that fell 42
inches and struck hard, smooth cardboard at 60 degrees. (b) Pattern of a
single drop of human blood that fell 42 inches and struck hard, smooth
cardboard at 10 degrees. Reprinted from Herbert L. MacDonell, *Flight
Characteristics and Stain Patterns of Human Blood* (Washington, D.C:
U.S. Government Printing Office, 1971), pp 44, 49.

PRESERVATION OF BLOOD EVIDENCE

As crime laboratories expand their capability to characterize blood, it is
important that field investigators become conscious of the precautions that
must be observed to preserve bloodstains in a stable and uncontaminated
state. Unnecessary exposure of blood to heat, moisture, and bacterial contamination will only serve to shorten the survival time of its antigens and
enzymes. It is important that all stained material be submitted without delay
to the crime laboratory; each day's delay contributes to a loss of antigen and
enzymatic activity and lessens the evidential value of blood.

Before the collection of blood evidence begins, it is important that the
bloodstains be photographed close up and their location relative to the entire

crime scene recorded through notes, sketches, and photographs. If it is determined that the shape and position of bloodstains may provide information about the circumstances of the crime, an expert must immediately be dispatched to the location for an on-the-spot evaluation of the blood evidence. The significance of the position and shape of bloodstains can best be ascertained when the expert has an on-site overview of the entire crime scene and can better reconstruct the movements of the individuals involved. No attempt should be made to disturb the blood pattern before this phase of the investigation is completed.

Blood has great evidential value when a transfer between victim and suspect can be demonstrated. For this reason, all clothing from both the victim and suspect should be collected and sent to the laboratory for examination. This procedure must be followed even when the presence of blood on a garment does not appear obvious to the investigator. Laboratory search procedures are far more revealing and sensitive than any that can be conducted at the crime scene. In addition, blood should also be searched for in the less than obvious places. For example, the criminal may have wiped his hands on materials not readily apparent to the investigator. Efforts must be made to find towels, handkerchiefs, or rags that may have been used and then hidden. There is always a possibility that blood shed on a floor may have been wiped or mopped to conceal the crime. Thus, careful attention should be given to examining floor cracks or other crevices that may have trapped a quantity of blood.

Wet blood can be typed much more quickly and easily in the laboratory than dried blood. If a sufficient quantity of liquid blood is found at the scene, it may be collected with a medicine dropper, placed in a glass tube and kept refrigerated until submission to the laboratory. When the quantity of moist blood is insufficient to be preserved in this manner, it is best to allow the material to thoroughly air-dry out of the presence of direct sunlight or heat. The packaging of bloodstained evidence in plastic or airtight containers must be avoided because the accumulation of residual moisture could contribute to the growth of blood-destroying bacteria and fungi. Preferably, each stained article should be packaged separately in a paper bag or in a well-ventilated box.

If feasible, the entire stained article should be packaged and submitted for examination. If this is not possible, the dried blood must be scraped off the surface with a disposable scalpel blade onto a clean sheet of paper. A portion of the unstained surface material near the recovered stain must likewise be removed and placed in a separate package. If it's not possible or feasible to remove the unstained surface material, then an apparent uncontaminated area close to the questioned stain should be swabbed with a clean cotton swab moistened with distilled water and the swab submitted to the laboratory. The forensic examiner will use the unstained material or swab as a control to confirm that the results of the tests performed were brought about by the stain and not by the material on which it was deposited. An alternative procedure is to absorb the dried blood onto a clean swab or filter paper dampened with distilled water. When stains are recovered in this manner, swabbing an unstained area adjacent to the stained area with clean, moistened cotton or filter paper is also necessary to provide the laboratory with a proper control.

A human bloodstain will only attain its full forensic value when an analyst can compare each of its blood factors to whole blood specimens collected from victims and suspects. For this purpose, at least 5 cc of whole blood should be drawn from individuals by a qualified medical person. The blood sample should be collected in a sterile tube. The addition of a preservative and anticoagulant should be avoided as it may interfere with some of the blood grouping tests performed in the laboratory. The blood must be kept refrigerated while awaiting transportation to the laboratory.

A word of caution is necessary concerning transfused blood. Blood transfusions can alter a person's blood chemistry and can obscure true blood types. In such cases it is necessary to wait at least 60 days after the transfusion is made to obtain a valid control blood sample. Where legal or other circumstances prevent the taking of a blood sample, the investigator should check hospital or military records for the individual's blood type.

PRINCIPLES OF HEREDITY

TRANSMISSION OF OUR TRAITS

All of the antigens and polymorphic enzymes and proteins that have been described in previous sections are genetically controlled traits. That is, they are inherited from parents and become a permanent feature of a person's biological makeup from the moment he or she is conceived. Determining the identity of these traits, then, not only provides us with a picture of how one individual agrees or differs from another, but it gives us an insight into the basic biological substances that determine our overall makeup as human beings and the mechanism by which they are transmitted from one generation to the next.

The transmission of hereditary material is accomplished by means of microscopic units called **genes**. The gene is the basic unit of heredity. Each gene by itself or in concert with other genes controls the development of a specific characteristic in the new individual; the genes determine the nature and growth of virtually every body structure.

The genes are positioned on **chromosomes**, threadlike bodies that appear in the nucleus of every body cell. All human cells contain 46 chromosomes, mated in 23 pairs. The only exceptions are the human reproductive cells, the egg and sperm, which contain only 23 unmated chromosomes. During fertilization, a sperm and egg combine so that each contributes chromosomes to form the new cell (*zygote*). Hence, the new individual begins life properly mated with 23 chromosome pairs. Because the genes are positioned on the chromosomes, the new individual inherits genetic material from each parent.

Actually, two dissimilar chromosomes are involved in the determination of sex. The egg cell always contains a long chromosome known as the *X chromosome*; but the sperm cell may contain either a short one, known as the *Y chromosome*, or a long X one. When an X-carrying sperm fertilizes an egg, the new cell is XX and develops into a female. A Y-carrying sperm produces an XY fertilized egg and develops into a male. Because it is the contribution of the sperm cell that ultimately determines the nature of the chromosome pair, we can say that the father biologically determines the sex of the child.

The discovery of a specific stain for the detection of the Y chromosome has made the sexing of human cells a distinct possibility in the forensic laboratory. Investigators can now visualize the Y chromosome by soaking cells in a solution of magnesium chloride and staining with the chemical quinacrine hydrochloride. Under these conditions, the Y chromosome is observed under a microscope as a fluorescent bright spot. Using this approach, criminalists have in some situations successfully differentiated male and female bloodstains; however, the technique requires experience and a very cautious approach.[4] Further experimentation along these lines will also hopefully bring nearer the possibility that the sexing of human hair will be a reliable technique performed in forensic laboratories in the future.[5]

Just as chromosomes come together in pairs, so do the genes they bear. Genes that govern a given characteristic are similarly positioned on the chromosomes inherited from the mother and father. Thus, a gene for eye color on the mother's chromosome will be aligned with a gene for eye color on the corresponding chromosome inherited from the father. Genes that influence a given characteristic and are aligned with one another on a chromosome pair are known as alleles. Another rather simple example of allele genes in man is that of blood types belonging to the A-B-O system. Inheritance of the A-B-O type is best described by a theory that utilizes three genes designated A, B, and O.

A gene pair made up of two similar genes—e.g., AA and BB—is said to be homozygous, and a gene pair made up of two different genes—e.g., AO— is said to be heterozygous. If the chromosome inherited from the father carried the A gene and the chromosome inherited from the mother carried

[4] R. Wigmore et al., "The Detection of Y Chromosomes in Bloodstains—A Reevaluation," *Journal of Forensic Sciences*, 24 (1979), 366.
[5] J. L. Mudd, "The Determination of Sex from Forcibly Removed Hairs," *Journal of Forensic Sciences*, 29 (1984), 1072.

the same gene, the offspring would have an AA combination. Similarly, if one chromosome contained the A gene and the other had the O gene, the genetic makeup of the offspring would be AO.

When an individual inherits two similar genes from his parents, there is no problem in determining the blood type of that person. Hence, an AA combination will always be type A, a BB type B, and an OO type O. However, when two different genes are inherited, one gene will be dominant. It can be said that the A and B genes are **dominant** and that the O gene is always **recessive**—that is, its characteristics remain hidden. For instance, with an AO combination, A is always dominant over O and the individual will be typed as A. Similarly, a BO combination is typed as B. In the case of AB, the genes are co-dominant and the individual's blood type will be AB. The recessive characteristics of O will only appear when both recessive genes are present. Hence, the combination OO is typed as O.

A pair of allele genes together constitutes the **genotype** of the individual. However, there is no laboratory test known that can determine an individual's genotype. For example, a person's outward characteristic or **phenotype** may be that of type A, but this does not tell us whether his genotype is AA or AO. The genotype can only be determined by studying the family history of the individual. If the genotypes of both parents are known, that of their possible offspring can be forecast.

An easy way of figuring this out is by constructing a so-called Punnet square. To do this, write along a horizontal line the two genes of the male parent, and in the vertical column the two kinds of female genes present, as shown below. In our example we'll assume the male parent is type O and therefore has to be an OO genotype; the female parent is type AB and can only be AB genotype:

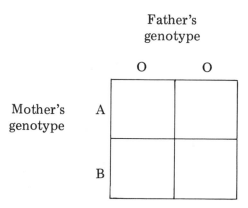

Next, write in each box the corresponding gene contributed from the female and then from the male. The result will be that the squares contain all the possible genotype combinations that the parents can produce in their offspring:

	O	O
A	AO	AO
B	BO	BO

Hence, in this case, 50 percent of the offspring are likely to be AO and the other 50 percent BO. These are the only genotypes possible from the above combination. Because O is recessive, 50 percent of the offspring will probably be type A and 50 percent type B. From this example we can see that no blood-group gene can appear in a child unless it is present in at least one of the parents.

In the same way, the genotypes of our parents determine the identity of all blood-group systems as well as the polymorphic enzymes and proteins of their offspring. For example, an individual whose blood carries the enzyme EAP-BA has two allelic genes determining this trait. One gene corresponds to EAP-B, the other to EAP-A. When paired these genes are codominant.

PATERNITY TESTING

Although the genotyping of blood factors has useful applications for studying the transmittance of blood characteristics from one generation to the next, it actually has no direct relevance to criminal investigations. It does, however, have important implications in disputed paternity cases, which are normally encountered in civil and not criminal courts.

Many cases of disputed paternity can be resolved when the suspected parents and the offspring are related according to their blood-group systems. For instance, in the above example, had the child been type AB, the suspected father would have been cleared. A type O father and a type AB mother cannot give rise to a type AB child. On the other hand, if the child had been type A or type B, the most that could be said is that the suspect *may* have been the father; this does not mean that he is in fact the father. Obviously, there are many other males who also have type O blood. Of course, the more blood-group systems that are tested, the better the chances of excluding an innocent male from involvement. Conversely, if no discrepancies are found between offspring and suspect father, the more certain one can be that the suspect is indeed the father.

Recently, a new and improved paternity testing technique has been developed. It is called the HLA (human leucocyte antigen) test. This test relies on identifying a complex system of antigens that exists on white blood cells. If a suspect cannot be excluded as fathering a child after this test is performed, the chances are better than 90 percent that he is the father. These odds can be raised to more than 95 percent by combining the HLA test with A-B-O and haptoglobin blood typing.[6]

FORENSIC CHARACTERIZATION OF SEMEN

A great number of cases received in a forensic laboratory involve sexual offenses, making it necessary to examine exhibits for the presence of seminal stains.

The normal male releases 2.5 to 6 milliliters of seminal fluid during an ejaculation. Each milliliter contains 100 million or more spermatozoa, the male reproductive cells. The forensic examination of articles for seminal stains can actually be considered a two-step process. First, before any tests can be conducted, the stain must be located. Considering the number and soiled condition of outergarments, undergarments, and possible bed clothing submitted for examination, this may in itself prove to be an arduous task. Once located, the stain will have to be subjected to tests that will prove its identity; possibly, it may even be tested for the blood type of the individual from whom it originated.

Often, seminal stains are readily visible on a fabric because they exhibit a stiff, crusty appearance. However, reliance on such appearance for locating the stain is at best unreliable and is only useful to a criminalist when the stain is present in a rather obvious area. Certainly, if the fabric has been washed or contains only minute quantities of semen, visual examination of the article will offer little chance of detecting the stain. The best way to locate and at the same time characterize a seminal stain is to perform the acid phosphatase color test.

Acid phosphatase is an enzyme that is secreted by the prostate gland into seminal fluid. Its concentrations in seminal fluid are up to 400 times greater than those found in any other body fluid. Its presence can easily be detected when it comes in contact with an acidic solution of sodium alpha-naphthylphosphate and Fast Blue B dye.

The utility of the acid phosphatase test is apparent when it becomes necessary to search numerous garments or large fabric areas for seminal stains. If a filter paper is simply moistened with water and rubbed lightly

---

[6] P. I. Terasaki et al., "Ninety-Five Percent Probability of Paternity with HLA, ABO and Haptoglobins," *Forensic Science International*, 12 (1978), 227.

over the suspect area, acid phosphatase, if present, will be transferred to the filter paper. Then, when a drop or two of the sodium alpha-naphthylphosphate and Fast Blue B solution are placed on the paper, the appearance of a purple color will be indicative of the acid phosphatase enzyme. In this manner, any fabric or surface can be systematically searched for seminal stains. If it is necessary to search extremely large areas—e.g., a bed sheet or carpet—the article can be tested in sections, narrowing the location of the stain with each successive test. A negative reaction can be interpreted as meaning the absence of semen. Although some vegetable juices (e.g., cauliflower and watermelon), fungi, contraceptive creams, and vaginal secretions do give a positive response to the acid phosphatase test, none of these substances normally reacts with the speed of seminal fluid. A reaction time of less than 30 seconds is considered a strong indication of the presence of semen.

Other tests for semen involve the detection of choline and spermine. Since choline and spermine are also present in other biological materials and since neither of these components is unique to semen, the finding of either or both of them is only an indication of the possible presence of semen. Procedures for the identification of choline and spermine utilize micro-crystalline tests. The Florence test for choline uses potassium triiodide and the Barberio test for spermine uses picric acid as the crystallizing reagents.

Semen can be unequivocally identified by the presence of spermatozoa. When spermatozoa are located through a microscope examination, the stain is definitely identified as having been derived from semen. Spermatozoa are slender, elongated structures 50 to 70 microns long, each with a head and a thin flagellate tail (see Figure 12-13). The criminalist can normally locate

Figure 12-13. Photomicrograph of human spermatozoa (420X).
Courtesy Linda Jankowski.

them by immersing the stained material in a small volume of water. Rapid stirring of the liquid will transfer any spermatozoa present into the water. A drop of the water is dried onto a microscope slide, then stained and examined under a compound microscope at a magnification of approximately 400×.

Considering the extremely large number of spermatozoa found in seminal fluid, one would think the chance of locating one would be very good; however, this is not always true. One reason is that spermatozoa are extremely brittle when dry and easily disintegrate if the stain is washed or when the stain is rubbed against another object, as can frequently happen in the handling and packaging of this type of evidence. Furthermore, sexual crimes may involve males who have an abnormally low sperm count, a condition known as **oligospermia**, or they may involve individuals who have no spermatozoa at all in their seminal fluid (**aspermia**). Significantly, aspermatic individuals are increasing in numbers due to the increasing popularity of vasectomies.

Often in forensic laboratories, analysts will be placed in the situation of examining stains or swabs which they suspect contain semen (because of the presence of acid phosphatase) but which yield no detectable spermatozoa. How then can one unequivocally prove the presence of semen? The solution to this problem came with the discovery in the 1970s of a protein called **p30**. Under the analytical conditions employed in forensic laboratories, p30 is unique to seminal plasma. When p30 is isolated and injected into a rabbit, it will stimulate the production of antibodies (anti-p30). The sera collected from these immunized rabbits can now be used to test suspected semen stains.

As shown in Figure 12-14, the stain extract is placed in one well of an electrophoretic plate and the anti-p30 in an opposite well. When an electric potential is applied, the antigens and antibodies will move toward each other. The formation of a visible line midway between the two wells shows the presence of p30 in the stain and hence proves that the stain was seminal in nature.

Semen extract and anti–p30 are added to their respective wells

Antigen and antibody are being moved toward each other

Formation of a visible precipitation line midway between the wells shows the presence of p30 in the stain and proofs the stain is seminal in nature.

Figure 12-14.

Once the material under examination is proven to be semen, the next endeavor will be to attempt to associate the semen as closely as possible to a single individual. Initial efforts in this area begin with a possible ABO blood-group determination. We have already observed that nearly 80 percent of the population are secretors having high concentrations of their blood-type antigens in most body fluids. Hence, for a substantial segment of the male population, seminal fluid and/or stains can yield the identity of an individual's blood type. Often this information can provide important corroborative evidence that supports a suspect's involvement in a sexual assault. Likewise, such an identification can serve to exonerate someone unjustly accused of committing such a crime. However, the determination of blood type from semen is not without its problems, especially under conditions that normally accompany a sexual assault. Often, the semen stains found on the victim's garments will be mixed with sweat and/or vaginal secretions. Since it is just as probable for a female victim to secrete her blood-type antigens as it is for the male suspect, it becomes important to establish whether the victim and suspect are both secretors and their respective blood types. This information can readily be obtained in the laboratory by a determination of the concentration levels of A, B, and H antigens present in saliva. The saliva of secretors will yield higher levels of blood antigens than that of nonsecretors. Naturally, if both the victim and suspect are secretors having the same blood type, the examiner must be especially cautious in typing a seminal stain, taking special care to make sure that the stain is free of any possible contaminants.

As with blood, forensic serologists have been successful in finding polymorphic enzymes in semen. Unfortunately, the list of readily identifiable enzymes in semen stains is far shorter than it is for blood. Two enzymes which lend themselves to ready detection in semen stains are PGM and Pep A. Hopefully with additional research this list will lengthen.

COLLECTION OF RAPE EVIDENCE

The finding of seminal constituents in a rape victim is important evidence for substantiating the fact that sexual intercourse has taken place, but their absence does not necessarily mean that a rape did not occur. Physical injuries such as bruises or bleeding tend to confirm the fact that a violent assault did take place. Furthermore, there is a distinct possibility that the forceful physical contact between victim and assailant will result in a transfer of physical evidence—i.e., blood, semen, hairs, and fibers. The presence of such physical evidence will help forge a vital link in the chain of circumstances surrounding a sexual crime.

To protect this kind of evidence, all the outer- and undergarments from the involved parties should be carefully removed and packaged separately in paper bags (not plastic bags). If it is deemed appropriate, bedding, or the object upon which the assault took place, should be submitted to the laboratory for processing. Items suspected of containing seminal stains must be handled carefully. Folding an article through the stain may cause it to flake off, as will the rubbing of the stained area against the surface of the packaging material. If, under unusual circumstances, it is not possible to transport the stained article to the laboratory, the stained area should be cut out and it should be submitted with an unstained piece acting as a control.

In cases relating to the typing of seminal stains, laboratory submissions must include saliva so that the secretor status of both the suspect and victim can be determined. To obtain saliva, the individuals in question should be asked to thoroughly saturate a clean paper towel or three or four cotton swabs with saliva. The saliva should then be air-dried out of direct sunlight or heat. It is best that the donor not have anything in his mouth for 30 minutes before giving this sample—this includes gum, cigarettes, cigars, etc. In addition, a sample of whole blood from both the victim and suspect should be obtained for blood typing.

The fact that individuals may secrete their blood-type antigens in body fluids can be a double-edged sword for the careless investigator. By needlessly touching the suspect area, the investigator may inadvertently transfer his own blood type to the stain through the medium of perspiration. In this respect, it is exceedingly important that stained articles be handled with care, minimizing direct personal contact. In some instances it may be desirable to wear disposable plastic gloves when such evidence must be touched.

The rape victim must be subject to a medical examination as soon as possible after the assault. At this time the following items of physical evidence are to be secured:

1. *Vaginal Swabs.* A minimum of four swabs are taken. One swab is to be smeared onto a microscope slide.
2. *Oral and Anal Swabs.* To be taken when warranted by case history.
3. *Pubic Combings.* Comb pubic area for loose or foreign hairs.
4. *Head and Pubic Hair Controls.* Pull out two dozen hairs from the pubic area and fifty hairs from the head.
5. *Saliva Sample.* Obtain as described above.
6. *Blood Sample.* Collect a minimum of 5 cc.
7. *Fingernail Scrapings.* Scrape the under surface of the nails with a dull object and retain for laboratory examination.
8. *All Clothing.* Package as described above.

If a suspect is apprehended, the following items are routinely collected:

1. *All Clothing.* Items believed to have been worn at time of assault.
2. *Pubic Hair Combings.*

3. *Pulled Head and Pubic Hair Controls.*
4. *Saliva and Blood Samples.*

The persistence of seminal constituents in the vagina may become a factor when trying to ascertain the time of an alleged sexual attack. While the presence of spermatozoa in the vaginal cavity provides evidence of intercourse, important information regarding the time of sexual activity can be obtained from the knowledge that motile or living sperm *may* generally survive up to 4-6 hours in the vaginal cavity of a living person. However, a successful search for motile sperm requires that a microscopic examination of a vaginal smear be conducted immediately after it is taken from the victim.

A more extensive examination of vaginal collections is later made at a forensic laboratory. Nonmotile sperm *may* be found in a living female for up to three days after intercourse and occasionally up to six days. The likelihood of finding seminal acid phosphatase in the vaginal cavity markedly decreases with time following intercourse, with little chance of identifying this substance 48 hours after intercourse.[7] Hence, taking into consideration the possibility of the prolonged persistence of both spermatozoa and acid phosphatase in the vaginal cavity after intercourse, investigators should seek information to determine when and if voluntary sexual activity last occurred prior to the sexual assault. This information will be useful for evaluating the significance of a find of these seminal constituents in the female victim.

Another significant indicator of recent sexual activity is p30. This protein usually is not found in the vaginal cavity beyond 8 hours following intercourse.[8]

REVIEW QUESTIONS

1. Karl Landsteiner discovered that blood can be classified by its
   _____ .
2. No two individuals, except for identical twins, can be expected to have the same combination of blood types or antigens. (True, False)
3. _____ is the fluid portion of unclotted blood.
4. The liquid that separates from the blood when a clot is formed is called the _____ .
5. _____ transport oxygen from the lungs to the body tissues and carry carbon dioxide back to the lungs.

---

[7] Anne Davies and Elizabeth Wilson, "The Persistence of Seminal Constituents in the Human Vagina," *Forensic Science*, 3 (1974), 45.

[8] N. A. Stubbing and P. J. Newall, "An Evaluation of Gamma-Glutamyl Transpeptidase (GGT) and p30 Determinations for the Identification of Semen on Postcoital Vaginal Swabs," *Journal of Forensic Sciences*, 30 (1985), 604.

6. On the surface of the red blood cells are chemical substances called _____. It is these substances that impart blood-type characteristics to the cells.

7. Type A individuals have _____ antigens located on the surface of their red blood cells.

8. Type O persons have (both, neither) A and B antigens on their cells.

9. It is the presence or absence of the _____ and _____ antigens on the red blood cells that determines a person's blood type in the A-B-O system.

10. The D antigen is also known as the _____ antigen.

11. Serum contains proteins known as _____, which destroy or inactivate antigens.

12. An antibody will react with (any, only a specific) antigen.

13. Agglutination describes the clumping together of red blood cells by the action of an antibody. (True, False)

14. Type B blood contains _____ antigens and anti-_____ antibodies.

15. Type AB blood has (both, neither) anti-A and anti-B.

16. A drug-protein complex can be injected into an animal to cause the formation of specific _____ for that drug.

17. The term _____ describes the study of antigen-antibody reactions.

18. Type AB blood will (be, not be) agglutinated by both anti-A and anti-B serum.

19. Type B red blood cells will agglutinate when added to type (A, B) blood.

20. Type A cells will agglutinate when added to type (AB, O) blood.

21. An immunological assay technique currently being used to detect the presence of minute quantities of drugs in blood and urine is _____.

22. The distribution of type A blood in the United States is approximately (42, 15) percent.

23. The distribution of type AB in the United States is approximately (12, 3) percent.

24. (All, Most) blood hemoglobin has peroxidaselike activity.

25. For many years the most commonly used color test for identifying blood was the _____ color test.

26. _____ reagent reacts with blood, causing it to luminesce.

27. Blood can be characterized as being of human origin by the _____ test.

28. Antigens and antibodies (can, cannot) be induced to move toward one another under the influence of an electrical field.

29. The _____ technique is the current method of choice for the indirect typing of bloodstains.

30. Approximately _____ percent of the population are classified as secretors.

31. _____ are proteins that have important functions in regulating many of the body's chemical reactions.

32. Enzymes that exist in different forms in a population are (polymorphic, monomorphic).

33. Protein and enzyme components can be separated and typed by the technique of _____ .

34. The shape of bloodstains may provide useful information regarding the direction, dropping distance, and angle of impact of splattered blood. (True, False)

35. Small amounts of blood are best submitted to a crime laboratory in a (wet, dry) condition.

36. Airtight packages make the best containers for blood-containing evidence. (True, False)

37. The basic unit of heredity is the _____ .

38. Genes are positioned on threadlike bodies called _____ .

39. All cells in the human body, except the reproductive cells, have _____ pair of chromosomes.

40. The sex of an offspring is always determined by the (mother, father).

41. Genes that influence a given characteristic and are aligned with one another on a chromosome pair are known as _____ .

42. When a pair of allelic genes are identical, they are said to be (homozygous, heterozygous).

43. A (phenotype, genotype) is an observable characteristic of an individual.

44. The combination of genes present in the cells of an individual is called the _____ .

45. A gene (will, will not) appear in a child when it is present in one of the parents.

46. A type B person may have the genotype _____ or the genotype _____ .

47. A type AB mother and type AB father will have offspring of what possible genotypes?

48. A type AB mother and type AB father will have offspring of what possible phenotypes?

49. The _____ color test is used to locate and characterize seminal stains.

50. Semen is unequivocally identified by the microscopic appearance of _____ .

51. Males having a low sperm count suffer from a condition known as (oligospermia, aspermia).

52. The protein _____ is unique to seminal plasma.

53. The blood type of a male secretor (can, cannot) be determined from a seminal stain.

54. If the typing of seminal stains is desired by an investigator, (saliva, urine) from the suspect and victim must be submitted to the laboratory.

55. Seminal constituents may remain in the vagina for up to six days after intercourse. (True, False)

FURTHER REFERENCES

Baechtel, F. S., "The Identification and Individualization of Semen Stains," in *Forensic Science Handbook*, Vol. 2, R. Saferstein, ed. Englewood Cliffs, N.J.: Prentice-Hall, Inc., 1987.

Baird, J. B., "The Individuality of Blood and Bloodstains," *The Canadian Society of Forensic Science Journal*, 11 (1978), 83.

Culliford, Bryan J., *The Examination and Typing of Bloodstains in the Crime Laboratory*. Washington, D.C.: U.S. Government Printing Office, 1971.

De Forest, Peter R., et al., *Forensic Science—An Introduction to Criminalistics*. New York: McGraw-Hill Book Company, 1983.

Gaensslen, R. E., *Sourcebook in Forensic Serology, Immunology and Biochemistry*. Washington, D.C.: U.S. Government Printing Office, 1983.

Melvin, Joseph R., Jr., et al., "Paternity Testing," in *Forensic Science Handbook*, Vol. 2, R. Saferstein, ed. Englewood Cliffs, N.J.: Prentice-Hall, Inc., 1987.

Sensabaugh, G. F., "Biochemical Markers of Individuality," in *Forensic Science Handbook*, R. Saferstein, ed. Englewood Cliffs, N.J.: Prentice-Hall, Inc., 1982.

Whitehead, P. H., L. A. King, and D. J. Werrett, "New Information from Bloodstains," *Naturwissenschaften*, 66 (1979), 446.

Willott, G. M., "The Role of the Forensic Biologist in Cases of Sexual Assault," *Journal of the Forensic Science Society*, 15 (1975), 269.

AUDIOVISUAL PRESENTATIONS

Laboratory Chemistry (filmstrip and audio tape). Robert J. Brady Co., Inc., Bowie, Md.

13

Fingerprints

HISTORY OF FINGERPRINTING

Since the beginnings of criminal investigation, police have sought an infallible means of human identification. The first systematic attempt at personal identification was devised and introduced by a French police expert, Alphonse Bertillon, in 1883. The Bertillon system relied on a detailed description (*portrait parlé*) of the subject, combined with full-length and profile photographs and a system of precise body measurements known as **anthropometry**.

The use of anthropometry as a method of identification rested on the premise that the dimensions of the human bone system remained fixed from the age of twenty until death. Skeleton sizes were thought to be so extremely diverse that no two individuals could have exactly the same measurements. Bertillon recommended the routine taking of eleven measurements of the human anatomy. These included height, reach, width of head, and the length of the left foot.

For two decades this system was considered the most accurate method of identification. It was only in the first years of the new century that police began to appreciate and accept a system of identification based on the classification of finger ridge patterns known as **fingerprints**. Today, the fingerprint is the pillar of modern criminal identification.

Evidence exists that the Chinese used the fingerprint to sign legal documents as far back as three thousand years ago. However, whether this practice was performed for ceremonial custom or as a means of personal identity

347

remains a point of conjecture lost to history. In any case, the examples of fingerprinting in ancient history are ambiguous, and the few that do exist certainly did not contribute to the development of fingerprinting techniques as we know them today.

Several years before Bertillon began work on his system, William Herschel, an English civil servant stationed in India, started the practice of requiring natives to sign their contracts with the imprint of a right hand that had been pressed against a stamp pad. The motives for Herschel's requirement remain unclear; it is debatable whether he envisioned fingerprinting as a means of personal identification or just as a method for utilizing the Hindu custom that a trace of bodily contact was more binding than a signature on a contract. In any case, he did not publish anything about his activities until after a Scottish physician, Henry Fauld, working in a hospital in Japan, published his views on the potential application of fingerprinting to personal identification.

In his communication to a scientific publication in 1880, Fauld suggested that skin ridge patterns could be important for the identification of criminals. He related an incident about a thief who left his fingerprint on a whitewashed wall, and how in comparing these prints with those of a suspect, he found that they were quite different. A few days later another suspect was found whose fingerprints compared with those on the wall. When confronted with this evidence, the individual confessed to the crime.

Fauld was convinced that fingerprints furnished infallible proof of identification. He even offered to set up at his own expense a fingerprint bureau at Scotland Yard to test the practicality of the method. But his offer was rejected in favor of the Bertillon system. This decision was reversed less than two decades later.

It was the extensive research into fingerprinting conducted by another Englishman, Francis Galton, that provided the needed impetus that made police agencies aware of its potential application. In 1892, Galton published his classic textbook *Finger Prints*, the first book of its kind on the subject. In his book he discussed the anatomy of fingerprints, and suggested methods for recording them. Galton also proposed assigning fingerprints to three pattern types—loops, arches, and whorls. Most importantly, the book convincingly demonstrated that no two prints were identical and an individual's prints remained unchanged from year to year. At Galton's insistence, the British government adopted fingerprinting as a supplement to the Bertillon system.

The next step in the development of fingerprint technology was the creation of classification systems capable of filing many thousands of prints in a logical and searchable sequence. Dr. Juan Vucetich, an Argentinian police officer fascinated by Galton's work, devised a workable concept in 1891. His classification system has been refined over the years and is still widely used today in most Spanish-speaking countries. In 1897, another classification system was proposed by an Englishman, Sir Edward Richard Henry. Four years later, Henry's system was adopted by Scotland Yard. Today, most English-speaking countries, including the United States, use some version of Henry's classification system to file fingerprints.

Early in the twentieth century, Bertillon's measurement system was beginning to fall into disfavor. It was becoming apparent that its results were highly susceptible to error, particularly when the measurements were taken by persons who were not thoroughly trained. The method was dealt its most severe and notable setback in 1903 when a convict Will West, arrived in Fort Leavenworth Prison. A routine check of the prison files startlingly revealed that a William West, already in the prison, could not be distinguished from the new prisoner by body measurements or even by photographs. In fact, the two men looked just like twins, and their measurements were practically the same. Subsequently, fingerprints of both prisoners clearly distinguished them.

In the United States, the first systematic and official use of fingerprints for personal identification was adopted by the New York City Civil Service Commission in 1901. Here the method was used for certifying all civil service applications. Several American police officials received instruction in fingerprint identification at the 1904 World's Fair in St. Louis from representatives of Scotland Yard. After the Fair and the Will West incident, fingerprinting began to be used in earnest in all major cities of the United States. In 1924, the fingerprint records of the Bureau of Investigation and Leavenworth Prison were merged to form the nucleus of the identification records of the new Federal Bureau of Investigation. Presently, the FBI has the largest collection of fingerprints in the world; currently, the criminal fingerprint file contains over 83 million cards representing over 22 million persons. By the beginning of World War I, England and practically all of Europe had adopted fingerprinting as their primary method of identifying criminals.

THE FUNDAMENTAL PRINCIPLES OF FINGERPRINTS

FIRST PRINCIPLE: A FINGERPRINT IS AN INDIVIDUAL CHARACTERISTIC; NO TWO FINGERS HAVE YET BEEN FOUND TO POSSESS IDENTICAL RIDGE CHARACTERISTICS

The acceptance of fingerprint evidence by the courts has always been predicated on the assumption that no two individuals have identical fingerprints. Early fingerprint experts consistently referred to Galton's calculation showing the possible existence of 64 billion different fingerprints to support this contention. Later, researchers questioned the validity of Galton's figures and attempted to devise mathematical models to better approximate this value. However, no matter what mathematical model one refers to, the conclusions are always the same: the probability for the existence of two identical fingerprint patterns in the world's population is extremely small.

Not only is this principle supported by theoretical calculations, but just as importantly, it is verified by the millions upon millions of individuals who have had their prints classified over the past 80 years—no two have ever been found to be identical.

The individuality of a fingerprint is not determined by its general shape or pattern but by a careful study of its **ridge characteristics** (also known as *minutiae*). It is the identity, number, and relative location of characteristics, such as those illustrated in Figure 13-1, that impart individuality to a fingerprint. If two prints are to compare, they will have to reveal characteristics that are not only identical but have the same relative location to one another in a print. In a judicial proceeding, a point-by-point comparison must be demonstrated by the expert, using charts similar to the one shown in Figure 13-2 in order to prove the identity of an individual.

If an expert were asked to compare the characteristics of the complete fingerprint, no difficulty would be encountered in completing such an assignment; there are as many as 150 individual ridge characteristics on the average fingerprint. However, in practice the vast majority of the prints recovered at crime scenes are partial impressions, showing only a segment of the entire print. Under these circumstances, the expert has to be prepared to compare only a small number of ridge characteristics from the recovered print to a known recorded print. For years, experts have debated the question of just how many ridge comparisons are necessary before two fingerprints can be identified as being the same. Numbers that range from 8 to 16 have been suggested as being sufficient to meet the criteria of individuality. However, the difficulty that arises in establishing such a minimum is that no comprehensive statistical study has ever been undertaken to determine the frequency

Figure 13-1. Ridge characteristics. *Courtesy* Police Science Services, Niles, Illinois.

1. *Bifurcation*
2. *Ridge ending*
3. *Enclosure*
4. *Ridge ending*
5. *Bifurcation*
6. *Bifurcation*
7. *Bifurcation*
8. *Ridge ending*
9. *Ridge ending*
10. *Short ridge*
11. *Bifurcation*
12. *Ridge ending*

Figure 13-2. A fingerprint exhibit illustrating the matching ridge characteristics between the crime-scene print and an inked impression of one of the suspect's fingers. *Courtesy* New Jersey State Police.

of occurrence of different ridge characteristics and their relative locations. Until such a study is undertaken and completed, no meaningful guidelines can be established for defining the uniqueness of a fingerprint.

In 1973, the International Association for Identification, after a three-year study of this question, concluded that "no valid basis exists for requiring a predetermined minimum number of friction ridge characters which must be present in two impressions in order to establish positive identification." Hence, the final determination must be based on the experience and knowledge of the expert, with the understanding that others may profess honest differences of opinion on the uniqueness of a fingerprint if the question of minimal number of ridge characteristics exists.

*SECOND PRINCIPLE: A FINGERPRINT WILL REMAIN
UNCHANGED DURING AN INDIVIDUAL'S LIFETIME*

Fingerprints are a reproduction of friction skin ridges found on the palm side of the fingers and thumbs. Similar friction skin can also be found on the surface of the palms and soles of the feet. Apparently, these skin surfaces have been designed by nature to provide our bodies with a firmer grasp and a resistance to slippage. A visual inspection of friction skin reveals a series of lines corresponding to hills (ridges) and valleys (grooves). It is the shape and form of the skin ridges that one sees as the black lines of an inked fingerprint impression.

Actually, skin is composed of layers of cells. Those nearest the surface make up the outer portion of the skin known as the **epidermis**, and the inner skin is known as the **dermis**. As one looks at a cross section of skin (Figure 13-3), a boundary of cells separating the epidermis and dermis is noted. It is the shape of this boundary, made up of **dermal papillae**, that determines the form and pattern of the ridges on the surface of the skin. Once the dermal papillae develop in the human fetus, the ridge patterns will remain unchanged throughout life except to enlarge during growth.

Each skin ridge is populated with a single row of pores that are the openings for ducts leading from the sweat glands. It is through these pores that perspiration is discharged and deposited on the surface of the skin. Once the finger touches a surface, perspiration along with oils that may have been picked up by touching the hairy portions of the body is transferred onto that surface, thereby leaving an impression of the finger's ridge pattern (a

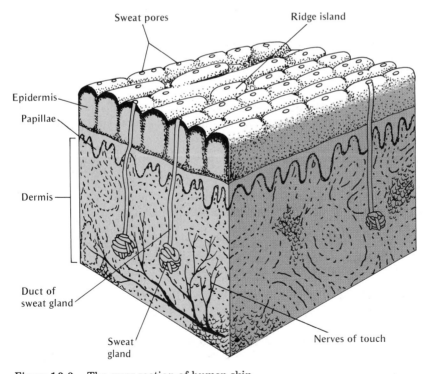

Figure 13-3. The cross section of human skin.

fingerprint). Prints deposited in this manner are invisible to the eye and are commonly referred to as *latent* or hidden fingerprints.

Although it is impossible to change one's fingerprints, there has been no lack of effort on the part of some criminals to obscure them. If an injury reaches deeply enough into the skin and damages the dermal papillae, a permanent scar will form. However, for this to happen, such a wound would have to penetrate 1 to 2 millimeters beneath the skin's surface. Indeed, efforts at intentionally scarring the skin can only be self-defeating, for it would be totally impossible to obliterate all the ridge characteristics on the hand, and the presence of permanent scars merely provides new characteristics for identification.

Perhaps the most publicized attempt at obliteration was that of the notorious gangster John Dillinger, who attempted to destroy his own fingerprints by applying a corrosive acid to them. Prints taken at the morgue after he was shot to death, compared with fingerprints recorded at the time of a previous arrest, proved that his efforts had been fruitless (see Figure 13-4).

THIRD PRINCIPLE: FINGERPRINTS HAVE GENERAL RIDGE PATTERNS THAT PERMIT THEM TO BE SYSTEMATICALLY CLASSIFIED

All fingerprints are divided into three classes on the basis of their general pattern: **loops, whorls, and arches.** Sixty to 65 percent of the population has loops, 30 to 35 percent have whorls, and about 5 percent has arches. These

Figure 13-4. The right index impression of John Dillinger before scarification on the left and afterwards on the right. Comparison is proved by the fourteen matching ridge characteristics. *Courtesy* Institute of Applied Science, New York.

three classes form the basis for all the ten-finger classification systems presently in use.

A typical loop pattern is illustrated in Figure 13-5. A loop must have one or more ridges entering from one side of the print, recurving, and exiting from the same side. If the loop opens toward the little finger, it is called an **ulnar loop**; if it opens toward the thumb, it is a **radial loop**. The pattern area of the loop is surrounded by two diverging ridges known as *type lines*. The ridge point nearest the type-line divergence is known as the *delta*. To many, a fingerprint delta resembles the silt formation that builds up as a river flows into the entrance of a lake; hence, the analogy to the geological formation known as a delta. All loops must have one delta. The *core*, as the name suggests, is the approximate center of the pattern.

Figure 13-5.   Loop pattern.

Whorls are actually divided into four distinct groups, as shown in Figure 13-6; plain whorl, central pocket loop, double loop, and accidental. All whorl patterns must have type lines and a minimum of two deltas. A plain whorl and the central pocket loop have at least one ridge that makes a complete circuit. This ridge may be in the form of a spiral, oval, or any variant of a circle. If an imaginary line is drawn between the two deltas contained within these two patterns, and if the line touches any one of the spiral ridges, the pattern is a plain whorl. If no such ridge is touched, the pattern is a central pocket loop.

As the name implies, the double loop is made up of two loops combined into one fingerprint. Any print classified as an accidental either contains two or more patterns (not including the plain arch) or is a pattern not covered by

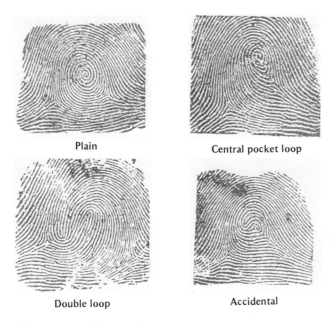

Plain   Central pocket loop

Double loop   Accidental

Figure 13-6.   Whorl patterns.

other categories. Hence, an accidental may consist of a combination loop and plain whorl, or a loop and tented arch.

Arches, the least common of the three general patterns, are subdivided into two distinct groups: plain arches and tented arches, shown in Figure 13-7. The plain arch is the simplest of all fingerprint patterns; it is formed by ridges entering from one side of the print and exiting on the opposite side. Generally, these ridges tend to rise in the center of the pattern, forming a wavelike

Plain   Tented

Figure 13-7.   Arch patterns.

pattern. The tented arch is similar to the plain arch except that instead of rising smoothly at the center, there is a sharp upthrust or spike, or the ridges meet at an angle that is less than 90 degrees.[1] Arches do not have type lines, deltas, or cores.

With a knowledge of basic fingerprint pattern classes, we may now begin to develop an appreciation for fingerprint classification systems. However, the subject is far more complex than can be described in a textbook of this nature. The student seeking a more detailed treatment of the subject would do well to consult references cited at the end of the chapter.

THE CLASSIFICATION OF FINGERPRINTS

The original Henry system, as it was adopted by Scotland Yard in 1901, converted ridge patterns on all ten fingers into a series of letters and numbers arranged in the form of a fraction. However, the system as it was originally designed could only accommodate files of up to 100,000 sets of prints; thus, as collections grew in size, it became necessary to expand the capacity of the classification system. In the United States the FBI, faced with the problem of filling ever-increasing numbers of prints, expanded its classification capacity by modifying and adding additional extensions to the original Henry system. These modifications are collectively known as the FBI system and are used by most agencies in the United States today.

THE PRIMARY CLASSIFICATION

Although we will not discuss all of the different divisions of the FBI system, a description of just one part, the primary classification, will provide an interesting insight into the process of fingerprint classification.

The primary classification is part of the original Henry system and provides the first classification step in the FBI system. Using this classification alone, all of the fingerprint cards in the world could be divided in 1024 groups. The first step in obtaining the primary classification is to pair up fingers, placing one finger in the numerator of a fraction, the other in the denominator. The fingers are paired in the following sequence:

R. Index	R. Ring	L. Thumb	L. Middle	L. Little
R. Thumb	R. Middle	R. Little	L. Index	L. Ring

The presence or absence of the whorl pattern is the basis for the determination of the primary classification. If a whorl pattern is found on any finger

---

[1] A tented arch is also any pattern that resembles a loop but lacks one of the essential requirements for classification as a loop.

of the first pair, it is assigned a value of 16, on the second pair, a value of 8, on the third pair, a value of 4, on the fourth pair, a value of 2, and on the last pair a value of 1. Any finger having an arch or loop pattern is assigned a value of 0.

After values for all ten fingers are obtained in this manner, they are totaled, and 1 is added to both the numerator and denominator. The fraction thus obtained is the primary classification. As an example, if the right index and right middle fingers are whorls and all the others are loops, the primary classification is:

$$\frac{16 + 0 + 0 + 0 + 0 + 1}{0 + 8 + 0 + 0 + 0 + 1} = \frac{17}{9}$$

Approximately 25 percent of the population falls into the 1/1 category—that is, all their fingers have either loops or arches.

A fingerprint classification system cannot in itself unequivocally identify an individual; it will merely provide the fingerprint examiner with a number of candidates, all of whom have an indistinguishable set of prints in the system's file. The identification must always be made by a final visual comparison of the questioned and file print's ridge characteristics; only these features can impart individuality to a fingerprint. Although ridge patterns impart class characteristics to the print, it is the type and position of ridge characteristics that give it its individual character.

The Henry and FBI classification systems are ten-finger classification schemes useful only for processing a full set of fingerprints. Unfortunately, it is a rarity when the crime scene yields anything more than a single partial print of a suspect. Under such circumstances, a ten-finger file will only be of value when the investigator has the names of known suspects in hand. In this case, by going through a name index, fingerprint cards of suspects on file can be removed and compared to the recovered crime-scene print. However, some police departments also have established a single-fingerprint collection to aid them in their search for suspects. Here, each fingerprint is filed on a separate card and is independently classified. Unfortunately, this approach becomes much too cumbersome when too many individuals are included in the file. Experience shows that single-print collections are only useful for agencies that restrict its members to active criminals who are most likely to engage in crimes that provide the best chance for recovery of fingerprints—e.g., house burglaries and car thefts.

COMPUTERIZED FINGERPRINT SEARCH SYSTEMS

Since the early 1960s, police agencies in most industrialized countries of the world have been trying to harness the power of the computer to classify and search their bulging fingerprint files. Police forces are now on the verge of making important technological breakthroughs that will make this goal a reality. Present plans call for a computer system in England that will automatically read, classify, and match against records, fingerprints found at crime scenes. The West German Bunderkriminalamt has started computer retrieval and matching of latent fingerprints against its collection of 17 million prints. The Canadian Mounted Police has completed the conversion of its file to a computer-based system, and Sweden's automated computerized fingerprint system became operational in 1975. In the United States, the FBI is proceeding with its ambitious program of developing a system to automatically read, classify, and match fingerprints.

The computerized systems being developed independently by the British Home Office and the FBI both incorporate automatic scanning devices that can read and code fingerprint characteristics directly from standard fingerprint cards. Both systems read the print with a flying spot scanner that measures light reflected from the print and converts the image into digital minutiae data. Minutiae data describe certain ridge characteristics by locating areas where ridges terminate (ridge endings) and where ridges branch into two ridges (bifurcations). The digital data are then transferred into a computer, where they are classified and held in storage for future matching against incoming fingerprints.

The FBI has begun work on an Automated Image Retrieval System which will be able to match incoming fingerprint cards or latent fingerprints with a fingerprint card in the FBI files. This system is capable of revealing minute characteristics (ridge endings and bifurcations) used by fingerprint examiners to identify an individual's fingerprints.

In 1983, the FBI initiated a new program to accomplish the automatic classification of fingerprints by developing an advanced computerized fingerprint reader. This new system will represent a significant improvement in a computer's ability to read poor quality fingerprints. It is expected that the searching and classification of incoming prints against the FBI files will be performed in a matter of minutes. The classification produced will be compatible with the current FBI system used by all the state and national data bases for criminal fingerprints in the United States. The computer will utilize software based on artificial intelligence concepts and will utilize rule-based systems to mimic the human decision process used in classifying a fingerprint. After testing of these developments, it is expected that these new fingerprint readers will become operational in the early 1990s.

A Japanese-designed system marketed by NEC Information Systems has recently been installed in the states of California and Alaska. Its principle of operation is based on matching fingerprint minutiae. The NEC system seems to be very effective for matching latent prints collected from crime scenes with file data originally obtained from ten-fingerprint cards. Where the FBI system matches the position and type of minutiae (ridge endings and bifurcations), the NEC system also determines the axis of a fingerprint by calculating ridge counts between each minutia and four neighboring minutiae. This added feature seems to overcome distortion problems and the uncertain orientation normally associated with partial latent fingerprints and significantly improves the capability of the computer to search a partial latent against file prints.

It seems quite certain that by the end of the twentieth century, the searching of latent fingerprints against voluminous state and federal fingerprint collections will be a routine operational procedure for all police investigators. The positive implications of this technology to criminal investigation will be immense.

METHODS OF DETECTING FINGERPRINTS

Through common usage, the term *latent fingerprint* has come to be associated with any fingerprint discovered at a crime scene. Sometimes, however, prints found at the scene of a crime are quite visible to the eye, and the word *latent* is a misnomer. Actually, there are three kinds of crime-scene prints: visible prints are made by fingers touching a surface after the ridges have been in contact with a colored material such as blood, paint, grease, or ink; plastic prints are ridge impressions left on a soft material such as putty, wax, soap, or dust; and true latent or invisible prints are impressions caused by the transfer of body perspiration or oils present on finger ridges to the surface of an object.

Locating visible or plastic prints at the crime scene normally presents little problem to the investigator because these prints are usually distinct and visible to the eye. Locating the latent or invisible print is obviously a much more difficult task and does require the utilization of techniques that will visualize the print. Although the investigator is presented with a number of alternate methods for visualizing a latent print, the method of choice will depend on the type of surface that is being examined.

Hard and nonabsorbent surfaces (e.g., glass, mirror, tile, and painted wood) require different development procedures from surfaces that are soft and porous (e.g., papers, cardboard, and cloth). Prints on the former are preferably developed by the application of a powder, whereas prints on the latter generally require treatment with a chemical.

Fingerprint powders are commercially available in a variety of compositions and colors. These powders, when applied lightly to a nonabsorbent surface with a camel's-hair brush, will readily adhere to perspiration residues and/or its deposits of body oils left on the surface. Experienced examiners find that gray and black powders are adequate for most latent print work; the examiner will select the powder that affords the best color contrast with the surface being dusted. Hence, the gray powder, composed of an aluminum dust, is used on dark-colored surfaces. It is also applied to mirrors and metal surfaces that are polished to a mirrorlike finish because these surfaces will photograph black. The black powder, composed basically of black carbon or charcoal, is applied to white or light-colored surfaces.

Other types of powders are available for developing latent prints. A magnetic-sensitive powder can be spread over a surface with a magnet in the form of a Magna Brush. Since the Magna Brush hasn't any bristles to come in contact with the surface, there is less chance that the print will be destroyed or damaged. The magnetic-sensitive powder comes in black and gray colors and is especially useful on such items as finished leather and rough plastics where the minute texture of the surface has a tendency to hold particles of ordinary powder. Fluorescent powders are also used to develop latent fingerprints. These powders will fluoresce under ultraviolet light. By photographing the fluorescence pattern of the developing print under UV light, it's possible to avoid having the color of the surface obscure the print.

Of the several chemical methods used for visualizing latent prints, iodine fuming is the oldest. Iodine is a solid crystal that, upon being heated, is transformed into a vapor without passing through a liquid phase; such a transformation is called **sublimation**. Most often, the suspect material is placed in an enclosed cabinet along with iodine crystals (see Figure 13-8). As the crystals are heated, the resultant vapors will fill the chamber and combine with constituents of the latent print to make it visible. The reasons why latent prints are visualized by iodine vapors are not yet fully understood. Many believe that the iodine fumes combine with fatty oils; however, there is also convincing evidence to show that the iodine may actually interact with residual water left on a print from perspiration.[2] Unfortunately, iodine prints are not permanent and begin to fade once the fuming process is stopped. It is necessary, therefore, for the examiner to photograph the prints immediately upon development in order to retain a permanent record. Also, iodine-developed prints can be fixed with a 1 percent solution of starch in water applied by spraying. The print will turn blue and can be expected to last for several weeks to several months.

Another chemical used for visualizing latent prints is ninhydrin. The development of latent prints with ninhydrin is dependent on its chemical reaction with amino acids and proteins present in trace amounts in perspiration. Ninhydrin (triketohydrindene hydrate) is commonly sprayed onto the porous surface from an aerosol can. A solution is prepared by mixing the ninhydrin powder with a suitable solvent such as acetone or ethyl alcohol; a 0.6 percent solution appears to be effective for most applications. Generally, prints begin to appear within an hour or two after ninhydrin application; however, weaker prints may be visualized after 24 to 48 hours. The develop-

---

[2] J. Almag, Y. Sasson, and A. Anati, "Chemical Reagents for the Development of Latent Fingerprints II: Controlled Addition of Water Vapor to Iodine Fumes—A Solution to the Aging Problem," *Journal of Forensic Sciences*, 24 (1979), 431.

Figure 13-8. A heated fuming cabinet. *Courtesy* Sirchie Laboratories, Inc., Raleigh, N. Carolina.

ment can be hastened if the treated specimen is heated in an oven or on a hotplate at a temperature of 80° to 100°C. The ninhydrin method has developed latent prints on paper as old as fifteen years.

Silver nitrate is a third chemical used for visualizing latent prints. After the moisture from perspiration has evaporated, a substantial portion of the latent print residue will consist of common salt (sodium chloride). In the presence of the chemical silver nitrate, the chloride ion of the salt will react to form silver chloride. Although silver chloride is colorless, it can be transformed by ultraviolet light into silver. Silver shows up the latent print as black or reddish-brown in color. Commonly, a 3 percent solution of silver nitrate in water is brushed onto a paper or cardboard object suspected of containing a print. The prints are then developed by being exposed to the light.

For most fingerprint examiners, the chemical method of choice is ninhydrin. Its extreme sensitivity and ease of application have all but eliminated the use of iodine for latent print visualization. However, in those instances in which ninhydrin fails, development with silver nitrate may provide identifiable results. Application of silver nitrate will wash away any traces of fatty oils and proteins from an object's surface: hence, if one wishes to utilize all of the above-mentioned chemical development methods on the same surface, it is necessary to first fume with iodine, follow this treatment with ninhydrin, and then apply silver nitrate to the object.

In the past, chemical treatment for fingerprint development was reserved for porous surfaces such as paper and cardboard. However, since 1982, a chemical technique known as Super Glue® fuming has gained wide popularity for developing latent prints on nonporous surfaces such as metals, electrical tape, leather, and plastic bags.[3] Super Glue is approximately 98 to 99 percent cyanoacrylate ester, and it's this chemical which actually interacts with and visualizes a latent fingerprint. Cyanoacrylate ester fumes are created when Super Glue is placed on absorbent cotton treated with sodium hydroxide. The fumes can also be created by heating the glue. The fumes and the evidential object are contained within an enclosed chamber for up to 6 hours. Development occurs when fumes from the glue adhere to the latent print, usually producing a white-appearing latent print. Interestingly, small enclosed areas, such as the interior of an automobile, have been successfully processed for latent prints with fumes from Super Glue. The fuming technique can be used before or after processing with fingerprint powders, and in fact, subsequent processing with powder of a latent print developed by fuming may even further enhance the print's image.

The use of powders and chemicals may interfere with physical and chemical analysis, particularly in the case of blood, fabrics, and documents. Therefore, in cases involving items with material adhering to their surfaces and/or which will require further laboratory examinations, fingerprint processing should not be performed at the crime scene. Rather, the items should be submitted to the laboratory where they can be processed for fingerprints in conjunction with other examinations that have to be undertaken.

A recent and most exciting development in fingerprint technology has been the discovery that latent fingerprints can be visualized by exposure to laser light. The laser method, developed jointly by the Ontario Provincial Police and Xerox Research Center of Canada, takes advantage of the fact that perspiration contains a variety of components that fluoresce when illuminated by an argon-ion laser. The light emitted by the print can either be

---

[3] F. G. Kendall and B. W. Rehn, "Rapid Method of Super Glue Fuming Application for the Development of Latent Fingerprints," *Journal of Forensic Sciences*, 28 (1983), 777.

viewed directly or recorded photographically through specially selected filters.[4]

Detection occurs when latent print residues absorb the laser light and re-emit it in wavelengths longer than the illuminating source (see Figure 13-9). The fingerprint examiner, wearing safety goggles containing optical filters, visually examines the specimen being exposed to the laser light. The filters absorb the laser light and permit the wavelengths at which latent print residues fluoresce to pass through to the eyes of the wearer. The filter also protects the operator against eye damage from scattered or reflected laser light. Likewise, latent print residue producing sufficient fluorescence can be photographed by placing this same filter across the lens of the camera. Examination of specimens and photography of the fluorescing latent prints are carried out in a darkened room. Additionally, the application of zinc chloride after ninhydrin treatment or the application of the dye rhodamine 6G after Super Glue fuming may increase the quality of previously developed prints upon their exposure to laser illumination.

The laser fingerprint detection technique has many desirable features. It's nondestructive and can be used on surfaces subjected to extremes in temperature and moisture as well as on surfaces that are not amenable to the use of powders or chemicals. Prints as old as forty years have been developed by the laser technique. Some insight into the effectiveness of latent fingerprint developing techniques is revealed by a recent FBI survey taken of crime-scene evidence submitted in connection with 3000 cases.[5] Latent prints were

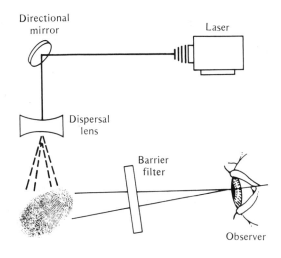

Figure 13-9. Schematic depicting latent print detection with the aid of a laser. *Courtesy Federal Bureau of Investigation, Washington, D.C.*

---

[4] B. E. Dalrymple, "Case Analysis of Fingerprint Detection by Laser," *Journal of Forensic Sciences*, 24 (1979), 586.

[5] J. E. Ridgely, Jr., "Latent Print Detection by Laser," *FBI Law Enforcement Bulletin*, 54 (6), 1985, 1.

$$\frac{RI}{RT} + \frac{RR}{Rm} + \frac{LT}{RL} + \frac{Lm}{LI} + \frac{LL}{LR}$$

developed in 242 cases with fingerprint powders, 930 cases with ninhydrin, 1 case with silver nitrate, and 1 case with iodine fumes. The laser detected prints in 214 cases. The latent prints in these cases were not developed in any instance by subsequent application of fingerprint powders or chemicals. From these numbers it's apparent that the laser represents a significant advancement in latent fingerprint development and complements other methods of latent fingerprint development.

PRESERVATION OF DEVELOPED PRINTS

Once the latent print has been visualized, it must be permanently preserved for future comparison and possible court evidence. A photograph must be taken before any further attempts at perservation are made. Actually, any camera equipped with a close-up lens will do; however, many investigators prefer to use a camera specially designed for fingerprint photography. Such a camera comes equipped with a built-in illuminator and a fixed focus to take photographs on a 1:1 scale when the camera's open eye is held exactly flush against the print's surface (see Figure 13-10). In addition, photographs must be taken to provide an overall view of the print's location with respect to other evidential items at the crime scene.

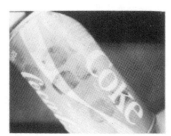

Figure 13-10. Fingerprint camera and its resultant photo. *Courtesy* Sirchie Laboratories, Inc., Raleigh, N. Carolina.

Once photographs have been secured, one of two procedures is to be followed. If the object is small enough to be transported without destroying the print, it should be preserved in its entirety; the print should be covered with cellophane so it will be protected from damage. On the other hand, prints on large immovable objects that have been developed with a powder can best be preserved by "lifting." The most popular type of lifter is a broad adhesive tape similar to scotch tape. If the powdered surface is covered with the adhesive side of the tape and pulled up, the powder will be transferred to the tape. Then the tape is placed on a properly labeled card that offers a good background contrast with the powder.

A variation of this procedure is the use of an adhesive-backed clear plastic sheet that is attached to a colored cardboard backing. Before it is applied to the print, a celluloid separator is peeled from the plastic sheet to expose the adhesive lifting surface. The tape is then pressed evenly and firmly over the powdered print and pulled up (see Figure 13-11). The sheet containing the adhering powder is now pressed against the cardboard backing to provide a permanent record of the fingerprint.

Figure 13-11. "Lifting" a fingerprint. *Courtesy* Sirchie Laboratories, Inc., Raleigh, N. Carolina.

REVIEW QUESTIONS

1. The first systematic attempt at personal identification was devised and introduced by _____.

2. A system of identification relying on precise body measurements is known as _____.

3. The fingerprint classification system used in most English-speaking countries was devised by _____.

4. The first systematic and official use of fingerprints for personal identification in the United States was adopted by the New York City Civil Service Commission. (True, False)

5. The individuality of a fingerprint (is, is not) determined by its pattern.

6. A point-by-point comparison of a fingerprint's _____ must be demonstrated in order to prove identity.

7. _____ are a reproduction of friction skin ridges.

8. The form and pattern of skin ridges are determined by the (epidermis, dermal papillae).

9. A permanent scar will form in the skin only when an injury damages the _____.

10. Fingerprints (can, cannot) be changed during a person's lifetime.

11. The three general patterns into which fingerprints are divided are _____, _____, and _____.

12. The most common fingerprint pattern is the _____.

13. Approximately 5 percent of the population have the _____ fingerprint pattern.

14. A loop pattern that opens toward the thumb is known as a(n) (radial, ulnar) loop.

15. The pattern area of the loop is enclosed by two diverging ridges known as _____.

16. The ridge point nearest the type-line divergence is known as the _____.

17. All loops must have (one, two) delta(s).

18. The approximate center of a loop pattern is called the _____.

19. If an imaginary line drawn between the two deltas of a whorl pattern touches any of the spiral ridges, the pattern is classified as a (plain whorl, central pocket loop).

20. The simplest of all fingerprint patterns is the _____.

21. Arches (have, have no) type lines, deltas, or cores.

22. The presence or absence of the _____ pattern is used as a basis for determining the primary classification in the Henry system.

23. The largest category (25%) in the primary classification system is (1/1, 1/2).

24. A fingerprint classification system (can, cannot) unequivocally identify an individual.

25. Computerized fingerprint search systems match prints by comparing the position of bifurcations and ridge endings. (True, False)

26. A fingerprint left by a person with soiled or stained fingertips is called a
    _____ .

27. _____ fingerprints are impressions left on a soft material.

28. Fingerprint impressions that are not readily visible are called _____ .

29. Fingerprints on hard and nonabsorbent surfaces are best developed by the application of a _____ .

30. Fingerprints on porous surfaces are best developed with _____ treatment.

31. _____ vapors will chemically combine with fatty oils or residual water to visualize a fingerprint.

32. The chemical _____ visualizes fingerprints by its reaction with amino acids.

33. Chemical treatment with _____ visualizes fingerprints by combining with the salt residues of perspiration.

34. A latent fingerprint is first treated with silver nitrate followed by ninhydrin. (True, False)

35. A chemical technique known as _____ is used for developing latent prints on nonporous surfaces such as metal and plastic.

36. Detection of latent fingerprints can occur when perspiration residues absorb _____ light and re-emit it in wavelengths longer than the illuminating source.

37. Once a fingerprint has been visualized, it must first be preserved by
    _____ .

FURTHER REFERENCES

Allison, Harrison C., *Personal Identification*. Boston: Holbrook Press, 1973.

Cowger, James E., *Friction Ridge Skin*. New York: Elsevier Science Publishing Co., 1983.

Hazen, Robert J., "Significant Advances in the Science of Fingerprints," in *Forensic Science*, 2nd ed., G. Davies, ed. Washington, D.C.: American Chemical Society, 1986.

Moenssens, André A., *Fingerprint Techniques*. Philadelphia: Chilton Book Co., 1971.

Neudorfer, Charles D., "Fingerprint Automation—Progress in the FBI's Identification Division," *FBI Law Enforcement Bulletin*, 55 no. 3 (1986), 3.

The Science of Fingerprints. Washington, D.C.: U.S. Government Printing Office, 1977.

AUDIOVISUAL PRESENTATIONS

Fingerprints (80 35-mm slides and audio tape). Police Science Services, Niles, Ill.

Macroscopic Examination (filmstrip and audio tape). Robert J. Brady Co., Inc., Bowie, Md.

14

Firearms, Tool Marks, and Other Impressions

Just as natural variations in skin ridge patterns and characteristics provide a key to human identification, minute random markings on surfaces can impart individuality to inanimate objects. Structural variations and irregularities caused by scratches, nicks, breaks, and wear permit the criminalist to relate a bullet to a gun, a scratch or abrasion mark to a single tool, or a tire track to a particular automobile. Individualization, a goal so vigorously pursued in all other areas of criminalistics, frequently becomes an attainable reality in firearm and tool mark examination.

Although a portion of this chapter will be devoted to the comparison of surface features for the purposes of bullet identification, a complete description of the services and capabilities of the modern forensic firearms laboratory cannot be restricted just to this one subject, important as it may be. The high frequency of shooting cases has necessitated that the science of firearms identification extend beyond the mere comparison of bullets to include knowledge of the operation of all types of weapons, the restoration of obliterated serial numbers on weapons, the detection and characterization of gunpowder residues on garments and around wounds, the estimation of muzzle-to-target distances, and the detection of powder residues on hands. Each of these functions will be covered in this chapter.

369

BULLET COMPARISONS

It is the inner surface of the barrel of a gun that leaves its markings on a bullet passing through it. These markings are peculiar to each gun. Hence, if one bullet found at the scene of a crime and another test-fired from a suspect's gun show the same markings, the suspect is linked to the crime. Because it is these inner surface striations that are so important for bullet comparison, it is important to know why and how they originate.

The gun barrel is produced from a solid bar of steel that has been hollowed out by drilling. The microscopic drill marks left on the barrel's inner surface are randomly irregular and would in themselves serve to impart a uniqueness to each barrel. However, the manufacture of a barrel requires the additional step of impressing its inner surface with spiral *grooves*, a step known as *rifling*. The surfaces of the original bore remaining between the grooves are called *lands* (see Figure 14-1). As a fired bullet travels through a barrel, it engages the rifling grooves; these grooves will then guide the bullet through the barrel, giving it a rapid spin. This is done because a spinning bullet will not tumble end over end on leaving the barrel but will remain instead on a true and accurate course.

The diameter of the gun barrel, sketched in Figure 14-2, measured between opposite lands, is known as the *caliber* of the weapon. Caliber is normally recorded in hundredths of an inch or in millimeters—e.g., .22, .38, and 9 mm. Actually, the term *caliber*, as it is commonly applied, is not an exact measurement of the barrel's diameter; for example, a 38 (.38 inches) caliber weapon might actually have a bore diameter that ranges from 0.345 to 0.365 inches.

Before 1940, barrels were rifled by having one or two grooves at a time cut into the surface with steel hook cutters. The cutting tool was rotated as it passed down the barrel so that the final results were grooves spiraling either to the right or left. However, as the need for increased speed in the manufacture of weapons became apparent, newer techniques were developed that were far more suitable for the mass production of weapons. The broach cutter, shown in Figure 14-3 consists of a series of concentric steel rings,

Figure 14-1. Interior view of a gun barrel showing the presence of lands and grooves.

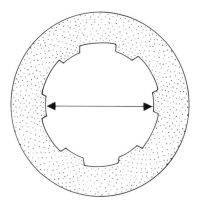

Figure 14-2. The cross section of a barrel with six grooves. The diameter of the bore is the caliber.

Figure 14-3. A segment of a broach cutter. *Courtesy* New Jersey State Police.

with each ring slightly larger than the preceding one. As the broach passes through the barrel, it simultaneously cuts all the grooves into the barrel at the required depth. The broach is rotated as it passes through the barrel, giving the grooves their desired direction and rate of twist.

In contrast to the broach, the button process involves no cuttings. Here, a steel plug or "button" impressed with the desired number of grooves is forced under extremely high pressures through the barrel. A single pass of the button down the barrel compresses the metal to create lands and grooves on the barrel walls that are negative forms of those on the button. The button is rotated to produce the desired direction and rate of twist (Figure 14-4).

Like the button process, the mandrel rifling process involves no cutting of metal. A mandrel is a rod of hardened steel machined so its form is the reverse impression of the rifling it is intended to produce. The mandrel is inserted into a slightly oversized bore, and the barrel is compressed with hammering or heavy rollers into the mandrel's form.

Every firearms manufacturer chooses a rifling process that is best suited to meet the production standards and requirements of its product. Once the choice is made, however, the class characteristics of the weapon's barrel will remain consistent; each will have the same number of lands and grooves with the same approximate width and direction of twist. For example, .32 caliber Smith & Wesson revolvers have five lands and grooves twisting to the right. On the other hand, Colt .32 caliber revolvers exhibit six lands and grooves twisting to the left. Although these class characteristics may prove to be of some value in permitting the examiner to distinguish one type or brand name weapon from another, they will certainly not impart individuality to any one barrel; no class characteristic can do this.

If one could cut a barrel open lengthwise, a careful examination of the interior would reveal the existence of fine lines or striations, many running

Figure 14-4. (Top) Cross section of a .22 caliber rifled barrel. (Bottom) A button used to produce the lands and grooves in the barrel. *Courtesy* New Jersey State Police.

the length of the barrel's lands and grooves. These striations are impressed into the metal as the negatives of minute imperfections found on the rifling cutter's surface, or they are produced by minute chips of steel pushed against the barrel's inner surface by a moving broach cutter. The fact is that the random distribution and irregularities of these markings are impossible to duplicate exactly in any two barrels. **No two rifled barrels, even those manufactured in succession, will have identical striation markings.** These striations form the individual characteristics of the barrel.

As the bullet passes through the barrel, its surface is impressed with the rifled markings of the barrel. The bullet emerges from the barrel carrying the impressions of the bore's interior surface; these impressions reflect both the class and individual characteristics of the barrel (see Figure 14-5). Because

Figure 14-5. A bullet is impressed with the rifling markings of the barrel after it emerges from the weapon. *Courtesy* New Jersey State Police.

there is no practical way of making a direct comparison between the markings on the fired bullet and those found within a barrel, the examiner must obtain test bullets fired through the suspect barrel for comparison. In order to prevent damage to the test bullet's markings and to facilitate the bullet's recovery, test firings are normally made into a recovery box filled with cotton or into a water tank.

The number of lands and grooves, and their direction of twist, are obvious points of comparison during the initial stages of the examination. Any differences in these class characteristics will immediately serve to eliminate the possibility that both bullets traveled through the same barrel. A bullet having five lands and grooves could not possibly have been fired from a weapon of like caliber having six lands and grooves, nor could one having a right twist have come through a barrel impressed with a left twist. Once it has been ascertained that both bullets carry the same class characteristics, the effort must begin to match the striated markings on both bullets. It is an effort that can only be made with the assistance of the comparison microscope (see Chapter 7).

It is no coincidence that modern firearms identification began with the development and utilization of the comparison microscope. This instrument is the single most important tool at the disposal of the firearms examiner. The test and evidence bullets are mounted on cylindrical adjustable holders beneath the objective lenses of the microscope, each pointing in the same direction (see Figure 14-6). Both bullets are observed simultaneously within the same field of view, and the examiner rotates one bullet until a well-defined land or groove comes into view. Once the striation markings are located, the other bullet is rotated until a matching region is found. Not only must the lands and grooves of the test and evidence bullet have identical widths, but the longitudinal striations on each must coincide. When a matching area is located, the two bullets are simultaneously rotated to obtain additional matching areas around the periphery of the bullets. Figure 14-7 shows a typical photomicrograph of a bullet match as viewed under a comparison microscope.

Unfortunately, the firearms examiner rarely encounters a situation in which a perfect match exists all around the bullet's periphery. The presence of grit and rust can to some degree alter the markings on bullets fired through the same barrel. More commonly, recovered evidence bullets may become so mutilated and distorted on impact as to yield only a small area with intact markings. Furthermore, striation markings on a barrel are not permanent structures; they are subject to continuing change and alteration through wear as succeeding bullets traverse the length of the barrel. Fortunately, in most cases, these changes are not dramatic ones and will not prevent the matching of two bullets fired by the same weapon. As with fingerprint comparison, there are no hard and fast rules governing the minimum number of points required for a bullet comparison. The final opinion must be based upon the judgment, experience, and knowledge of the expert.

Figure 14-6. Bullet holder beneath the objective lens of a comparison microscope. *Courtesy* Ernst Leitz.

Frequently, the firearms examiner is presented with a spent bullet without any accompanying suspect weapon and is requested to provide information with regard to the caliber and possible make of the weapon. If a bullet appears not to have lost its metal, its weight may be one factor in determining its caliber. In some instances, the number of lands and grooves, the direction of twist, and the width of lands and grooves are useful class characteristics for eliminating certain makes of weapons from consideration. For example, a bullet that has 5 lands and grooves and twists to the right could not come from a weapon manufactured by Colt because Colts are not manufactured with these class characteristics. Sometimes a bullet will have rifling

Figure 14-7. Photomicrograph of two bullets through a comparison microscope. Test bullet is on the right; the questioned bullet is on the left. *Courtesy* Philadelphia Police Dept. Laboratory.

marks that set it apart from most other manufactured weapons, as in the case of Marlin rifles. These weapons are rifled by a technique known as "microgrooving," and may have 8 to 24 grooves impressed into their barrels; few other weapons are manufactured in this fashion. In most cases, however, the firearms examiner will be more successful at eliminating a weapon from consideration rather than identifying a weapon's make or model solely from class characteristics.

Unlike rifled firearms, a shotgun has a smooth barrel. It therefore follows that projectiles passing through a shotgun barrel will not be impressed with any characteristic markings that can later be related back to the weapon. Shotguns generally fire small lead balls or pellets contained within a shotgun shell (see Figure 14-8). A paper or plastic wad pushes the pellets through the barrel upon ignition of the cartridge's powder charge. By weighing and measuring the diameter of the shot recovered at a crime scene, the examiner can usually determine the size of shot used in the shotshell. The size and shape of the recovered wad may also reveal the gauge of the shotgun used and, in some instances, indicate the manufacturer of the fired shotshell.

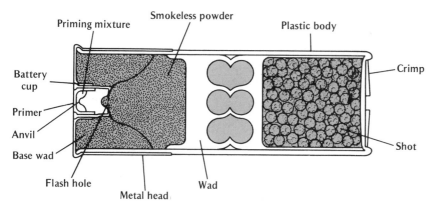

Figure 14-8. Cross section of a loaded shotgun shell.

The diameter of the shotgun barrel is expressed by the term *gauge*.[1] The higher the gauge number, the smaller the barrel's diameter. For example, a 10-gauge shotgun has a bore diameter of 0.775 inches as contrasted to 0.662 inches for a 16-gauge shotgun. The exception to this rule is the .410-gauge shotgun, which refers to a barrel .410 inches in diameter.

CARTRIDGE CASES

The act of pulling a trigger serves to release the weapon's firing pin, causing it to strike the primer, which in turn ignites the powder. The expanding gases generated by the burning gunpowder propel the bullet forward through the barrel, simultaneously pushing the spent cartridge case or shell back with equal force against the breechblock. As the bullet is marked by its passage through the barrel, the shell is also impressed with markings by its contact with the metal surfaces of the weapon's firing and loading mechanisms. As with bullets, these markings can be reproduced in test-fired cartridges to provide distinctive points of comparison for individualizing a spent shell to a rifled weapon or shotgun.

The shape of the firing pin will be impressed into the relatively soft metal of the primer on the cartridge case, revealing the minute distortions of the firing pin. These imperfections may be sufficiently random to individualize the pin impression to a single weapon. Similarly, the cartridge case in its rearward thrust is impressed with the surface markings of the breechblock. The breechblock, like any machined surface, is populated with random stria-

---

[1] Originally the number of lead balls with the same diameter as the barrel would make a pound. For example, a 20-gauge shotgun is one having an inside diameter equal to the diameter of a lead ball that weighs 1/20 of a pound.

tion markings that become a highly distinctive signature for individualizing its surface. Other distinctive markings that may appear on the shell as a result of metal-to-metal contact are caused by the ejector and extractor mechanism and the magazine or clip, as well as by imperfections on the fire chamber walls. Photomicrographs in Figure 14-9 (a) and (b) reveal a comparison of the firing pin and breechblock impressions between evidence and test-fired shells.

Firing pin, breechblock, extractor, and ejector marks may also be impressed onto the surface of the brass portion of shells fired by a shotgun. These impressions provide just as valuable points for individualizing the shell to a weapon as do cartridge cases discharged from a rifled firearm. Furthermore, in the absence of a suspect weapon, the size and shape of a firing pin impression and/or the position of ejector marks in relationship to extractor and other markings may provide some clue as to the type or make of the weapon that may have fired the questioned shell, or at least may eliminate a large number of possibilities.

GUNPOWDER RESIDUES

In incidents involving gunshot wounds, it is often necessary to determine the distance from which the weapon was fired. Frequently, in incidents involving a shooting death, the individual apprehended and accused will plead self-

(a)   (b)

Figure 14-9. Comparison microscope photomicrograph showing a match between (a) firing pin impressions and (b) the breechblock markings on two shells. *Courtesy* New Jersey State Police.

defense as the motive for the attack. Such claims are fertile grounds for firing-distance determinations because finding the proximity of the parties involved in the incident is necessary to establish the true facts of the incident. Similarly, a careful examination of the wounds of suicide victims usually reveals characteristics associated with a very close-range gunshot wound. The absence of such characteristics is a strong indication that the wound was not self-inflicted and signals the possibility of foul play.

Modern ammunition is propelled toward a target by the expanding gases created by the ignition of smokeless powder or nitrocellulose in a cartridge. Under ideal circumstances, it would be expected that all of the powder would be consumed in the process and would be converted into the rapidly expanding gases. However, in practice this is not the case because the powder is never totally burned. When a firearm is discharged, unburned and partially burned particles of gunpowder in addition to smoke are propelled out of the barrel along with the bullet toward the target. If the muzzle of the weapon is sufficiently close, these products will be deposited onto the target. It is the distribution of gunpowder particles and other discharge residues around the bullet hole that permits an assessment of the distance from which a handgun or rifle was fired.

The accuracy of a distance determination varies according to the circumstances of the case. In instances in which the investigator is unable to recover a suspect weapon, the best that the examiner can do is to state whether or not a shot could have been fired within some distance interval from the target. More exact opinions are possible only when the examiner has the suspect weapon in hand and has knowledge of the type of ammunition used in the shooting.

The precise distance from which a handgun or rifle has been fired must be determined by means of a careful comparison of the powder-residue pattern located on the victim's clothing or skin against test patterns made when the suspect weapon is fired at varying distances from a target. A white cloth or a fabric comparable to the victim's clothing may be used as a test target (see Figure 14-10). Because the spread and density of the residue pattern will vary widely between weapons and ammunition, such a comparison is only significant when it is made with the suspect weapon and ammunition, or ammunition of the same type and make. By comparing the test and evidence patterns, the examiner may find enough similarity in shape and density upon which to base an opinion as to the distance from which the shot was fired.

Without the benefit of a weapon, the examiner is restricted to looking for recognizable characteristics around the bullet hole. Such findings are at best approximations made as a result of general observations and knowledge that the examiner has accumulated over an extended period of time spent in firearms examination. However, there are some noticeable characteristics to be looked for. For instance, in the case in which the weapon is held in contact with or is less than 1 inch from the target, a heavy concentration of smokelike vaporous lead usually surrounds the bullet entrance hole. Often

(a)   (b)

(c)   (d)

Figure 14-10.   The test powder patterns were made with a .38 Special Smith & Wesson revolver. The muzzle of the weapon was fired at the following distances from the target: (a) contact, (b) 6 inches, (c) 12 inches, (d) 18 inches. *Courtesy* New Jersey State Police.

loose fibers surrounding a contact hole will show scorch marks from the flame discharge of the weapon, and some synthetic fiber may show signs of being melted as a result of the heat from the discharge. Furthermore, the blowback of muzzle gases may produce a stellate (star-shape) tear pattern around the hole. Such a hole will invariably be surrounded by a rim of a smokelike deposit of vaporous lead (see Figure 14-11).

A halo of vaporous lead (smoke) deposited around a bullet hole is normally indicative of a discharge 12 to 18 inches or less from the target. The presence of scattered specks of unburned and partially burned powder grains without any accompanying soot can often be observed at distances up to approximately 25 inches. However, occasionally, scattered gunpowder particles will be noted at a firing distance as far out as 36 inches. With ball powder ammunition this distance may be extended to 6 to 8 feet. Finally, a weapon that has been fired more than 3 feet from a target will usually not deposit any powder residues onto the target's surface. In these cases, the only visual indication to characterize the hole as being made by a bullet is a dark ring, known as *bullet wipe*, around the perimeter of the entrance hole. Bullet wipe consists of a mixture of carbon, dirt, lubricant, primer residue, and lead wiped off the bullet's surface as it passes through the target. Again, it must be emphasized that in the absence of a suspect weapon, the above observations are general guidelines for *estimating* target distances. It must be

Figure 14-11. A contact shot. *Courtesy* New Jersey State Police.

kept in mind that numerous factors—i.e., barrel length, caliber, type of ammunition, and the type and condition of the weapon fired—all influence the amount of gunpowder residue deposited on a target.

When garments or other evidence relevant to a shooting are received in the crime laboratory, the surfaces of all items are first examined microscopically for the presence of gunpowder residue. These particles may be identifiable by their characteristic color, sizes, and shapes. However, the absence of visual indications does not preclude the possibility that gunpowder residue is present. Sometimes the lack of color contrast between the powder and garment or the presence of heavily encrusted deposits of blood can obscure the visual detection of gunpowder. Often, an infrared photograph of the suspect area will overcome the problem. Such a photograph may enhance the contrast, thus revealing vaporous lead and powder particles deposited around the hole; see Figure 14-12 (a) and (b). In other situations this may not help, and the analyst will need to use chemical tests to detect gunpowder residues.

Nitrites are one type of chemical product that results from the incomplete combustion of smokeless (nitrocellulose) powder. One test method for locating powder residues involves transferring particles embedded on the target surface to chemically treated gelatin-coated photographic paper. The

(a)   (b)

Figure 14-12. (a) A shirt bearing a powder stain, photographed under normal light. (b) Infrared photograph of the same shirt. *Courtesy* New Jersey State Police.

examiner presses the photographic paper onto the target with a hot iron; once the nitrite particles are on the paper, they are made easily visible by chemical treatment.[2] In addition, comparing the developed nitrite pattern to nitrite patterns obtained from test firings at known distances can be a useful technique for determining the shooting distance from the target. A second chemical test is then performed for the detection of any trace of lead residue which might be around the bullet hole. The procedure is accomplished by spraying the questioned surface with a solution of sodium rhodizonate followed by a series of oversprays with acid solutions. This treatment will cause lead particles to exhibit a pink color followed by a blue-violet color.

The determination of firing distances involving shotguns must again be related to test firings performed with the suspect weapon, using the same type of ammunition known to be used in the crime. In the absence of a weapon, the muzzle-to-target distance can be estimated by measuring the spread of the discharged shot. With close-range shots varying in distance up to 4 or 5 feet, the shot charge enters the target as a concentrated mass, producing a hole somewhat larger than the bore of the barrel. As the distance increases, the pellets progressively separate and spread out. Generally speaking, the spread in the pattern made by a 12-gauge shotgun is increased 1 inch for each yard of distance. Thus, a 10-inch pattern would be produced at approximately 10 yards. Of course, this is only a rule of thumb; normally there are a great number of variables that can affect the shot pattern. Other factors to be taken into consideration include the barrel length, the size and quantity of the pellets fired, the quantity of powder charge used to propel the pellets, and the choke of the gun under examination. *Choke* is the degree of constriction placed at the muzzle end of the barrel. The greater the choke, the narrower will be the shotgun pattern and the faster and further the pellets will travel.

PRIMER RESIDUES ON THE HANDS

The firing of a weapon not only propels residues toward the target; gunpowder and primer residues are also blown back in the direction of the shooter. As a result, traces of these residues are often deposited on the firing hand of the shooter, and their detection can provide valuable information as to whether or not an individual has recently fired a weapon.

Early efforts at demonstrating powder residues on the hands centered on chemical tests that could detect the presence of unburned gunpowder or nitrates. For many years the "dermal nitrate test" enjoyed popularity as such a test. It required the application of hot paraffin or wax to the suspect's

---

[2] P. C. Maiti, "Powder Patterns around Bullet Holes in Bloodstained Articles," *Journal of the Forensic Science Society*, 13 (1973), 197.

hand with a paint brush. After drying into a solid crust, the paraffin was removed and tested with the chemical diphenylamine. The presence of a blue color was taken as an indication of a positive reaction for nitrates (see Table 11-3). However, during recent years the dermal nitrate test has fallen into disfavor with law enforcement agencies owing mainly to its lack of specificity. Common materials such as fertilizers, cosmetics, urine, and tobacco are all known to give positive reactions that are indistinguishable from that obtained for gunpowder by this test.

Current efforts to identify a shooter are now centered on the detection of primer residues deposited on the hand of a shooter at the time of firing. With the exception of most .22 caliber ammunition, primers presently manufactured contain a blend of lead styphnate, barium nitrate, and antimony sulfide. Residues from these materials are most likely to be deposited on the thumb web and the back of the firing hand of a shooter because these areas are in closest proximity to gases escaping along the side or back of the gun during discharge. In addition, individuals who handle a gun without firing it may have primer residues deposited on the palm of the hand coming in contact with the weapon.

Determination of whether or not a person has fired or handled a weapon is normally made by measuring the amount of barium and antimony on the relevant portions of the suspect's hands. A variety of materials and techniques are now utilized for removing these residues. The most popular approach, and certainly the most convenient from the field investigator's point of view, is to remove any residues present by swabbing both the firing and nonfiring hands with cotton that has been moistened with 5 percent nitric acid. The front and back of each hand are separately swabbed. All four swabs, along with a moistened control, are then forwarded to the crime laboratory for analysis (see Appendix II for a detailed description of residue collection procedures). Another approach involves hand washing by dipping each hand into a plastic bag containing dilute nitric acid.

In any case, once the hands have been treated for the collection of barium and antimony, the collection medium must be analyzed for the presence of these elements. The demonstration of high barium and antimony levels on the suspect's hand(s) is a strong indication that that person fired or handled a weapon. Because these elements are normally present after a firing only in small quantities (less than 10 micrograms), only the most sensitive of analytical techniques can be used for their detection.

Unfortunately, even though most specimens submitted for this type of analysis have been from individuals strongly suspected of having fired a gun, there has been a low rate of positive findings. The major difficulty appears to be the short time that primer residues remain on the hands. These residues are readily removed by the intentional or unintentional washing, rubbing, or wiping of hands. In fact, one study convincingly demonstrated that it is very difficult to detect primer residues on cotton hand swabs that were taken as recently as 2 hours after firing a weapon.[3] Hence, as a matter of policy, some laboratories will not accept cotton hand swabs taken from living subjects 6 or more hours after a firing has occurred. On the other hand, it is interesting to note that significant levels of barium and antimony have been found in washings collected from hands dipped into dilute nitric acid up to 24 hours after firing.[4] Yet, in spite of the time limitations, as noted above, the hand swabbing approach continues to be the most popular collection technique in the United States. It should be noted, however, that both hand swabbing and washing cannot be used to detect firings with most 0.22 rim-fire ammunition. Such ammunition may contain only barium or neither barium nor antimony in its primer composition.

Until recently, neutron activation analysis (see Chapter 6) was the only method available that demonstrated a sensitivity sufficiently high to be suitable for detecting barium and antimony in gunshot residues. However, the necessity for having access to a neutron source and expensive counting equipment limited this technique to a small number of crime laboratories. Recently, the advent of flameless atomic absorption spectrophotometry has changed this situation (see page 145). Flameless atomic absorption has a sensitivity comparable to that of neutron activation for detecting barium and antimony in hand swabs or washings. Furthermore, the instrument can be purchased at a cost well within the budgets of most crime laboratories. As a result of this development, the immediate future promises to see more crime laboratories expanding their capabilities to perform primer-residue determinations on hands utilizing the atomic absorption technique.

A rather novel approach to primer-residue detection has been suggested by researchers at Aerospace Corporation in California.[5] Their analysis procedure requires the application of adhesive tape to the hand's surface in order to remove any adhering residue particles. Microscopic size primer and gunpowder particles on the tape are then located with the aid of a scanning electron microscope (SEM). These particles have a characteristic size and shape that readily distinguish them from other contaminants present on the hands (see Figure 7-12). When the SEM is linked to an X-ray analyzer (see page 169), an elemental analysis of the particles can be conducted. A finding of a select combination of elements (e.g., lead, barium, and antimony) confirms that the particles were indeed primer residue.

The major advantage of the SEM approach for primer-residue detection

---

[3] J. W. Kilty, "Activity After Shooting and Its Effect on the Retention of Primer Residues," *Journal of the Forensic Sciences*, 29 (1975), 219.

[4] S. S. Krishnan, "Detection of Gunshot Residues on the Hands by Trace Element Analysis," *Journal of Forensic Sciences*, 22 (1977), 304.

[5] G. M. Wolten et al., "Particle Analysis for the Detection of Gunshot Residue, I: Scanning Electron Microscopy/Energy Dispersive X-Ray Characterization of Hand Deposits from Firing," *Journal of Forensic Sciences*, 24 (1979), 409.

is its enhanced specificity over either swabbing or hand washing. The SEM characterizes primer particles by their size and shape as well as by their chemical composition. Nevertheless, whether this approach represents a practical alternative to existing procedures remains a question still to be answered.

SERIAL NUMBER RESTORATION

Today many manufactured items, including automobile engine blocks and firearms, are impressed with a serial number for identification. Increasingly, the criminalist is requested to restore such a number when it has been removed or obliterated by grinding, rifling, or punching.

Serial numbers are usually stamped on a metal body or frame, or on a plate, with hard steel dies. These dies strike the metal surface with a force that allows each digit to sink into the metal at a prescribed depth. Restoration of serial numbers can be accomplished because the metal crystals in the stamped zone are placed under a permanent strain that extends a short distance beneath the original numbers. When a suitable etching agent is applied, the strained area will dissolve at a faster rate as compared to the unaltered metal, thus permitting the etched pattern to appear in the form of the original numbers. However, if the zone of strain has been removed, or if the area has been impressed with a different strain pattern, it is usually not possible to restore the number.

Before any treatment with the etching reagent, the obliterated surface must be thoroughly cleaned of dirt and oil and polished to a mirrorlike finish. The reagent is best applied when the polished metal is swabbed with a moistened cotton ball. The choice of etching reagent will depend on the type of metal surface being worked on. A solution consisting of hydrochloric acid (120 ml), copper chloride (90 g), and water (100 ml) generally works well for steel surfaces.

COLLECTION AND PRESERVATION OF FIREARM EVIDENCE

Firearms. The Hollywood image of an investigator picking up a weapon by its barrel with a pencil or stick in order to protect fingerprints is one that must be avoided. This practice will only serve to disturb powder deposits, rust, or dirt lodged in the barrel, and consequently may alter the striation markings on test-fired bullets. If the recovery of latent fingerprints is a primary concern, it is best to hold the weapon by the edge of the trigger guard or by the checkered portion of the grip, which usually does not retain identifiable fingerprints.

The most important consideration in handling a weapon is safety. Before any weapon is sent to the laboratory, all precautions must be taken to prevent an accidental discharge of a loaded weapon in transit. In most cases, it will be necessary to unload the weapon. If this is done, a record should first be made of the weapon's hammer and safety position; likewise, the location of all fired and unfired ammunition in the weapon must be recorded. When a revolver is recovered, the chamber position in line with the barrel should be indicated by a scratch mark on the cylinder. Each chamber is designated with a number on a diagram, and as each cartridge or casing is removed, it should be marked to correspond to the numbered chambers in the diagram. Knowledge of the cylinder position of a cartridge casing may be useful for later determining the sequence of events, particularly in shooting cases, when more than one shot was fired. Place each round in a separate box or envelope. If the weapon is an automatic, the magazine must be removed, checked for prints, and the chamber then emptied.

Just like any other type of physical evidence recovered at a crime scene, firearm evidence must be marked for identification and a chain of custody must be established. Therefore, when a firearm is recovered, an identification tag should be attached to the trigger guard. The tag should be marked to show appropriate identifying data, including the weapon's serial number, make, model, and the investigator's initials. The firearm itself may be further identified by being marked directly with a sharp-pointed scriber in an inconspicuous area of the weapon—e.g., the inside of the trigger guard. This practice will avoid any permanent defacement of the weapon.

When a weapon is recovered from an underwater location, no effort must be made to dry or clean it. Instead, the firearm should be transported to the laboratory in a receptacle containing enough of the same water necessary to keep it submerged. This procedure will prevent rust from developing during transport.

Ammunition. The protection of class and individual markings on bullets and cartridge cases must be the primary concern of the field investigator who is handling such evidence. Thus, extreme caution is to be exercised when a lodged bullet must be removed from a wall or other object. If the bullet's surface were accidentally scratched during this operation, valuable striation markings could be obliterated. It is best to free bullets from their target by carefully breaking away the surrounding support material while avoiding direct contact with the projectile.

Bullets recovered at the crime scene are scribed with the investigator's initials either on the base or on the nose of the bullet (Figure 14-13). Again, the obliteration of striation markings that may be present on the bullet must be scrupulously avoided. If the bullet is badly deformed and there is no apparent place for identification, it should just be placed in a container that is appropriately marked for identification. In any case, the investigator must protect the bullet by wrapping it in tissue paper before placing it in a pillbox

Figure 14-13. Discharged evidence bullets should be marked on the base or nose. When there is more than one bullet, a number should accompany the initials. NEVER mark bullets on the side.

or an envelope for shipment to the crime laboratory. In handling the bullet, the investigator should be conscious of the possibility that minute traces of evidence, i.e., paint and fibers, may be adhering to the bullet. Care must be taken to leave these trace materials intact. Similarly, a fired casing must be identified in a manner that will avoid the destruction of marks impressed on it from the weapon. The investigator's initials should be placed either near the outside or inside mouth of the shell (see Figure 14-14). Discharged shells from shotguns are initialed with ink or indelible pencil on the paper or plastic tube remaining on the shell, or on the metal nearest the mouth of the shell. In addition, in situations where semiautomatic or automatic weapons have been fired, the ejection pattern of the casings can help establish the relationship of the suspect to his victim. For this reason, the exact location of the place a shell casing was recovered is important information that must be noted by the investigator.

In incidents involving shotguns, any wads recovered are to be packaged and sent to the laboratory. An examination of the size and composition of the wad may reveal information about the type of ammunition used and the gauge of the shotgun.

Figure 14-14. Discharged evidence shells should be marked on the outside or inside as close to the mouth of the shell as possible. Discharged shotgun shells should be marked on the brass close to the paper or plastic. NEVER mark the shells where the firing pin strikes the primer.

Gunpowder Deposits. The clothing of a firearm victim must be carefully preserved so as to prevent damage or disruption to powder residues deposited around a bullet or shotshell hole. The cutting or tearing of clothing in the area of the holes must be avoided as the clothing is being removed. As a matter of routine, all wet clothing should be air-dried out of direct sunlight and then folded carefully so as not to disrupt the area around the bullet hole. Each item should be placed in a separate paper bag.

TOOL MARKS

A tool mark is considered to be any impression, cut, gouge, or abrasion caused by a tool coming into contact with another object. Most often, tool marks are encountered at burglary offenses that involve the forcible entry into a building or safe. Generally, these marks occur in the form of indented impressions into a softer surface or as abrasion marks caused by the tool cutting or sliding against another object.

Typically, an indented impression is left on the frame of a door or window as a result of the prying action of a screwdriver or crowbar. A careful examination of these impressions can reveal important class characteristics—i.e., the size and shape of the tool. However, they rarely reveal any significant individual characteristics that could permit the examiner to individualize the mark to a single tool. Such characteristics, when they do exist, usually take the form of discernible random nicks and breaks that the tool has acquired through wear and use (Figure 14-15).

Just as the machined surfaces of a firearm are impressed with random striations during its manufacture, the edges of a pry bar, chisel, screwdriver, knife, and cutting tool will likewise display a series of microscopic irregularities having the appearance of ridges and valleys. Such markings are left as a result of the machining processes used to cut and finish tools. The shape and pattern of such minute imperfections are further modified by damage and wear during the life of the tool. Considering the unending variety of patterns that the hills and valleys can assume, it is highly unlikely that any two tools will be identical. Hence, it is the presence of these minute imperfections that imparts individuality to each tool.

If the edge of a tool is scraped against a softer surface, it may cut a series of striated lines that reflect that pattern of the tool's edge. Markings left in this manner are compared in the laboratory through a comparison microscope with test tool marks made from the suspect tool. The result can be a positive comparison, and hence a definitive association of the tool with the evidence mark, when a sufficient quantity of striations match between the evidence and test markings.

One of the major problems associated with tool mark comparisons is the difficulty in duplicating in the laboratory the tool mark left at the crime

Figure 14-15. A comparison of a tool mark with a suspect screwdriver. Note how the presence of nicks and breaks on the tool's edge helps individualize the tool to the mark. *Courtesy* New Jersey State Police.

scene. A thorough comparison requires the preparation of a series of test marks obtained by applying the suspect tool at various angles and pressures to a soft metal surface (lead is commonly used). This approach gives the examiner ample opportunity to duplicate many of the details of the original evidence marking. A photomicrograph of a typical tool mark comparison is illustrated in Figure 14-16.

Whenever it is practical, the entire object or the part of the object bearing a tool mark should be submitted to the crime laboratory for examination. When removal of the tool mark is impractical, the only recourse left to the field investigator is to photograph the marked area to scale and make a cast of the mark. Under these circumstances, liquid silicone casting material or dental plaster has been found to be the most satisfactory for reproducing most of the fine details of the mark. However, even under the most optimum conditions, the clarity of many of the tool mark's minute details will be lost or obscured in a photograph or cast. Of course, this will reduce the possibility that the criminalist could individualize the mark to a single tool.

Under no circumstances must the crime-scene investigator attempt to fit the suspect tool into the tool mark. Any contact between the tool and

Figure 14-16. A photograph of a tool mark comparison seen under a comparison microscope. *Courtesy* Ernst Leitz, New Jersey.

the marked surface may alter the mark and will, at the least, raise serious questions about the integrity of the evidence. The suspect tool and mark must be packaged in separate containers, with every precaution taken to avoid contact between the tool or mark with another hard surface. Failure to properly protect the tool or mark from damage could result in the destruction of their individual characteristics. Furthermore, the investigator must bear in mind that the tool or its impression may contain valuable trace evidence. Chips of paint adhering to the mark or tool provide perhaps the best example of how the transfer of trace physical evidence can occur as a result of using a tool to gain forcible entry into a building. Obviously, the presence of trace evidence greatly enhances the evidential value of the tool or its mark and requires that special care be taken in the handling and packaging of the evidence to avoid the loss or destruction of these items.

OTHER IMPRESSIONS

From time to time, impressions of another kind are left at a crime scene. This evidence may take the form of a shoe, tire, or fabric impression and may be as varied as a shoe impression left on a piece of paper at the scene of a burglary (Figure 14-17), a hit-and-run victim's garment that has come into

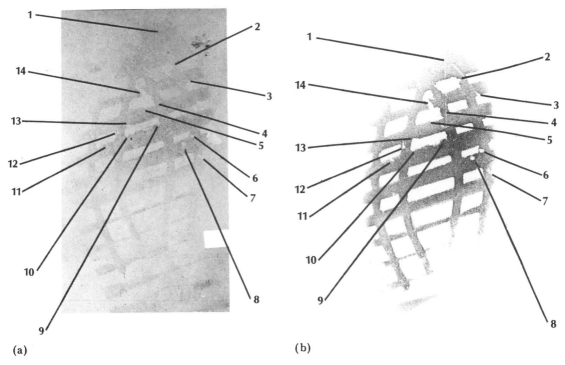

Figure 14-17. (a) Impression of shoe found at the crime scene. (b) Test impression made with suspect shoe. A sufficient number of points of comparison exist to support the conclusion that the suspect shoe left the impression at the crime scene. Both photos *courtesy* New Jersey State Police.

violent contact with an automobile (Figure 14-18), or the impression of a bloody shoe print left on a floor or carpet at a homicide scene (Figure 14-19).

The primary consideration in collecting impressions at the crime scene is the preservation of the impression or its reproduction for later examination in the crime laboratory. Before any impression is moved or otherwise handled, it must be photographed (a scale should be included in the picture) to show all the observable details of the impression. Several shots should be taken directly over the impression as well as at various angles around the impression. The skillful use of side lighting for illumination will help highlight many ridge details that might otherwise remain obscured. Photographs should also be taken to show the position of the questioned impression in relation to the overall crime scene.

Although photography is an important first step in preserving an impression, it still must only be considered as a backup procedure that is available to the examiner if the impression is damaged before reaching the crime laboratory. Naturally, it is preferable for the examiner to receive the

Figure 14-18. A small child was found dead at the edge of a rural road near a railroad crossing, the victim of a hit-and-run driver. A local resident was suspected; however, he denied any knowledge of the incident. The investigating officer noted what appeared to be a fabric imprint on the bumper of the suspect's automobile. The weave pattern of the clothing of the deceased was compared with the imprint on the bumper and was found to compare. When the suspect was confronted with this information, he admitted his guilt. *Courtesy* Centre of Forensic Sciences, Toronto, Canada.

original impression for comparison to the suspect shoe, tire, garment, etc. In most instances where the impression is on a readily recoverable item, such as glass, paper, or floor tile, little or no difficulty is presented in transporting the evidence intact to the laboratory.

If an impression is encountered on a surface that cannot be submitted to the laboratory, the investigator may be able to preserve the print in a manner that is analogous to lifting a fingerprint. This is especially true of impressions made in light deposits of dust or dirt. Here, it is desirable that a lifting material large enough to lift the entire impression be used. One prod-

(a)   (b)

Figure 14-19.   A bloody imprint of a shoe was found on the carpet in the home of a homicide victim (b). The suspect's shoe shown in (a) made the impression. Note the distinctive impression of the hole present in the shoe's sole. *Courtesy* Dade County Crime Laboratory, Miami, Florida.

uct that is excellent for lifting impressions is called "handprint" and is available from the Kinderprint Co., Martinez, Calif. Carefully place the lifting material over the entire impression. Use a fingerprint roller to eliminate any air pockets before lifting the impression off the surface.

Another and more exotic approach to lifting and preserving dust impressions involves the use of a portable electrostatic lifting device.[6] The principle employed is similar to creating an electrostatic charge on a comb and using the comb to lift small pieces of tissue paper. A plastic film is placed on top of the dust mark and charged with a corona discharge or a hand-held probe from a voltage power supply (see Figure 14-20). A charge difference develops between the lifting film and the surface below the dust mark so that the dust is attracted to the film. In this manner, dust prints off chairs, walls, floors, and the like can be transferred to the plastic film. The dust is not permanently attached to the lifting film and the best method for retaining the mark permanently is to photograph it. The electrostatic lifting tech-

---

[6] This instrument is manufactured by Foster & Freeman, England.

Figure 14-20. Electrostatic lifting of a dust impression off a carpet. *Courtesy* New Jersey State Police.

nique is particularly helpful in recovering barely visible dust prints off colored surfaces.

When shoe and tire marks are impressed into soft earth at a crime scene, their preservation is best accomplished by photography and casting. Class I dental stone and plaster of Paris are two forms of gypsum which can be used for making casts of shoe and tire impressions.[7] The cast should be allowed to air-dry for 24 to 48 hours before it is shipped to the forensic science laboratory for examination. If soil or debris from the impression area is adhering to the cast, no attempt should be made at the crime scene to clean it. An aerosol product known as Snow-Print-Wax is available for casting snow impressions.[8] The recommended procedure is to spray three light coats of the wax at an interval of 1 to 2 minutes between layers, and then let it dry for 10 minutes. A viscous mixture of Class I dental stone or plaster of Paris is then poured onto the wax-coated impression. After the casting material has hardened, the cast can be removed.

Whatever the circumstances, the laboratory procedures used for examining any type of impression remain the same. Of course, a comparison is only possible when an item suspected of having made the impression is recovered. Test impressions may be necessary to compare the characteristics of the suspect item with the evidence impression. The evidential value of the impression will be determined by the number of class and individual char-

---

[7] W. J. Bodziak, "Shoe and Tire Impression Evidence," *FBI Law Enforcement Bulletin*, 53 (7) (1984), 3.

[8] Available from Kinderprint Co., P.O. Box 16, Martinez, Calif. 94553.

acteristics that the examiner finds. Agreement with respect to size, shape, or design may permit the conclusion that the impression *could* have been made by a particular shoe, tire, or garment; however, one cannot entirely exclude other possible sources from having the same class characteristics. More significant is the existence of individual characteristics arising out of wear, cuts, gouges, or other damage. A sufficient number or the uniqueness of such points of comparison will support a finding that both the evidence and test impressions originated from one and only one source.

In situations where tire tread impressions are left at a crime scene, the laboratory can examine the design of the impression and possibly determine the style and/or manufacturer of the tire. This may be particularly helpful to investigators in situations where a suspect tire has not yet been located.

Human bite mark impressions on skin and foodstuffs have proven to be important items of evidence for convicting defendants in a number of homicide and rape cases in recent years. If a sufficient number of points of similarity between test and suspect marks are present, a forensic odontologist may conclude that a bite mark was made by one particular individual.

In one case illustrative of the value of bite marks, a wad of used chewing gum was found at a murder site.[9] Examination of the gum revealed the presence of teeth marks. Dental impressions of the victim and two suspects arrested in connection with the murder were then taken. From these, a forensic odontologist was able to make test impressions in silicone for comparison to the chewing gum. Sufficient points of similarity existed to allow the examiner to eliminate the victim and one suspect and to conclude that the gum had been imprinted by the second suspect's teeth.

Tests were also undertaken to determine the blood type of the individual who had chewed the gum. Laboratory tests on the saliva residues on the gum showed that it had been chewed by a secretor with the blood type AB. This type appears in approximately 4 percent of the population and coincided with the blood type of the same suspect selected above.

There was no trial in this case because shortly after these findings were established, a guilty plea of murder was entered by the suspect.

REVIEW QUESTIONS

1. The _____ is the original part of the bore left after rifling grooves are formed.
2. The diameter of the gun barrel is known as its _____.
3. The number of lands and grooves is a(n) (class, individual) characteristic of a barrel.

---

[9] H. D. Sperber, "Chewing Gum—An Unusual Clue in a Recent Homicide Investigation," *Journal of Forensic Sciences*, 23 (1978), 792.

4. The (individual, class) characteristics of a rifled barrel are formed by striations impressed into the barrel's surface.

5. The single most important instrument for comparing bullets is the _____.

6. If bullets were fired in succession from the same weapon, all the individual characteristics would always be identical. (True, False)

7. It is (always, sometimes) possible to determine the make of a weapon by examining a bullet it fired.

8. A shotgun has a (rifled, smooth) barrel.

9. The diameter of a shotgun barrel is expressed by the term _____.

10. Shotgun pellets can be individualized to a single weapon. (True, False)

11. A cartridge case (can, cannot) be individualized to a single weapon.

12. The shape of the indentation caused by the firing pin may be a characteristic peculiar to a firearm. (True, False)

13. The distribution of gunpowder particles and other discharge residues around a bullet hole permits an approximate determination of the distance from which the gun was fired. (True, False)

14. Without the benefit of a weapon, an examiner can make an exact determination of firing distance. (True, False)

15. A halo of vaporous lead (smoke) deposited around a bullet hole is normally indicative of a discharge _____ to _____ inches from the target.

16. An _____ photograph may help visualize gunpowder deposits around a target.

17. One test method for locating powder residues involves transferring particles embedded on the target surface to chemically treated photographic paper. (True, False)

18. As a rule of thumb the spread in the pattern made by a 12-gauge shotgun is increased 1 inch for every _____ of distance from the target.

19. Current methods for identifying a shooter rely on the detection of (primer, gunpowder) residues on the hands.

20. Determining whether or not an individual has fired a weapon is done by measuring the elements _____ and _____ present on the hands.

21. Firings with all types of ammunition can be detected by hand swabbings with nitric acid. (True, False)

22. Restoration of serial numbers is possible because in the stamped zone the metal is placed under a permanent strain that extends beneath the original numbers. (True, False)

23. It (is, is not) proper to insert a pencil into a barrel in picking up the weapon.
24. Recovered bullets are initialed either on the _____ or _____ of the bullet.
25. Cartridge cases are best marked at the base of the shell. (True, False)
26. The clothing of the victim of a shooting must be handled so as to prevent disruption to _____ around bullet holes.
27. A _____ is any impression caused by a tool coming into contact with another object.
28. Tool marks compare only when a sufficient number of _____ match between the evidence and test markings.
29. A wear pattern can impart (class, individual) characteristics to a shoe.
30. When shoe and tire marks are impressed into soft earth at a crime scene, their preservation is best accomplished by _____ and _____.

FURTHER REFERENCES

Abbott, J. R., and A. C. Germann, *Footwear Evidence*. Springfield, Ill.: Charles C. Thomas, Publisher, 1964.

Barnes, F. C., and R. A. Helson, "An Empirical Study of Gunpowder Residue Patterns," *Journal of the Forensic Sciences*, 19 (1974), 448.

Cassidy, Michael J., *Footwear Identification*. Ottawa, Canada: Royal Canadian Mounted Police, 1980.

Davis, J., *Tool Marks, Firearms and the Striagraph*. Springfield, Ill.: Charles C. Thomas, Publisher, 1958.

Kirk, Paul L., *Crime Investigation*, 2nd ed. John I. Thornton, ed. New York: John Wiley & Sons, 1974.

Kinard, W. D., and C. R. Midkiff, Jr., "Developments in Firearms Residue Detection," in *Forensic Science*, 2nd ed., G. Davies, ed. Washington, D.C.: American Chemical Society, 1986.

Krishnan, S. S., "Detection of Gunshot Residue: Present Status," in *Forensic Science Handbook*, R. Saferstein, ed. Englewood Cliffs, N.J.: Prentice-Hall, Inc., 1982.

Moenssens, A. A., F. E. Inbau and J. E. Starrs, *Scientific Evidence in Criminal Cases*, 3rd ed., Mineola, N.Y.: Foundation Press, 1986.

Rowe, Walter F., "Firearms Identification," in *Forensic Science Handbook*, Vol. 2, R. Saferstein, ed. Englewood Cliffs, N.J.: Prentice-Hall, Inc., 1987.

Treptow, Richard S., *Handbook of Methods for the Restoration of Obliterated Serial Numbers*, National Aeronautics and Space Administration Contract Report CR-135322. Washington, D.C.: NASA, 1978.

Wilhelm, Russell M., "General Consideration of Firearms Identification and Ballistics," in *Medicolegal Investigation of Death*, 2nd ed., Werner U. Spitz and Russell S. Fisher, eds. Springfield, Ill.: Charles C. Thomas, Publisher, 1980.

AUDIOVISUAL PRESENTATIONS

Comparative Micrography (filmstrip and audio tape). Robert J. Brady Co., Inc., Bowie, Md.

15

Document and Voice Examination

Ordinarily, the work of the document examiner involves the examination of handwriting and typewriting to ascertain the source or authenticity of a questioned document. However, document examination is not restricted to a mere visual comparison of words and letters. The document examiner must know how to utilize the techniques of microscopy, photography, and even such analytical methods as chromatography to uncover successfully all efforts, both brazen and subtle, designed to change the content or meaning of a document. Alterations of documents through overwritings, erasures, or the more obvious crossing out of words must be recognized and be characterized by the examiner as efforts intended to alter or obscure the original meaning of a document. It is the special skills of the document examiner that are relied upon to reconstruct the written contents of charred or burned paper, or to uncover the meaning of indented writings found on a paper pad after the top sheet has been removed.

Any object that contains handwritten or typewritten markings whose source or authenticity is in doubt may be referred to as a "questioned document." Such a broad definition certainly covers all of the written and printed materials that are normally encountered in our daily, social, and business activities. Letters, checks, drivers' licenses, contracts, wills, voter registrations, passports, petitions, and even lottery tickets are the more common specimens received in crime laboratories to be examined. However, we need not restrict our examples to paper documents. Questioned documents may

400

include writings or other markings found on walls, windows, doors, or on any other objects.

It must be emphasized that document examiners possess no mystical powers or scientific formulas for identifying the authors of writings. Their success is predicated on applying knowledge gathered through years of training and experience to recognizing and comparing the individual characteristics of questioned and known authentic writings. For this purpose, the gathering of documents of known authorship or origin is critical to the outcome of the examination. Collecting known writings may entail considerable time and effort, and their collection may be further hampered by uncooperative or missing witnesses. However, the uniqueness of handwriting makes this type of physical evidence, like fingerprints, one of few definitive individual characteristics available to the investigator, a fact that certainly justifies an extensive investigative effort.

HANDWRITING COMPARISONS

Document experts continually testify to the fact that no two individuals write exactly alike. This is not to say that there cannot be marked resemblances between two individuals' handwritings, for there are many factors that comprise the total character of a person's writing. Perhaps the most obvious feature of handwriting to the layman is its general style. As children we all learn to write by attempting to copy letters that match a standard form or style shown to us by our teachers. The style of writing acquired by the learner is that which is fashionable for the particular time and locale. In the United States, for example, the two most widely used systems are the Palmer, first introduced in 1880, and the Zaner-Blosser, introduced in about 1895. To some extent, both of these systems are taught in nearly all of the 50 states.

The early stages that accompany the learning and practicing of penmanship are characterized by a conscious effort on the part of the student to copy standard letter forms. It is not surprising that many pupils in a handwriting class tend at first to have writing styles that are similar to each other, with minor differences attributable to skill in copying. However, as initial writing skills improve, a child normally reaches the stage where the nerve and motor responses associated with the act of writing become subconscious efforts. The individual's writing now begins to take on innumerable habitual shapes and patterns that distinguish it from all others. It is precisely these unique writing traits that the document examiner looks for.

The unconscious handwriting of two different individuals can never be duplicated. Individual variations associated with mechanical, physical, and mental functions make it extremely unlikely that all these factors can be exactly reproduced by any two people. Thus, variations are expected in angularity, slope, speed, pressure, letter and word spacings, relative dimensions of letters, connections, pen movement, writing skill, and finger dexterity. Furthermore, many other factors besides pure handwriting characteristics are to be considered. The arrangement of the writing on the paper may be as distinctive as the writing itself. Margins, spacings, crowding, insertions, and alignment are all results of personal habits. Spelling, punctuation, phraseology, and grammar can be personal, and if so, combine to individualize the writer.

In a problem involving the authorship of handwriting, all characteristics of both the known and questioned documents must be considered and compared. Dissimilarities between the two writings are a strong indication of two writers, unless these differences can logically be accounted for by the fact surrounding the preparation of the documents. Because any single characteristic, even the most unique one, may be found in the handwriting of other individuals, no one single handwriting characteristic can by itself be taken as basis for a positive comparison. The final conclusion must be based on a sufficient number of common characteristics between the known and questioned writings to effectively preclude the change of their having originated from two different sources.

What constitutes a sufficient number of personal characteristics? Here again, there are no hard and fast rules for making such a determination. This is a judgment that can only be made by the expert examiner in the context of each particular case.

When the examiner is presented with a reasonable amount of known handwriting for comparison, there is usually little difficulty in finding sufficient evidence to determine the source of a questioned document. Frequently, however, circumstances may prevent a positive conclusion, or may only permit the expression of a qualified opinion. Such situations usually develop when an insufficient number of known writings are made available for comparison. Although nothing may be found that definitely points to the questioned and known handwriting being of a different origin, there may not be enough personal characteristics present in the known writings that are consistent with the questioned materials.

Difficulties may also arise when the examiner is presented with questioned writings containing only a few words, all deliberately written in a crude unnatural form, or all very carefully written and thought out so as to disguise the writer's natural style—this is a situation usually encountered with threatening or obscene letters. It is extremely difficult to compare a handwriting that has been very carefully prepared to a document written with such little thought for structural details that it only contains the subconscious writing habits of the writer. However, although it may be relatively easy to change one's writing habits for a few words or sentences, the task of maintaining such an effort grows more difficult with each additional word. When there is an adequate amount of writing available to the examiner, the attempt at total disguise may fail. This was illustrated in the attempt by Clifford Irving to forge letters in the name of the late industrialist Howard Hughes in order to obtain lucrative publishing contracts for Hughes's life story. Figure 15-1 shows the forged signatures of Howard Hughes along with Clifford Irving's known writings. By comparing these signatures, document examiner R. A. Cabbane of the U.S. Postal Inspection Service detected many examples of Irving's personal characteristics in the forged signatures. For example, note the formation of the letter *r* in the word *Howard* on lines 1 and 3, as compared with the composite on line 6. Observe the manner in which the terminal stroke of the letter *r* has a tendency to terminate with a little curve at the baseline of writing on Irving's writing and the forgery. Notice the way the bridge of the *w* drops in line 1 and also in line 6. Also, observe the similarity in the formation of the letter *g* as it appears on line 1 as compared with the second signature on line 5.

The document examiner must also be aware of the fact that writing habits may be altered beyond recognition by the influence of drugs or alcohol. Under these circumstances, it may be impossible to obtain known

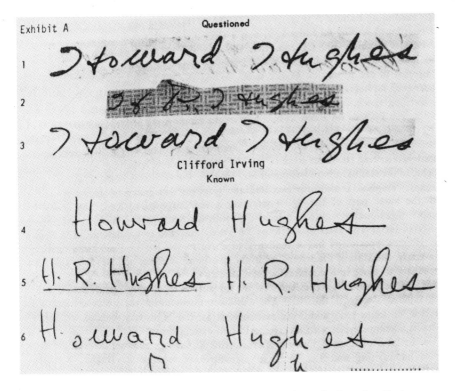

Figure 15-1. Reprinted by permission of the American Society for Testing and Materials from *The Journal of Forensic Sciences*, 1975.

writings of a suspect written under conditions comparable to those in existence at the time the questioned document was prepared.

THE COLLECTION OF HANDWRITING EXEMPLARS

It should be fairly obvious by now that the collection of an adequate number of known writings is most critical for determining the outcome of the comparison. Generally, known writings of the suspect furnished to the examiner should be as alike as possible to the questioned document. This is especially true with respect to the writing implement and paper. Styles and habits may be somewhat altered if a person switches from a pencil to a ballpoint pen or to a fountain pen. The way the paper is ruled, or the fact that it is unruled, may also affect the handwriting of a person who has become particularly accustomed to one type or the other. Known writings should also contain some of the words and combinations of letters present in the questioned document.

The known writings must be adequate in number to show the examiner the range of natural variations in a suspect's writing characteristics. No two specimens of writing prepared by one person are ever identical in every detail. Variation is an inherent part of natural writing. In fact, a signature forged by the tracing of an authentic signature can often be detected even if the original and tracing are shown to coincide exactly because no one ever signs two signatures exactly alike.

There are a great many sources that the investigator can use in establishing the authenticity of the writings of a suspect. One hundred and six common sources of handwriting specimens are listed in Appendix I, "Guide to the Collection of Physical Evidence." An important consideration in selecting sample writings is the age of the genuine document relative to the questioned one. It is important to try to find standards that date closely in time to the questioned document. For most typical adults, basic writing changes are comparatively slow. Therefore, material written within two or three years of the disputed writing are usually found satisfactory for comparison; but, as the age difference between the genuine and unknown specimens becomes greater, the standard has a tendency to become less representative.

Despite the many potential sources of handwriting exemplars, it may be difficult or impossible to obtain an adequate set of collected standards. In these situations, handwriting may have to be obtained voluntarily or under court order from the suspect. There is ample case law to support the constitutionality of taking handwriting specimens. In the case of *Gilbert* v. *California*[1] the Supreme Court upheld the taking of handwriting exemplars before the appointment of counsel. The Court also reasoned that handwriting samples are identifying physical characteristics that lie outside the protection privileges of the Fifth Amendment. Furthermore, in the case of *United States*

---

[1] 388 U.S. 263 (1967).

v. *Mara*[2] the Supreme Court ruled that the taking of handwriting did not constitute an unreasonable search and seizure of a person and hence was not in violation of Fourth Amendment rights.

As opposed to nonrequested specimens (written without the thought that they may someday be used in a police investigation), requested writing samples may be consciously altered by the writer. However, the investigator can take certain steps to minimize attempts at deception. The requirement of several pages of writing will normally provide the examiner with enough material that is free of attempts at deliberate disguise or nervousness to permit a valid comparison to be made. In addition, the writing of dictation yields exemplars best representative of the suspect's subconscious style and characteristics.

Other steps that can be taken to minimize a conscious writing effort, as well as to ensure conditions approximating those of the questioned writing, can be summarized as follows:

1. The writer should be allowed to write sitting comfortably at a desk or table and without distraction.

2. The suspect should not under any conditions be shown the questioned document or be provided with instructions on how to spell certain words or what punctuation to use.

3. The suspect should be furnished a pen and paper similar to those used in the questioned document.

4. The dictated text should be the same as the contents of the questioned document, or at least should contain many of the same words, phrases, and letter combinations as found in the document. In hand-printing cases, the suspect must not be given any instruction on whether to use upper-case (capital) or lower-case (small) lettering. If after writing several pages the writer fails to use the desired type of lettering, he can then be instructed to include it. Altogether, the text must be no shorter than a page.

5. Dictation of the text should take place at least three times. If the writer is making a deliberate effort to disguise his writing, noticeable variations should appear between the three repetitions. Discovering this, the investigator must insist upon continued repetitive dictation of the text.

6. Signature exemplars can best be obtained when the suspect is required to combine other writings with a signature. For example, instead of compiling a set of signatures alone, the writer might be asked to fill out completely 20 to 30 separate checks or receipts, each of which includes a signature.

7. Before requested exemplars are taken from the suspect, a document examiner should be consulted and shown the questioned specimens.

---

[2] 410 U.S. 19 (1973).

TYPEWRITING COMPARISONS

The most common mechanical writing device the document examiner encounters is the typewriter. The two requests most often made of the examiner in connection with the examination of these machines are: (1) Can the make and model of the typewriter used to type the questioned document be identified? and (2) Can a particular suspect typewriter be identified as having prepared the questioned document?

To answer the first request, the examiner must have access to a complete reference collection of past and present typefaces used by typewriter manufacturers. The two most popular typeface sizes are *pica* (ten letters to the inch) and *elite* (twelve letters to the inch). Although there may be a dozen manufacturers utilizing a pica or an elite typeface, many of these are readily distinguishable when a comparison is made of the individual type character's style, shape, and size.

As is true for any mechanical device, use of a typewriter will result in wear and damage to the machine's moving parts. These changes will occur in a fashion that is both random and irregular, thereby imparting individual characteristics to the typewriter. Variations in vertical and horizontal alignment (characters are too high or low or too far left or right of their correct position) and perpendicular misalignment of characters (characters leaning to the left or to the right), as well as defects in each typeface, are most valuable for proving the identity of a typewriter (see Figure 15-2).

The method of associating a particular typewriter with a typewritten document requires the comparison of the questioned document to exemplars prepared from the suspect typewriter. As with handwriting, the collection of proper standards is the foundation of such comparisons. In this respect, it is

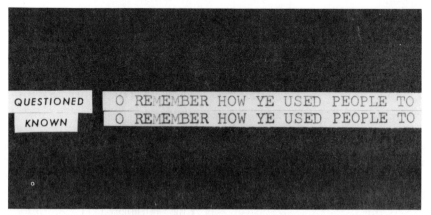

QUESTIONED   O REMEMBER HOW YE USED PEOPLE TO
KNOWN   O REMEMBER HOW YE USED PEOPLE TO

Figure 15-2. A portion of a typewriting comparison points to the conclusion that the same machine typed both specimens. Besides the similarity in the design and size of type, note the light impression consistently made by *M*. Also *E* slants to the right almost touching *D* in the word *USED* in both specimens. *Courtesy* New Jersey State Police.

preferable if the investigator can directly supply the document examiner with the questioned typewriter. This arrangement gives the examiner the opportunity to prepare an adequate number of exemplars as well as allowing for a direct examination of the machine's typefaces. In the case of IBM Selectric typewriters, the problem of securing the entire typing mechanism is made more difficult because of the interchangeability of type-head spheres. Here the typewriter as well as the suspect sphere must be secured for examination.

If the investigator has to prepare standards from the questioned machine, a minimum of one copy in full word-for-word order of the questioned typewriting must be obtained. In preparing standards from a machine with an adjustable touch control, partial copies of the questioned text should be typed in light, medium, and heavy touches, respectively. One point that should not be overlooked by either the investigator or the document examiner is the condition of the ribbon. Replacing a worn ribbon with a fresh one makes a significant difference in the typewritten copy. A lightly inked ribbon tends to emphasize slight defects; a well-inked ribbon is likely to obscure them. If exemplars prepared with the ribbon in use differ substantially from the questioned document with respect to inkings, additional standards that more nearly duplicate the questioned document may have to be prepared after consultation with a document examiner. In addition, samples of each character on the keyboard should be typed without the ribbon. To do this, the investigator should set the typewriter in the stencil position and type directly on carbon paper placed over bond paper. This step eliminates any apparent type deformities that may be caused by the condition of the ribbon.

Another area of investigation relates to the ribbon. An examination of the type impressions left on a ribbon may make it possible to find the portion of the ribbon on which a particular text was typed.

In situations in which apprehension of the suspect typewriter is not possible, the investigator must set about gathering known writings that have been typed on the suspect machine. Ideally, material should be selected that contains many of the same combinations of letters and words found on the questioned document. The individual defects that may characterize a typewriter develop and change as the machine is used; some may have altered during the period of time between the preparation of the questioned and standard material. Hence, if a large quantity of specimens is available, those prepared near the time of the disputed document should be collected.

ALTERATIONS, ERASURES, AND OBLITERATIONS

On many occasions, documents are altered or are changed after preparation so that their original intent may be hidden, or so a forgery may be perpetrated. Documents can be changed in several ways, and for each, the application of a special discovery technique is necessary.

One of the most common ways to alter a document is to try to erase parts of it, using an India rubber eraser, sandpaper, razor blade, or knife to remove writing or type, by abrading or scratching the paper's surface. All such attempts at erasure disturb the upper fibers of the paper. These changes are readily apparent when the suspect area is examined under a microscope using direct light or by allowing the light to strike the paper obliquely from one side (side lighting). Although microscopy may reveal whether or not an erasure has been made, it will not necessarily indicate the original letters or words present. Sometimes so much of the paper has been removed that it is impossible to identify the original contents.

In addition to abrading the paper, the perpetrator may also choose to obliterate words with a chemical erasure. In this case, strong oxidizing agents are placed over the ink, and a reaction occurs that produces a colorless reaction product. Although such an attempt may not be noticeable to the normal eye, examination under the microscope will reveal a discoloration on the treated area of the paper. Sometimes examination of the document under ultraviolet or infrared lighting will reveal the chemically treated portion of the paper.

Some inks when exposed to blue-green light will absorb the radiation and will reradiate infrared light. This phenomenon has become known as "infrared luminescence." Thus, if an alteration is made to a document with ink differing from the original, it can sometimes be detected by illuminating the document with blue-green light and using infrared-sensitive film to record the light emanating from the document's surface. In this fashion, any differences in the luminescent properties of the inks will be observed; see Figures 15-3(a) and (b). Infrared luminescence has also been used successfully to reveal writing that has been erased. Such writings may be recorded by virtue of the fact that invisible residues of the original ink remain embedded in the paper even after an erasure.

Another important application of infrared photography arises from the observation that inks may differ in their ability to absorb infrared light. Thus, by illuminating a document with infrared light and recording the light reflected off the document's surface with infrared-sensitive film, one may be able to differentiate inks of a dissimilar chemical composition. (See Figure 15-4).

The intentional obliteration of writing by overwriting or crossing out is seldom used for fraudulent purposes because of its obviousness. Nevertheless, such cases may be encountered in all types of documents. Success at permanently hiding the original writing will depend on the material that is used to cover the writing. If it is done with the same ink as was used to write the original material, recovery will be difficult if not impossible. However, if the two inks are of a different chemical composition, photography with infrared-sensitive film may reveal the original writing. Infrared radiation may pass through the upper layer of writing while being absorbed by the underlying area, see Figure 15-5(a) and (b).

(a)

(b)

Figure 15-3. A number of checks were stolen from a government agency and altered by an employee. Part of one check as it appears to the naked eye is shown in (a). An infrared luminescence photograph was prepared of the amount figures at a magnification of 10X in (b). This clearly shows that the number "2" was added with a different ink. The accused pleaded guilty. *Courtesy* Centre of Forensic Sciences, Toronto, Canada.

Close examination of a questioned document sometimes reveals crossing strokes or strokes across folds of perforations in the paper that are not in a sequence that is consistent with the natural preparation of the document. Again, these differences can be shown by microscopic and/or photographic scrutiny.

Infrared photography is sometimes successfully used to reveal the contents of a document that has been accidentally or purposely charred in a fire.

(a)

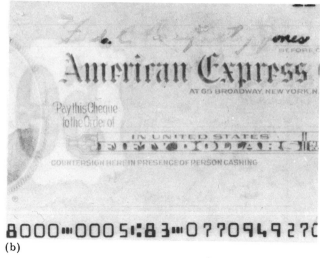

(b)

Figure 15-4. (a) This photograph, taken under normal illumination, shows the owner of an American Express check to be "Freda C. Brightly Jones." Actually this signature was altered. The check initially bore the signature "Fred C. Brightly Jr." (b) Taken under infrared illumination, using infrared-sensitive film, this photograph clearly shows that the alteration was accomplished by the addition of "a" to Fred and "ones" to Jr. The ink used to commit these changes is distinguishable since it absorbs infrared light while the original ink does not. *Courtesy* New Jersey State Police.

(a)

(b)

Figure 15-5. The top photograph (a) shows an area of a document that has been blacked out with a heavy layer of ink overwriting. In the bottom photograph (b), the covering ink has been penetrated by infrared photography to reveal the original writing. *Courtesy* Centre of Forensic Sciences, Toronto, Canada.

Figure 15-6. Decipherment of charred papers seized in the raid of a suspected bookmaking establishment. The charred documents were photographed with reflected light. *Courtesy* New Jersey State Police.

Another way to decipher charred documents involves reflecting light off the paper's surface at different angles in order to contrast the writing against the charred background (see Figure 15-6).

OTHER DOCUMENT PROBLEMS

Indented writings are the partially visible depressions appearing on a sheet of paper underneath the one on which the visible writing was done. Such depressions are due to the application of pressure on the writing instrument and would appear as a carbon copy of a sheet if carbon paper had been inserted between the pages.

In certain situations, indented writings have proved to be valuable evidence. For example, the top sheet of a bookmaker's records may have been removed and destroyed, but it still may be possible to determine the writing by the impressions left on the pad. These impressions may contain incriminating evidence supporting the charge of illegal gambling activities. When paper is studied under oblique or side lighting, its indented impressions are often readable; see Figure 15-7(a) and (b). A recent, innovative approach to visualizing indented writings has been developed at the London College of

(a)

(b)

Figure 15-7. A suspect forger was arrested. In his car were found written lists of the victims he intended to defraud. Some of these writings are shown in (a). A writing pad found in his house had indentations on the top page of the pad (b). These indentations corresponded to the writings found in the car, further linking the suspect to the writings. *Courtesy* Centre of Forensic Sciences, Toronto, Canada.

Printing in close consultation with the Metropolitan Police Forensic Science Laboratory.[3] The method involves applying an electrostatic charge to the surface of a polymer film that has been placed in close contact with a questioned document. Indented impressions on the document are revealed by applying a toner powder to the charged film. For many cases examined by this process, clearly readable images have been produced from impressions which could not be seen or were barely visible under normal illumination.

An instrument that develops indented writings by electrostatic detection is now commercially available and is attracting widespread interest and use by document examiners.

A study of the chemical composition of writing ink present on documents may verify whether or not known and questioned documents were prepared by the same pen. A nondestructive approach to comparing ink lines is accomplished with a visible microspectrophotometer (see pp. 165–167).[4] A case example illustrating the application of this approach to ink analysis appears in Figure 7-9. Thin-layer chromatography is also suitable for ink comparisons. Most commercial inks, especially ballpoint inks, are actually mixtures of several organic dyes. These dyes can readily be separated on a properly developed thin-layer chromatographic plate. The separation pattern of the component dyes is distinctly different for inks having different dye compositions, and thus provides many points of comparison between a known and a questioned ink.

Ink can be removed from paper with a hypodermic needle with a blunted point to punch out a small sample from a written line. About ten plugs or microdots of ink are sufficient for chromatographic analysis. For several years, the Bureau of Alcohol, Tobacco, and Firearms Laboratory in the U.S. Treasury Department has been actively engaged in gathering a complete library of all commercial pen inks. These inks have been systematically catalogued according to dye patterns developed by thin-layer chromatography (see Figure 15-8). On several occasions this approach has been used to prove that a document has been fraudulently backdated. For example, in one instance, it was possible to establish that a document dated 1958 was backdated because a dye identified in the questioned ink had not been synthesized until 1959.

To further aid forensic chemists in ink dating matters, several ink manufacturers at the request of the Bureau of Alcohol, Tobacco, and Firearms have voluntarily been tagging their inks during the manufacturing process. The tagging program allows inks to be dated to the exact year of manufacture by changing the tags annually.

---

[3] D. M. Ellen, D. J. Foster, and D. J. Morantz, "The Use of Electrostatic Imaging in the Detection of Indented Impressions," *Forensic Science International*, 15 (1980), 53.

[4] P. W. Pfefferli, "Application of Microspectrophotometry in Document Examination," *Forensic Science International*, 23 (1983), 129.

Figure 15-8 Chart demonstrating different TLC patterns of blue ballpoint inks. *Courtesy* Alcohol, Tobacco, and Firearms Laboratory, U.S. Treasury Department.

415

VOICE EXAMINATION

THE SOUND SPECTROGRAPH

In this era of telephone, radio, and tape-recorder communications, the human voice may often prove to be valuable evidence for associating an individual with a criminal act. The telephoned bomb threat, obscene phone call, or tape-recorded kidnap ransom messages have all become frequent enough occurrences to warrant the interest of law enforcement officials in scientific techniques capable of transforming the voice into a form suitable for personal identification. To this end a good deal of research and casework has been generated as a result of the development of the sound spectrograph; this is an instrument that converts speech into a visual graphic display.

The sound spectrograph was first developed at Bell Telephone Laboratories in 1941 during research devoted to studying speech signals as they related to communication services. During the years of World War II, the instrument was used to identify for intelligence purposes the voices broadcast by German military communications. Following the war and during his employment with the company, a Bell System engineer, Lawrence Kersta, worked with this new technique and became convinced that voice spectrograms, or "voiceprints," as he called them, could provide a valuable means of personal identification.

Kersta contended that each voice has its own unique quality and character arising out of individual variations in the vocal mechanism (see Figure 15-9). The probability that any two individuals will have the same size vocal cavities (throat, nasal, and two oral cavities formed by positioning the tongue) and will coordinate their articulators (lips, teeth, tongue, soft palate, and jaw muscles) in a like manner is so small as to make the human voice a unique personal trait. According to Kersta, the voiceprint is simply a graphic display of the unique characteristics of the voice.

As a result of Kersta's claim, the sound spectrograph has attracted great interest among criminal investigators. Since 1966, many law enforcement laboratories have purchased the instrument, and various courts have been asked to accept its results as evidence of an individual's participation in a crime. However, at this time, there are still conflicting opinions in the courts as to whether the voiceprint has gained a sufficient degree of "general acceptance" within the scientific community to satisfy the Frye criteria (see page 13) for admissibility as scientific evidence. A detailed report on voice prints by the National Academy of Science concluded that "the degree of accuracy and the corresponding error rates of aural-visual voice identification vary widely from case to case, depending upon several conditions including the properties of the voices involved, the conditions under which the voice samples were made, the characteristics of the equipment used, the skill of

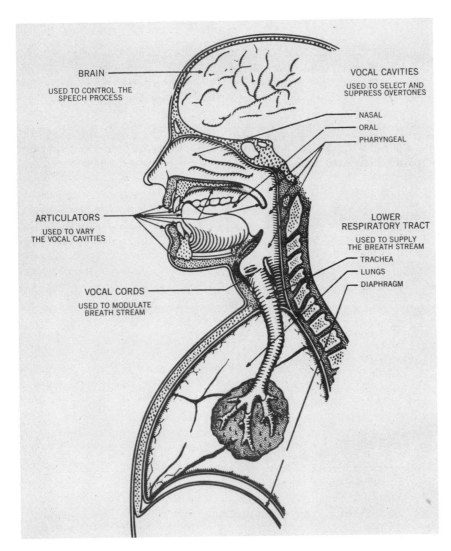

Figure 15-9. Schematic of the vocal mechanism. *Courtesy* Base Ten Systems, Inc.

the examiner making the judgments, and the examiners knowledge about the case."[5]

The sound spectrograph is shown in Figure 15-10. It converts the sound of a voice into a visual display called a *voiceprint*. The first step in making

[5] *On the Theory and Practice of Voice Identification* (Washington, D.C.: National Academy of Sciences, 1979).

Figure 15-10. The sound spectrograph. *Courtesy* New Jersey State Police.

the identification is to obtain tape recordings of both the suspect and known voices for comparison. The magnetic tape containing the message to be analyzed is fastened to a scanning drum that holds a 2.5-second segment of tape time. With each revolution of the drum, a variable electronic filter permits only a certain band of frequencies to be recorded. The selected frequencies are converted into electrical energy and are recorded by a stylus onto specially prepared chart paper. As the drum revolves, the variable filter moves to higher and higher frequencies while the stylus simultaneously records the intensity of each selected frequency range. Upon completion of the analysis, a print is produced that represents 2.5 seconds of tape time and contains a pattern of closely spaced lines showing all the audible frequencies in the tape segment.

Figure 15-11 demonstrates a typical voiceprint. The spectrum portrays three parameters of speech: time (horizontal axis), frequency (vertical axis), and the relative intensity or volume of the different frequencies. Intensity is proportional to the degree of darkness within each spectrographic region. Hence, in this manner, frequency patterns of identical or like-sounding words are obtained from both the questioned and the known voice for visual comparison. When sufficient similarity exists between the two, a positive conclusion is justified that both voices may have emanated from the same person.

The voiceprints depicting the word *you* are shown in Figure 15-12. As an exercise in voiceprint comparison, the reader can attempt to match the questioned voiceprint on the upper left to the voice of one of the five suspects.

Recent notable applications of voiceprint technology have served to increase the public awareness of this technique. For example, voiceprints played a part in Howard Hughes's refutation of Clifford Irving's purported autobiography of Hughes. A few days after McGraw-Hill and *Life Magazine* announced their intent to publish Irving's work, Hughes Tool Company officials arranged for a telephone interview between the reclusive Howard Hughes in the Bahamas and a group of newspaper, radio, and TV reporters

Figure 15-11.   A voiceprint. *Courtesy* New Jersey State Police.

Figure 15-12. Voiceprints of five male speakers uttering *You.* Match the questioned voiceprint on the upper left to the voiceprint of one of the five suspects. (The upper left and lower right voiceprints are of the same person.) *Courtesy* Base Ten Systems, Inc.

assembled in Los Angeles. At the request of one of the major TV networks, spectrographic comparisons of the voice from the Bahamas were made against a known sample of Hughes's voice recorded in 1947. The results proved beyond a doubt that the reporters had been conversing with Howard Hughes and not with an imposter. Irving was eventually found guilty of forging the "Hughes autobiography."

In another case, a perpetrator called the police to report that he had killed a woman and to reveal the location of the body. He gave his name as that of an acquaintance. During the course of the investigation, the man whose name was used was eliminated as the caller and the perpetrator was identified through voiceprint comparisons. Based on that identification, the imposter was found guilty and was sentenced to prison.

REVIEW QUESTIONS

1. Any object that contains handwriting or typewriting and whose source or authenticity is in doubt is referred to as a _____.

2. Variations in mechanical, physical, and mental functions make it (likely, unlikely) that the writing of two different individuals can be distinguished.

3. In a problem involving the authorship of handwriting, all characteristics of both the _____ and _____ documents must be considered and compared.

4. A single handwriting characteristic can by itself be taken as a basis for a positive comparison. (True, False)

5. Normally, known writings need not contain words and combination of letters present in the questioned document. (True, False)

6. As the age difference between genuine and unknown specimens becomes greater, the standard has a tendency to become (more, less) representative of the unknown.

7. In the case of _____, the Supreme Court held handwriting to be nontestimonial evidence not protected by Fifth Amendment privileges.

8. When requested writing is being given by a suspect, care must be taken to minimize a _____ writing effort.

9. Random wear and damage to a typewriter will impart it with _____ characteristics.

10. Examination of a document under _____ or _____ lighting may reveal chemical erasures of words or numbers.

11. Some inks when exposed to blue-green light will absorb this radiation and emit _____ light.

12. Handwriting containing inks of different chemical compositions may be distinguished by photography with _____ film.

13. _____ writings are partially visible impressions appearing on a sheet of paper underneath the one on which the visible writing was done.

14. Many ink dyes can be separated by the technique of _____ chromatography.

15. The _____ was first developed at Bell Telephone Laboratories in 1941.

16. The sound spectrograph converts sound into a visual display called a
    _____ .

17. Presently, voices analyzed by the sound spectrograph have been widely
    accepted as evidence in United States courts. (True, False)

FURTHER REFERENCES

Brohier, Geoffry, "Document Examination," in *An Introduction to Modern Criminal Investigations*, S. S. Krishnan, ed. Springfield, Ill.: Charles C. Thomas, Publisher, 1978.

Brunelle, Richard L., "Questioned Document Examination," in *Forensic Science Handbook*, R. Saferstein, ed. Englewood Cliffs, N.J.: Prentice-Hall, Inc., 1982.

Brunelle, Richard L., and Robert W. Reed, *Forensic Examination of Ink and Paper*. Springfield, Ill.: Charles C. Thomas, Publisher, 1984.

Crown, D. A., R. L. Brunelle, and A. A. Cantu, "The Parameters of Ballpen Ink Examination," *Journal of Forensic Sciences*, 21 (1976), 917.

Harrison, W. R., *Suspect Documents*. New York: Praeger, 1958.

Hilton, Ordway, *Scientific Examination of Questioned Documents, rev. ed.* New York: Elsevier North-Holland, Inc., 1982.

Moenssens, André A., and Fred E. Inbau, *Scientific Evidence in Criminal Cases*, 2nd ed. Mineola, N.Y.: Foundation Press, 1978.

On the Theory and Practice of Voice Identification. Washington, D.C.: National Academy of Sciences, 1979.

Tosi, Oscar, *Voice Identification: Theory and Legal Applications*. Baltimore, Md.: University Park Press, 1979.

AUDIOVISUAL PRESENTATION

Questioned Documents (80 35-mm slides and audio tape). Police Science Services, Niles, Ill.

16

The Future

In 1949, Charles O'Hara and James Osterburg, noted authors of criminalistics, wrote: "The present position of criminalistics among the sciences may properly be compared with that of chemistry in the nineteenth century." Certainly the changes that have taken place since this observation was made are nothing short of revolutionary. Forensic science may still have many shortcomings, but it has successfully shed the distinction of being a nineteenth-century science.

Crime laboratories have now become the major benefactors of enormous advancements in scientific technology. Chromatography and spectrophotometry have already had a tremendous impact on forensic methodology. The future promises even more progress. Mass spectrometry, atomic absorption, and high-performance liquid chromatography, among other developments, are rapidly gaining recognition as essential forensic tools. The scanning electron microscope is already enhancing the application of microscopy to the examination of trace physical evidence. An even more promising tool is the scanning electron microscope linked to an X-ray microanalyzer. This combination gives forensic scientists the ability to examine very small samples nondestructively while plotting the elemental composition of the specimen in view.

Not only will the practitioners of forensic science continue to see the development of new instruments and techniques suitable for solving their unique problems, but the old workhorses of the crime laboratory—i.e., the gas chromatograph and the spectrophotometer—are in store for a major face-

423

lift thanks to a revolutionary development in electronics called the *microprocessor*. The microprocessor contains thousands of microscopic transistors, diodes, capacitors, and the like—all hooked together on a quarter-inch chip. The electronic components of a computer that once filled a room can now be reduced to the size of a few microprocessor chips. Already, instrument manufacturers are taking advantage of this development to link minicomputers to many types of analytical instrumentation. This will help to further automate and speed the collection of data in the crime laboratory.

However, the unabated progress of analytical technology must not obscure the fact that the profession of forensic science has reached a critical junction in its history. The preoccupation with equipping a crime laboratory with elaborate and sophisticated hardware has left a wide gap between the skill of the scientist and the ability of the criminal investigator to recognize and preserve physical evidence at the crime scene. The crime scene is the critical first step in the process of utilizing scientific services in a criminal investigation. All the expertise and instrumentation that any crime laboratory can muster will be rendered totally impotent if evidence has been left lying unrecognized or ignored on the ground, or if the evidence has been inadvertently destroyed by careless investigators or curiosity seekers. Yet studies confirm that this is precisely what is happening to evidence at many crime scenes (refer to references 1, 3, 4, 5, and 6 at the end of this chapter).

The theme that there is a need for trained and knowledgeable evidence collectors at crime scenes has been a recurring one throughout this text. Once again this requirement must be reiterated. How is the evidence collector or investigator to gain the skill and appreciation for recognizing the value of physical evidence? The trend of events seems to be one of conceding past failings and acknowledging the need for creating specialists to perform evidence collection functions. In growing numbers, police agencies are training and equipping "evidence-collection technicians" to assist criminal investigators in retrieving evidence at the crime scene.

If this program is to have any significant impact on investigative procedures, immediate steps will have to be taken that go beyond the mere designation of an evidence-collection unit within a police agency's table of organization. The effectiveness of such a program should not be measured by the number of oversized and overequipped mobile vans at the unit's disposal; instead, a staff of dedicated operators and administrators trained and experienced in evidence collection has to be assembled. This unit must be recognized as the essential first step in forensic analysis and must become an integral part, both administratively and functionally, of the total forensic service offered by a law enforcement agency.

The education of evidence collectors and investigators is a very critical factor in improving the quality of the crime-scene investigation. Although continued in-depth training of the investigators by forensic scientists is an essential ingredient for the success of such a program, many agencies, for lack of space, time, or desire, have not implemented this training. It is there-fore gratifying that colleges and universities are emerging as centers of educa-tion for law enforcement personnel. Criminal justice or law enforcement programs offer themselves as viable forums for teaching the philosophy and theory of criminal investigation and forensic science. However, academia must strive to supplement, not supplant, police in-service training. Police administrators now have the responsibility for selecting the personnel to perform investigative function. These administrators cannot abdicate their responsibility to create and foster training programs that will assure the com-petent performance of the investigator's mission.

Whether a college degree will some day be required by all police is still a subject of debate, but the trend is certainly in that direction. Already, nearly 750 higher-education institutions in the United States offer some kind of law enforcement program. It is from the ranks of these students that future generations of criminal investigators and police administrators will be recruited. For the forensic scientist, participation in these programs offers a unique opportunity to teach, develop, and put into practice the philosophy that science is an integral part of criminal investigation.

Of course education alone will not guarantee the success of the criminal investigator or evidence collector. Experience, perceptive skill, persistence, and precise judgment are all ingredients essential to the makeup of the suc-cessful investigator and evidence collector. Combine all these with a careful selection process designed for choosing only those who qualify for this role, and the end result will be a substantial enhancement of the quality of crim-inal investigative services.

I don't want to leave the reader with the impression that crime labora-tories are not being used, or that forensic scientists have difficulty in justify-ing a full day's work. On the contrary, these facilities are overworked and understaffed. Just the demand imposed on them to complete the examination of drug evidence and blood alcohol is enough to inundate and preoccupy all but the larger crime laboratories. Most facilities can barely keep their heads above water and are literally drowning in a "sea" of drugs. Furthermore, the disproportionate burden placed on the skills, time, and equipment of the laboratory by drug and blood-alcohol evidence has had a detrimental effect on the capacity of the law enforcement system to process physical evidence generated by more serious crimes.

The solution to the problem may seem obvious: more people, larger facilities, and, of course, more money. In this respect, the crime laboratories must stand in line with other components of the criminal justice system. For the simple truth of the matter is that skyrocketing crime rates have over-burdened our police, courts, and correctional institutions. In light of public and political outcries, criminal justice administrators have sought programs geared to producing quick and dramatic reductions in crime rates. In this kind of atmosphere, hiring more scientists or buying a mass spectrometer or a gas chromatograph may hardly seem to many to be the best solution to the problem of crime reduction.

I am not advocating a crash program for building crime laboratories, or, for that matter, a crash program aimed at improving the lot of any one segment of the criminal justice community at the expense of the others. The reduction of crime will only come about with a balanced approach to criminal justice, as well as the alleviation of social injustices. In this respect, we must keep the future role of the crime laboratory in its proper perspective while examining the goals and performance that we expect from all components of our criminal justice system.

It must be emphasized to criminal justice planners and administrators that the size and effectiveness of a crime laboratory directly mirror the capability of the investigative agencies that it services. If all or even most of the burglaries, homicides, assaults, rapes, and other types of major offenses were investigated with the thoroughness expected of a proper criminal investigation, the quantity of physical evidence collected would require the existence of better staffed and better equipped crime laboratories.

I need only illustrate this point by observing that the single most important impetus behind the expansion of crime laboratory services in the United States since 1966 has been the large influx of drug specimens. A required chemical analysis of these confiscated materials has made the laboratory's participation in prosecution proceedings mandatory. The criminal justice system, faced with the prospect of unreasonable delays due to understaffed laboratories, quickly moved to expand these facilities in order to keep pace with the ever-increasing number of drug seizures. Unfortunately, this same kind of pressure has not yet developed in relation to the collection and analysis of other types of physical evidence related to crimes just as serious as drug offenses if not more so.

Although the commitment of police to improve the quality of the crime-scene investigation is essential, it must be accompanied by a simultaneous effort to improve the caliber of crime laboratory services. Certainly the thorough collection of crime-scene evidence will necessitate the employment of more forensic scientists to handle the increasing caseloads. However, it would be a mistake for forensic scientists to be lulled into a false sense of security by believing that the tremendous strides made in the development of analytical instruments and techniques during the past thirty years are alone sufficient to meet the needs and goals of their profession. In truth, progress can be expected in the future only if crime laboratories are assured of staffs composed of trained and knowledgeable scientists. Unfortunately, because the rapid expansion of criminalistic services has created unprecedented demands for more forensic scientists, it has become exceedingly difficult to locate, train, and assimilate competent individuals into existing crime laboratory operations.

At present, few colleges and universities offer courses or degree prorefractive index data collected by all of the British forensic regional laboratories are transmitted to a central computer located at the Central Research Establishment, where they are compiled and stored. Forensic scientists at the regional laboratories can now query the computer and receive within minutes the frequency of occurrence of a particular type glass of a given refractive index or a range of indices.

Because the responsibility for providing forensic services is spread among more than 319 independent government laboratories in the United States, the task of accumulating meaningful statistical data applicable to the entire country or to large regions is exceedingly difficult. Future progress will depend on the willingness of all crime laboratories to enter into cooperative programs that will ensure uniform standards of analysis as well as provide for the collection and dissemination of analytical and statistical data.

The FBI's Forensic Science Research and Training Center is a key ingredient in the development of criminalistics in the United States. The FBI has made a substantial commitment to the Center in terms of manpower and equipment. This facility has established a research program concentrated in the areas of biochemistry, immunology, chemistry, and physics. This program is directed toward the development of new methods for forensic science. The research staff interacts with researchers from academia, industry, and other government and forensic science laboratories. Furthermore, the staff also participates in specialized scientific courses offered by the FBI to state and local crime laboratory personnel. These courses have not only improved the quality of forensic science practices in the United States but have encouraged the standardization of many of the scientific procedures utilized by forensic laboratories throughout the United States.

A foundation of cooperation has been laid; much now remains to be accomplished. How successful our profession will be in fulfilling its present and future obligations to justice will be dependent on the skill, dedication, and ingenuity of its practitioners.

FURTHER REFERENCES

Gurgin, V. A., B. Parker, and S. J. Betsch, "Criminalistics: Today and Tomorrow," *Journal of Forensic Sciences*, 19 (1974), 518.

Kind, S. S., "Forensic Science in the United Kingdom," *Journal of the Forensic Science Society*, 19 (1979), 117.

Kingston, C. R., and J. L. Peterson, "Forensic Science and the Reduction of Crime," *Journal of Forensic Sciences*, 19 (1974), 417.

Parker, B., and J. L. Peterson, *Physical Evidence Utilization in the Administration of Criminal Justice*. Washington, D.C.: U.S. Government Printing Office, 1972.

430 *THE FUTURE*

Peterson, Joseph L., *The Utilization of Criminalistics Services by the Police.* Washington, D.C.: U.S. Government Printing Office, 1974.

Peterson, Joseph L., Steven Mihajlovic, and Michael Gilliand, *Forensic Evidence and the Police: The Effects of Scientific Evidence on Criminal Investigations.* Washington, D.C.: U.S. Government Printing Office, 1984.

Saferstein, Richard, "Criminalistics—A Look Back at the 1970's, a Look Ahead to the 1980's," *Journal of Forensic Sciences*, 24 (1979), 925.

Walls, H. J., "What Is 'Reasonable Doubt'? A Forensic Scientist Looks at the Law," in *Forensic Science*, Joseph L. Peterson, ed. New York: AMS Press, Inc., 1975.

Case
Readings

R. v PAYNE

J. M. Cameron, MD, PhD, MRCPath, DMJ

Reader in Forensic Medicine at the London Hospital Medical School

The case which we are about to relate is one illustrating brilliant detective work finally clinched by indisputable forensic scientific evidence. It is our intention to describe the scene and background of this ghastly "motiveless" murder, and then to produce the scientific evidence which triumphantly settled the case beyond all reasonable doubt.

On 23 November 1947, Claire Jacqueline Parvin was born. Twenty years later on 30 September 1967, she married Bernard Daniel Josephs. At 8:05 P.M. on Wednesday, 7 February 1968, after approximately five months of married bliss, Bernard returned home to Flat 15, Deepdene Court, Kingswood Road, Shortlands, Bromley, Kent, where they had lived since 25 October, 1967, to find his bride brutally murdered in the bedroom. She was wearing among other clothing a cerise woollen dress. This had been a Christmas present from her husband in 1966.

Approximately 18 months prior to her marriage, Claire Josephs became friends at work with a young girl who subsequently married Roger John

Reprinted by permission from the *Medico-Legal Journal*, Vol. 40, Part I, 1972.

Payne on 7 October 1966—a marriage which Claire and her mother attended. The two girls continued their friendship by correspondence, Claire getting advice concerning matters in connection with her forthcoming marriage—on one occasion Claire could well have met Roger John Payne. On 7 January 1968, Mrs. Payne visited Claire at Deepdene Court and Roger Payne was shown around the flat when he came to pick up his wife. On this occasion Claire was wearing a brown skirt and green jumper. The significance of this will be appreciated when reference is made later to the scientific evidence of certain fibres found on Payne's overcoat. A week after the visit of Mr. and Mrs. Payne to the Josephs' flat, namely January 15, 1968, Claire Josephs started work as a telephonist at West Wickham. Again the significance of this will become apparent when reference is made to the scientific evidence, for only after this date did Claire start to wear the cerise woollen dress which had been kept in a suitcase since mid-1967 and in which she was found dead.

On the morning of Wednesday, February 7, 1968, Bernard Josephs and his wife Claire had breakfast together before setting off to their respective jobs. Bernard helped his wife tidy up the flat and put away their breakfast dishes and generally tidy up the kitchen. Claire Josephs was driven to and from her work by a girl friend who on February 7 picked up Claire at 9.05 A.M.; both girls left work at 5.30 P.M. Claire dressed in a pink dress, blue raincoat and chiffon scarf, being dropped off at approximately 5.40 P.M. So it would be reasonable to assume that she arrived at her flat at about 5.45 P.M. This was confirmed by Claire's mother-in-law who phoned at 5.30 P.M. and got no reply but when she phoned at 5.45 P.M. she spoke to Claire for 12-15 minutes giving her instructions as how to make a lemon soufflé. This was the last occasion on which Claire Josephs is known to have been alive. As far as Claire's husband is concerned, he finished work in Barking at 6.00 P.M., went to a nearby public house with a friend where he drank until 7.00 P.M. when both men and his friend's fiancée commenced the journey home. At 7.50 P.M. the three went to a public house in Shortlands where they bought six bottles of beer before driving Bernard Josephs to Deepdene Court. His friend remarked that all the lights in the flat were out and, thinking that Claire might be at her parents' address, offered to wait and drop Mr. Josephs there. His offer was declined and Bernard made his way to the flat.

He let himself in, to find the house in darkness. He switched on the lights, and put his raincoat and briefcase on the settee—so far all was neat, tidy and undisturbed. He looked into the kitchen, walked into the hall and then into the bedroom. Switching on the light he saw his wife's legs protruding beyond the end of the bed, the curtains were drawn to leave a small gap. She was lying face downwards slightly turned to the right. He gently lifted her head and saw a ghastly wound across her neck. Horrified, he ran from the bedroom and in a distressed state telephoned his wife's parents, and his own parents, but failed to call the police or ambulance. His father-in-law was the first to arrive and notified at 8.13 P.M. the police and ambulance who arrived at 8.18 P.M. Among the next to arrive at 8.25 P.M. was the family doctor who certified the girl to be dead. It was approximately 10 minutes later at 8.35 P.M. on the arrival of Detective Sergeant Peck that any order was put into practice, for it must be appreciated that before 8.35 P.M. some twelve or more people were milling about the flat, thus reducing the possibility of finding fingerprints or other useful clues. There can be no recrimination or justifiable criticism of Bernard Josephs' initial action on finding his wife.

Det. Supt. John Cummings arrived at 9.15 P.M. to take charge of the inquiry into what was to be his final and probably most successful case. He noted that the flat revealed little or no evidence of disorder or disturbance and there had been no forcible entry. The deceased's right slipper was by the wall between the kitchen and the lounge doors, an indication of its having dropped off while she ran or stumbled. In the kitchen a mixing machine still set at No. 2 was plugged in but switched off at the point. In the bowl a soufflé mixture was partly made with eggs, butter and lemons on the right side, and a recipe lying on the left side. This indicated that she had probably been interrupted by a call at the door. On the draining board was a cup and saucer containing coffee, while on the sill was a matching plate containing six shortbread biscuits taken from a packet which had been broken open and was lying on the sideboard. This suggested to Det. Supt. Cummings that the caller was not well known, hence the more formal offer of a biscuit on a plate rather than from a packet. No weapon was found at the flat but the next morning a "Peerage" bread-knife with a 4½ in. plastic handle and an 8 in. blade with a serrated cutting edge was noted to be missing. Despite diligent and exhaustive searches, the bread-knife was never found.

At autopsy later that night she was found to have fourteen incised wounds in front of the neck, partially undercut from below up, and four stab wounds of the neck—one of which penetrated muscles on the right side of neck through the right side of the base of the tongue to reach the right side of the front of the spine (2nd cerebral vertebra). Over the voice-box were areas of bruising and marks intermittently extending round the neck which in conjunction with fine petechiae were suggestive of constriction of the neck with a degree of asphyxia at or shortly before death. Marks on the right side of the mouth could have been caused by fingernails. If assaulted from behind they would be consistent with having been caused by the left hand, leaving the right hand free. The linear incised wounds in front of the neck were consistent with having been caused by a knife with a serrated edge. The marks could have been caused either by a left-handed person from in front or a right-handed person from behind or by a right-handed person from above the head with the body on the floor. The defence type wounds on the right hand are also consistent with having been caused by a similar serrated knife. Superposition of such a knife on scale photographs and a cast of the right hand showed identical markings, particularly the wound in the first web of the hand and tip of [the] right little finger.

None of the numerous linear wounds in the front of the neck were fatal as they were either partial or full skin thickness extending only as far as underlying muscle. There were four stab wounds directly inwards and slightly upwards in direction, which could have been caused by an assault from behind with the victim upright or above the head if the body lay on the ground. These stab wounds had penetrated the neck vessels with the introduction of air into the circulation with the development of air embolism and subsequent haemorrhage, death being rapid thereafter. The cause of death was attributed to air embolism and haemorrhage due to wounds of the neck. Taking into consideration the various factors the time of death would centre on 7.15 P.M. approximately. There was no evidence of a sexual assault.

As there had been no forcible entry to the flat, inquiries were concentrated on relatives, friends and acquaintances who could have been entertained by Mrs. Josephs. This necessitated long and laborious routine inquiry which eventually resulted in Roger John Payne being interviewed for the first time on February 12. Payne was a 26-year-old bank clerk living near Maidstone, Kent. When seen there were numerous scratches on both his hands and a bruise on his forehead. He alleged they had been produced by his wife during a quarrel over a cat on Sunday, February 4. On February 7 Payne had to appear in London for a medical examination and interview in connection with his work. He commenced work at 9 A.M., left at 11.30 A.M., changed into a newly pressed suit straight from the cleaners and drove in his motor car (a pale blue Morris 1100) to London for his medical examination. At about 3.30 P.M. he left his interview and went to an address in Sutton arriving about 4.20 P.M. and leaving about 5.15 P.M. He next apparently went to a fish and chip shop, although no evidence to support this statement could be found, before driving to his mother's home (approximately 2¼ miles away). On the way his car broke down and whilst repairing it the bonnet apparently fell on his head. His mother stated initially he only stayed a few minutes between 6 and 7 P.M., although in a second statement he said he arrived about 6.30 P.M. and left about 7.30 P.M. He then drove home and again his car broke down when he alleged he got mud on his overcoat. When he arrived home about 9.15 P.M., his wife saw blood on his head. The next day Payne again took his suit to the cleaners. Payne was arrested on February 24, he appeared at Bromley Magistrate's Court on March 18 and 19, 1968, when the case for the DPP was put by Mr. Nugent, and Payne was represented by his counsel Mr. Gordon Graeme. He was committed to the Central Criminal Court where on May 15 before Mr. Justice Cooke, Payne pleaded not guilty. The case for the Crown was put by Mr. John Bussard,

QC, assisted by Mr. W. Richardson while for the defence appeared Mr. Wilfred Fordham, QC, and Mr. Gordon Graeme. After the defence objected to one woman juror, the case commenced. He was found guilty of the murder on May 24, by a majority of 11 to 1 after a retirement of 3¾ hours, and sentenced to life imprisonment. After the jury had returned their verdict, it was stated Payne had a number of previous convictions. In November 1959, at the age of 17, he was placed on probation for three years at Surrey Assizes for breaking into a girl's house armed with a knife, placing a hand over her mouth and attempting sexual intercourse with her. In April 1965, at Maldon and Surbiton Magistrates Court he was sentenced to 3 month's imprisonment for assault occasioning actual bodily harm, when at 2.45 A.M. he entered the bedroom of a middle-aged woman. He held her by the wrists, placed his hand over her mouth and injured her as she struggled (*Daily Express* 25.5.68).

Leave to appeal was rejected when Mr. Roger Frisby, QC, put his case before Lord Justice Salmon who sat with Lord Justice Megaw and Mr. Justice O'Connor.

Miss Margaret Pereira, BSc

Senior Principal Scientific Officer, Metropolitan Police Forensic Science Laboratory

The Metropolitan Police Forensic Science Laboratory became involved in this case on Friday, February 9, 1968, when clothing and post-mortem samples from the deceased were brought to the laboratory. At the same time, items were received from a suspect who was soon to be eliminated from the case as the result of police inquiries. Contrary to reports in certain newspapers, the dead girl's husband had been eliminated before the laboratory became involved in the case. Three days later, garments were accepted from a second suspect and, on February 13, a number of items were received relating to Roger John Payne. These included a hat, overcoat, suit and a blood sample. There was a request from the police for urgent examination of apparent bloodstains on the hat and overcoat. The following day it was reported that these stains were of the same group as Payne himself and different from that of Claire Josephs. Attention was then given to the clothing of the second suspect and nothing of an incriminating nature was found.

On Monday, February 19, the coffee cup from the kitchen was brought to the laboratory. It was felt that, in the absence of fingerprints, useful evidence might be obtained if saliva on the rim could be grouped. The following day the presence of saliva of Group A was reported. This was of the same group as Payne but was not of great significance as 42% of the British population are of this group. However, on the same day the examination for evidence of contact between the clothing of the dead girl and Payne was started.

It was found that the dress Claire was wearing was of a fluffy woollen fabric and was of an exceptionally bright cerise color. A few fibres exactly matching those of this dress were found on the hat and overcoat of Payne. This information was quickly reported to Bromley C.I.D.

After this, Det. Supt. Cummings asked that the clothing of the deceased should be examined for fibres which might have come from Payne's clothing and this aspect was given special attention. Both his overcoat and suit contained a variety of colours and neither was of pure wool. Because of the variety of types of fibre present in these garments this examination took several days but resulted in the detection, on Claire's raincoat, of a number of fibres which could have come from Payne's overcoat and others which matched his suit. All of the fibres matching these garments were of fairly common occurrence. Because of the fluffy nature of the dress it was unsuitble for examination for contact fibres.

Priority was also given to a man's handkerchief which was found at the flat and was not the property of Bernard Josephs. It was bloodstained and tests revealed the presence of blood of two different groups, AB, MN (Claire Josephs's group) and A, M (Payne's group and present in approximately 12% of the British population). Fibres were also found on this handkerchief matching Payne's overcoat, his suit and Claire's dress. This information was given to Det. Supt. Cummings on Friday, February 23, and it was decided that it was necessary to know the blood group of Bernard Josephs. A sample was obtained and tested that evening and found to be group O, N. Clearly, the blood present on the handkerchief did not originate from him.

Superintendent Cummings said that he intended to arrest Payne on the following day and also to search his house. During the examination of the clothing of Payne and Claire and also of the handkerchief, it had become apparent that there were fibres in all these items which probably had a common source. These were rayon fibres and the majority were plain red and others were combinations and permutations of red, black, pale yellow and blue. It was obvious that these fibres came from a rayon printed fabric in which the background was red. It was therefore suggested that there might be an item of this nature, perhaps a tie, at Payne's home.

On the following Monday, many items belonging to Payne were received. These included several ties, a cravat and a scarf. The latter was in a very frayed condition and was of red printed rayon. The fibres matched exactly with those found previously. In addition, there were eight red wool fibres on the scarf which matched those of Claire's dress. Also amongst the items received was a man's handerkerchief of the same pattern as the one found in the flat. It was however slightly larger but was woven in a similar manner.

Payne's Morris 1100 was also brought to the laboratory. Det. Supt. Cummings thought it highly likely that when the murderer left the flat, he took the knife away with him and disposed of it later. If the person was driving away in a Morris 1100, the most likely place to have secreted the weapon would be inside the pocket on the driver's door. Accordingly, this was the first part of the car to be examined and blood staining was found in the bottom corner of the pocket. It was later tested and found to be of group AB but MN grouping failed. However, in the PGM system, the blood-stain was also the same type as Claire Josephs (PGM 2-1) and the combination of AB, PGM 2-1 is found in approximately one person in eighty. It was apparent that the inner surface of the driver's door had been washed, but very faint human blood staining was detected in various places in the washed area. At a later stage, the debris on the floor of the car was examined and several fibres matching the nylon carpet in the girl's flat were found together with a few fibres matching her dress.

Further work on Payne's clothing revealed a total of sixty-one fibres matching Claire's dress on his overcoat, twenty-two on his hat, six on his jacket and none on his trousers. As previously stated, the suit had been cleaned and it was interesting that the fibres found on the jacket were not lying on the surface but were embedded in the interstices of the cloth. Fortunately, these fibres were brilliantly fluorescent and were easily detected by examining the garments under ultraviolet light.

Twenty rayon fibres matching Payne's scarf were found on Claire's raincoat and eight were present on the handkerchief found in the flat. There was also a single red and black rayon fibre matching the scarf on the left thumb nail of the deceased.

Evidence of these findings was given at the committal at Bromley Magistrates Court, and later Dr. Barbara Dodd attended the Metropolitan Police Laboratory when she took samples of the significant blood stains and subsequently examined them on behalf of the defence. Dr. Julius Grant also came to the laboratory on behalf of the defence and examined all of the fibres which were of relevance. Neither of these two experts gave evidence at the trial.

The trial commenced on May 15, 1968, and on May 17, Mr. Norman Roper carried out a further examination of the fibres on behalf of the defence. Later, he gave evidence at the trial where he agreed in principle with the prosecution witness about the similarity of the fibres concerned but disagreed as to their significance.

From a forensic scientist's point of view this was a case in which Locard's principle that "Every contact leaves its trace" was borne out to a remarkable degree. It was of course a matter of pure chance that there were fibres involved which shed rapidly and were very characteristic as was the fact that the dead girl's blood group was relatively uncommon. However, the possibility of obtaining such evidence of contact purely by chance must be infinitesimal.

THE ATTEMPTED ASSASSINATION OF ARCHBISHOP MAKARIOS: A FORENSIC SCIENCE CASE STUDY

Julius Grant, MSc, PhD, FRIC

At about 7.05 A.M. on the morning of Sunday, March 8, 1970, the President of the Republic of Cyprus, Archbishop Makarios, boarded his personal helicopter in the courtyard of the archbishop's palace in Nicosia, in order to fly to Macheras Monastery to officiate at a memorial service. He sat on the left of the pilot, Major Zacharias Papadoyiannis. The helicopter took off, and when it had attained the height of the Archbishopric, it made a turn of 150 degrees, still climbing. At a point about 10 metres above the roof of the Archbishopric Fig. I-1), a shot was heard from the left and rear, and a burst of machine-gun fire came from the same direction. The Archbishop was not hit, but his pilot sustained a severe wound in the abdomen. With great difficulty in view of his wound, the damage caused to the helicopter and the proximity of buildings and electric cables, the pilot managed to land on an open space on the corner of two neighbouring streets, out of range of the firing (Fig. I-2). The Archbishop and pilot dismounted from the helicopter and ran away from it, having in mind the possibility of an explosion. However, the pilot collapsed and was taken to a hospital where, after a critical illness, he eventually recovered.

The Presidential Guard at the Archbishopric was conscious that the firing came from the roof of the Pancyprian Gymnasium opposite the Archbishop's palace, and they fired in that direction (Fig. I-1). Shortly after the firing occurred, early risers in Thysseos and Othellos Streets, which adjoin the high side wall of the Pancyprian Gymnasium, saw four men climbing over the wall of the school into Thysseos Street. One spectator asked what was happening, but received no reply; he called out to the men to stop or he would shoot them. One then held his hands to his face, and turned back and said to one of the others who was coming up behind him and was holding a pistol, "They are shooting at us." All four then turned into Othellos Street. The spectator and other onlookers then saw the four men board a car waiting nearby and drive off. The first spectator telephoned the police and subsequently identified the car by appearance, although he was unable to note the number. Other spectators were able to provide confirmatory evidence regarding the car, although the evidence of identification of the four persons was weak. However, eventually it seems to have been established that the car was of a light blue colour with a white line and was a Fiat, Model 850, registration number ZDR 320. In the meantime the police had been informed of

Reprinted by permission from the *Medico-Legal Journal*, Vol. 40, Part 2, 1972.

Figure I-1

Figure I-2

the incident. They entered the Pancyprian Gymnasium, and took possession of the firearms and other exhibits found on the roof.

In another part of Nicosia, at a distance of about a mile from the scene of the attempt, a merchant opening his shop at about 8.30 in the morning noticed a self-drive car having the above description. As this had not been moved by 11.30 A.M. he telephoned the police. On Sunday, March 8, the day of the attempt, at 8.30 in the morning, one G. A. Taliadoros went to the Larnaca Road police station and reported that the car which he had hired on February 12 had been stolen from a parking place. His agitated condition and confused replies to questions aroused suspicion, and he was questioned about the circumstances of the theft of his car as well as about his own movements. In due course two associates of Taliadoros were also detained. They were questioned as to their whereabouts at the relevant time, and as their answers were deemed to be unsatisfactory, they were held in custody. Further arrests were made subsequently, and six persons, as follows, were ultimately detained, namely (Fig. I-3):

Adamos Haritonos, 23, student; and associate of Taliadoros
Georghios Alexandrou Taliadoros, 33, estate agent
Antonakis Prokopi Solomonodos, 32, former inspector of police
Antonakis Petrou Yenagritis, 28, police constable
Costas Polykarpou Ioannides, 32, newspaper editor
Polikarpos Antoni Polykarpou, 32, police constable

Monday, March 9, was a holiday and when on Tuesday, the 10th, Maria Constantinou, a cleaner of the Pancyprian school unlocked the toilets, she found below an aperture in the wall two dirty blankets in a heap. One was light grey in colour and the other a darker colour, rather brownish. These also were taken by the police for examination.

The police force acted with great promptitude and efficiency under the direction of Chief Supt. G. Hadjiloizou of the C.I.D. They took possession of the weapons found on the roof of the Pancyprian school and a number of other articles from the school roof, and also the blankets referred to above. At about the same time a shepherd found a cache of arms, also wrapped in two blankets, hidden in a ditch near Nicosia; and these were taken by the Police. They were similar to the arms found on the roof of the Gymnasium and fingerprints were obtainable from them.

Shortly after the above events, I received a telephone call from the High Commissioner for Cyprus in London asking me if I could fly to Cyprus at once; he hinted at the reason. A few days later I attended a Cabinet meeting at the Presidential Palace, where I met the President, and I was formally invited to be responsible for the forensic investigation of the assassination attempt. The resources of the police force and Government Analyst were

Figure I-3

placed at my disposal, and I take pleasure in paying tribute to the assistance
and hospitality I received.

The activities of the police had resulted in the following list of articles
of potential importance to be investigated:

From the school: weapons; two blankets; cigarette ends; button; faecal
matter.

From the arms cache: weapons; two blankets.

From the car: dust from the floor; dust from boot; fingerprints; cigarette
ends.

From the persons detained: all outer clothing; also some 50 articles of
other miscellaneous clothing; dust from a car and blankets from the
homes of the persons detained.

Miscellaneous: revolver holster; newspapers; car cover; etc.

The forensic examination of the above is now dealt with in order of
importance. The jacket worn by Taliadoros, when he was arrested, bore a

smear of white dust on the right shoulder approximately 3 X 2 cm. in dimensions, and similar in colour to that of the whitewashed walls of the school. Taliadoros said that he picked it up while sitting on a bench and leaning against the wall of the police station where he was originally detained. The police had assiduously taken samples of plaster from the walls of the school along the escape route of the gunmen from the roof to the wall of Thysseos Street, but it was apparent that the mark on the jacket was a surface rubbing, and was a top coat of whitewash and not plaster. In view of the importance of this smear and the lack of wholly positive other forensic evidence concerning Taliadoros, I thought it advisable to make a fresh examination of the scene. Surface rubbings were, therefore, first taken from the areas from which the plaster had been removed. An attempt was then made to reconstruct the early stages of the escape after the shots had been fired.

It will be seen from Fig. I-1 that the gunmen must have climbed down from the flat roof where they had fired at the President on to an open air passage flanked on the right by the high whitewashed wall shown in Fig. I-4. Free passage down the area was prevented on the left by the pitched skylights (four in number) which serve the classroom below and which are apparent in the photograph. It was found that the most convenient way of travelling along this passage in a hurry was to pass between the wall and the

Figure I-4

skylight, a distance of only 40 cm. This is too small to accommodate a man facing the direction in which he was running. Indeed there was a natural instinct, I found, to half-turn to the left, i.e., away from the wall, on passing between the narrow gaps. If this was done, the right shoulder did not necessarily touch the wall but, as a runner emerged from the gap, there was a distinct probability that his right shoulder would rub against the square-section vertical drainpipes from the roof, which project from the wall to the extent of about 10 cm. When this happened, a smear could be produced on the shoulder of the same size and type and in the same location as that found on Taliadoros's jacket.

A surface rubbing was, therefore, taken from one of the drainpipes at shoulder level, and it was found that the superficial coating was apparently unlike ordinary whitewash but was consistent with a mixture of whitewash and a white emulsion paint. A likely explanation of this is that it had been found that the whitewash would not cover the metal drainpipe, as well as on the actual wall, and a topcoating of emulsion paint had, therefore, been applied over it. The claim that the smear had come from the police station was easily disposed of, because the bench on which Taliadoros had sat had a wooden back separating the sitter from the wall; and moreover, the whitewash on the wall was not pure white but a pale yellow colour. Below are shown in tabular form the spectroscopic analysis of all the powders collected, from which it will be seen that the powder from the coat and that from the drainpipe matched perfectly; moreover they have no counterpart in any of the other samples, which are characteristic of an ordinary lime wash. The presence of both calcium and titanium is consistent with the use of a paint of good covering power, with the limewash on the pipe; and this occurs also on the coat.

Sample	J	1	2	3	4	5
Aluminum	Minor	Absent	Trace	Minor	Trace	Minor
Barium	Minor	Major	Trace	Minor	Trace	Major
Calcium	Major	Major	Major	Major	Major	Major
Chromium	Trace	Trace	Trace	Trace	Trace	Trace
Iron	Trace	Minor	Trace	Trace	Trace	Trace
Magnesium	Minor	Major	Major	Minor	Major	Major
Silicon	Major	Minor	Trace	Major	Trace	Minor
Titanium	Major	Absent	Absent	Major	Absent	Absent
Zinc	Absent	Minor	Absent	Absent	Trace	Trace

Key
J—Taliadoros's jacket.
1—Landing outside classroom door.
2—Lavatory outside wall.
3—Drainpipe on roof.
4—Lavatory wall where blankets were found.
5—Column at foot of staircase near classroom.

In the course of the hearing the defence pointed out that in Nicosia all the drainpipes of the houses are of this rectangular type, so that the rubbing could have come from one of hundreds in the town. Having foreseen this argument I had spent nearly two hours roaming the streets of the town and rubbing my jacket against drainpipes—often to the mystification of passers-by! Out of many in various parts of the town I found that about 60% were whitewashed, with the whitewash often partly rubbed off, and the remainder were painted with a gloss paint which could not be rubbed off. I did not find one which had the appearance or effect of the drainpipes in the roof corridor at the school. The Court regarded this as significant, according to the Presiding Judge in his summing-up.

Coming now to the two blankets found by the lavatories, these consisted of a grey blanket, torn, with bloodstains and dark stains resembling grease. There was also a brown blanket with several holes, also with dark stains resembling grease. The majority of the fibres comprising it were of wool, and were of a rather unusual shade of brown. The grease stains were extracted, and it was possible to show that the substance present was similar to a type of greasy lubricant in the stores of the Police Department; and that both were similar to the grease on the weapons, which doubtless was used to prevent them from rusting. Infra-red spectroscopy was used for this purpose. There was nothing characteristic about this grease, and this evidence, though contributory, was not in itself conclusive. However, an interesting fact noted was that the grease stains on the blanket and the grease on the weapons, while alike, were completely dissimilar from four other types of oil or grease also kept in the police store. Thus, although the weapons were not police weapons, the grease on them could have come from the police store.

It has been mentioned that bloodstains were found on the grey blanket. These were of human blood. It was thought at first that they were associated with the observation that one of the fugitives seen climbing over the wall had his hand against his face. However, none of the men arrested had any wounds, and examination of the bloodstains showed that they were of the drop rather than of the smear type to be expected from a wound. Medical examination showed no evidence of recent nose-bleeding from any of the men detained. As the stains were old, it was not possible to carry out a grouping test. It was felt that they could have been produced before the relevant date, and this aspect of the evidence was not pursued further.

So far as the weapons found on the scene were concerned, these are shown in Fig. I-1. They comprised a Bren gun, a Lee Enfield rifle, and an M6 rifle; 39 spent cartridges were found, and there were about the same number unused. The only features of importance were the grease referred to above, and fingerprints in the grease. On the weapons were found two prints each having 13 points of diagnostic identity with the right forefinger of Haritonos; one was on the magazine of the Bren gun. On some ammunition was found a print which had 16 points of diagnostic identity with the print from the right forefinger of Yenagritis. On other ammunition was found a print which had 16 points of identity with a print from the left thumb of Solomonodos. On further items of ammunition was found a print which had 16 points of diagnostic identity with a print from the left thumb of Yenagritis. Other prints were found, but were not produced in evidence. On the loaded Bren gun magazine and ammunition found on the roof of the Gymnasium were two prints having 16 points of diagnostic identity with a print from the right thumb of Solomonodos. Other fingerprint evidence attributable to Taliadoros, Haritonos and Yenagritis was found on the car. Some of these were found near the top edge and on the outside of one of the windows; indicating that the door had been pulled shut, using the partly opened window, by the owner of the print who was sitting inside.

In England 16 points of identity are taken as conclusive evidence of the identity of origin of two fingerprints. In Cyprus, in general the courts accept the same standards as in this country. It will be seen that except in one case the requisite 16 points were obtained. In the case of Haritonos only 13 such points per print were obtained, but points from different parts of more than one print from the same finger can be added together to make the necessary 16. It could be claimed that the lack of further points of identity was due to the poor character of the prints found on the scene in this instance and that there were no dissimilarities between the two prints which could not be accounted for in the same way. Solomonodos, who had been a police officer, accepted that the prints found could have been his. Both he and Yenagritis were in the National Guard in 1963-67, and they stated that they had been in the habit of handling arms and ammunition. In mid-1969 the police authorized the collection of arms surrounded by civilians. Yenagritis and Solomonodos claimed to have been involved in this operation; no Bren guns were among the arms then collected. Haritonos was in the National Guard in 1968 and said that he had handled Bren guns within nine months of the assassination attempt.

This gave rise to a lively controversy as to the age of the fingerprints, which is always difficult to determine with certainty. Supt. Dekatris, the capable fingerprint expert of the Cyprus C.I.D., held the view that the sharpness of the prints indicated recent origin. This was contested by the defence, but I felt that I could support the prosecution's argument because the prints were made in grease, which in the hot climate of Cyprus tends to run; and under these conditions fingerprints become blurred rapidly. An experiment in which prints made in grease on metal were kept at $20°C$ and $30°C$ (the summer temperature in Cyprus) for a few days showed a distinct difference in sharpness when developed.

The defence called an expert, formerly of the Greek police force, but he was unable to convince the Court that the fingerprints were old or that the blurring on ageing theory was untenable, especially bearing in mind that at least nine months had elapsed since the alleged handling of the weapons and the discovery of the arms. In any case this referred only to the presence of the fingerprints of Solomonodos and Yenagritis, and not to those of their associates.

Fingerprint evidence was also sought from the cigarette ends. These were found on the scene, in the car, and in the police station after detention. Practically all were of the same make and had been smoked in the same way, i.e., to the extent of two-thirds of their length. They were then stubbed out in a similar way by being bent almost at right-angles. It was hoped that the stubbing-out operation would have left a fingerprint on the cigarette paper, but unfortunately nothing that could be satisfactorily used as evidence was found when we used the ninhydrin test. On the other hand, experiments in which we produced similar stubs did leave fingerprints. The reason for this difference may have been the greater heat of burning in the case of the cigarette ends believed to have been associated with the accused; or because the smoker was one of the few people whose fingerprints do not respond to the ninhydrin test. It would have been interesting to have tested the fingerprints of the six men on paper to check this. A saliva grouping test on the cigarette ends might also have been helpful, but facilities were not available.

Much of the forensic work concerned fibres. The objective was to link the fibres from one or more blankets with one or more of the accused. This applied both to the fibres of which the blankets were made and to adventitious fibres found on the blankets. To this end a large collection from the wardrobes of the six men was seized and thoroughly examined, including the pocket linings—since the latest style in trousers can apparently contain as many as seven pockets! In all some 60 outer garments, including shoes, were tested; also included were contents of cars and blankets from the homes of the accused, which the defence alleged were the source of certain of the fibres found. This was extremely laborious work but was fully justified. The connecting links in the evidence were small in number but important. In my evidence on this aspect I thought it advisable to make clear the significance and limitation of evidence based on fibres. This disarmed some anticipated cross-examination.

In making a comparison between fibres found on a suspect and fibres found at the scene of a crime or on an article associated with it, there are three principal criteria to be taken into account, namely:

(a) the material of which the fibre is made;
(b) the colour of the fibre;
(c) its dimensions, i.e., shape and size.

1. Now, if one has two single fibres, one from the scene and one from the

suspect, and they are alike in all the three above respects, then one can say that the fibres could have come from the same source, but that there is no certainty that they did so.

2. On the other hand if the fibres being compared are unusual in some respect as well as being alike, then the chance that they come from the same source is greater.

3. Finally, if one is examining groups of fibres, i.e., tufts of fibres of different kinds and different colours, then if the two groups contain the same fibres in the same proportions, then the possibility that they come from the same source is very high indeed; but one still cannot say with absolute certainty that they did so.

On the jacket belonging to Taliadoros, which had the white smear referred to above, I found a number of fibres which were not part of the composition of the jacket, i.e., extraneous fibres. On the left shoulder of the jacket was such a brown fibre, which matched closely the principal fibres of the brown blanket found at the scene of assassination attempt. Since this was an unusual fibre, I placed it in category 2 above. This could not be regarded as conclusive evidence because the brown fibre could have come from some other source. However, as stated, the shade of the colour was unusual and it is interesting to note that although some hundreds of fibres from various items of clothing, car dust, etc. were examined, in no case did a brown fibre similar to that from the blanket occur except on the left shoulder of Taliadoros's jacket. It should be added that the police took a multi-coloured blanket from the home of Taliadoros. It contained brown fibres, which were said to have accounted for the fibre on his jacket; there was a superficial resemblance, but microscopical methods showed the fibres to be quite different.

In the right-hand pocket of the trousers of Taliadoros I found a tuft of fibres which was similar to the fibres comprising one of the blankets used to wrap the weapons. Since this consisted of no less than four fibres of different colours and types in each case, I placed this in the third category, representing the strongest possibility of identity.

On a pullover belonging to Yenagritis I found a human hair which was similar to a human hair which I found on one of the blankets from the school lavatory. It is impossible to say with complete certainty that two human hairs are or are not identical. However, these were alike in colour; they were both relatively long, too long for a male hair, even in these days; and I felt that the possibility that they came from the same source was strong. This was another link between Yenagritis and the blanket.

On the left arm of the jacket of Polykarpou I also found a tuft of fibres similar to those of one of the blankets, and the nature of these was such as to put them in the third category, of the strongest possibility. I also examined debris I collected from the body and boot of the car of Solomonodos and here I found a tuft of fibres similar to those of one of the blankets presumably used to wrap the guns. Here again the nature and the proportions of the fibres placed them in the category of maximum possibility.

The forensic evidence established links as follows:

Linking:

>   Arms to blankets—grease.
>   Arms to accused—fingerprints.
>   Blanket to accused—fibres.
>   Scene to accused—white smears (Taliadoros).
>   Car to accused—fingerprints and fibres.

The preliminary enquiry was heard in Nicosia starting April 15, 1970, with Mr. A. Frangos, Senior Counsel of the Republic, for the prosecution. Ninety-five witnesses were called by the prosecution; cross-examination was reserved.

The subsequent trial was held in the assize court room of Nicosia in October 1970. The prosecution was conducted by Mr. Talarides, Senior Counsel, and Mr. Frangos. In Cyprus legal procedure resembles that of England except that there is no jury, the verdict resting with the three presiding Judges. In a small country such as Cyprus this is regarded as a more desirable procedure. Apart from the prosecution forensic evidence, testimony was largely concerned with the actions, behaviour and alleged alibis of the accused. The Defence sought to establish alibis and to prove reasonable doubt as to the forensic evidence, but the combined effect of the latter apparently convinced the Judges. The charge against Polykarpou was withdrawn at the first hearing due to lack of evidence; only that from the fibres being available. Ioannides was acquitted owing to insufficient evidence; he was expelled from Cyprus. The remaining four were sentenced to 14 years' imprisonment in Nicosia and, according to the press, they subsequently confessed that theirs was one of several plots which were due to take place at the time of the attempted assassination and which undoubtedly would have done so had it not been for the prompt action of the authorities. The accused instructed their respective Counsel not to place any factors in mitigation before the Court; Haritonos stated that he did not pray for leniency.

The author is indebted to the Government of Cyprus for permission to reproduce the illustrations; and to Chief Supt. Hadjiloizou for his co-operation in the preparation of this paper.

TEAMWORK IN THE FORENSIC SCIENCES:
REPORT OF A CASE

L. W. Bradford and A. A. Biasotti

*Director and Supervising Criminalist, respectively, Laboratory of
Criminalistics, San José, California*

The scene in which the following events occurred is a single story dwelling in a quiet residential neighborhood where the victim lived. The victim was a 45-year-old woman who lived in the second house on a particular cul-de-sac street next to a red house on the corner (which is of later significance). A street light is situated here.

The investigative events began with the discovery of the victim lying face up over the foot of her bed with the top of her head completely blown off. Tissue debris covered both walls and the ceiling surrounding the victim. The gruesome discovery was made and reported immediately at 2:30 A.M. by an elderly male boarder who rented one bedroom in the victim's house. The boarder had entered the house, using his key, at about 1:15 A.M. after working as a bartender since 4 P.M. the previous day. He went directly to his bedroom and read for about an hour. When ready to retire, he noticed lights in the victim's bedroom and kitchen. Investigating, he discovered the victim. The first patrol unit arrived at the scene within minutes. The patrol officer found no weapon and, after a quick search for a possible intruder on the premises, called for assistance.

The detective team arrived at the scene within ten minutes and was followed within the hour by a team of four investigators who were immediately deployed to interview neighbors for possible leads. A more detailed search of the scene revealed that:

1. All doors were locked and there were no signs of forced entry.
2. The victim's clothing was neatly arranged on a chair next to her bed.
3. There was no indication of a struggle prior to the fatal shot.
4. Valuables appear to be intact and undisturbed.

After photographing the victim and the scene, the body was removed; and a search was made for the projectile which caused the extensive trauma to the victim. A high-velocity weapon was assumed to be the cause of death.

The major portion of a 150 grain, military type, jacketed bullet was

Reprinted by permission of the American Society for Testing and Materials from the *Journal of Forensic Sciences*, 18, no. 1 (1983), 31-9, copyright 1973.

recovered in the wall space back of the headboard of the victim's bed. A projection of the bullet path through the mattress, headboard, and wall, in conjunction with the position of the body, an apparent "defense" type wound on the lower right wrist of the victim, and the lack of powder residues indicated that the victim was shot while sitting on the end of the bed, leaning back at about a 30-degree angle, and holding her right arm in defensive fashion over her face. Class characteristics of the rifle impressed on the .30 caliber bullet indicated the possibility of Remington Rifles, Model numbers 721 to 760.

This fatal bullet was destined to be the vital link in connecting the suspect with the victim, but in a very unusual manner. The second vital link, discovered later in the investigation, was a cancelled check, which will be discussed separately.

Canvassing of the immediate neighbors developed several witnesses who on the evening before:

1. Heard a loud "bang" or "back fire" between 10:15 P.M. and 10:30 P.M.
2. Saw a red station wagon with white top, round tail lights, and loud muffler start up and drive out of cul-de-sac within a few minutes after hearing the "loud bang." The license number was not obtained.
3. Described the driver of the vehicle as a male—without further details.

It was also learned from persons in the neighborhood that a vehicle similar to the described station wagon had been parked near the scene on several occasions.

Careful and methodical interrogation of all the neighbors, known friends, and former husband (amicably separated) of the victim continued until such time that a conference was called by the detective-in-charge to summarize and evaluate the information assembled. Logical suspects, including the boarder, the former husband, and several known acquaintances, were quickly eliminated because alibis were confirmed by investigation. One lead, however, needed to be followed. It was learned from friends that the victim frequented a local commercial dance studio. Questioning of persons present during Wednesday afternoon at the dance studio indicated that most of the victim's dancing lessons had been with a part-time instructor who would be in a position to give more information about the victim's acquaintances and habits than anyone else.

Through further leads and contacts, the address of this man was found to be an apartment in an adjacent city. The instructor was 23 years old and married with two children. Two detectives, upon arriving at the suspect's apartment, noted a red and white 1955 Ford station wagon parked in the stall of the apartment. Upon knocking and identifying themselves they were invited into the living room by the instructor. While questioning him about the victim, her acquaintances, and his actions the night of the murder, the detectives noted a marble topped coffee table, end table, and lamp which fitted the description of furniture taken in a burglary of the victim's residence several months prior. When asked about this furniture, the instructor said that he had purchased it somewhere at a department store. He later changed his story indicating that it was given to him by a friend. The suspect further stated that he had visited the victim the previous week to borrow $50; but instead he sold her a painting for $140. He denied any knowledge of the murder or of owning a .30 caliber rifle.

He had a good alibi for the night of the murder. He had taken his wife (a waitress) to work early Wednesday evening, taking their children (girl, age 5; boy age 3) with them and returned home to baby-sit, clean house, and watch TV until about 12:30 A.M. when he departed, leaving the children at home alone, to pick up his wife at work.

As the result of this initial questioning, during which the suspect had changed some of his story, and considering the presence of the stolen furniture, the investigators asked the suspect to go to police headquarters for further questioning, which he did willingly. Further interrogation of the suspect at headquarters, and interrogation of his wife, separately, strengthened the investigators' suspicions that the suspect was not telling the truth and knew more about the murder than he had admitted. At the conclusion of these interviews, the man and wife accepted the police opinion that the furniture was stolen property and allowed it to be taken from their apartment. The man was released at this time after agreeing to a polygraph examination the following day.

Shortly after midnight when the investigators arrived at the suspect's apartment to recover the furniture, they learned from a neighbor adjacent to the suspect's apartment that their apartment had been burglarized about three weeks earlier while she and her husband were away for that weekend. This burglary had been investigated and revealed a forced entry by cutting a screen over the bathroom window and entry through an unlocked window. Reported stolen were a Remington .30-'06 Model 760 Gamemaster rifle and $10 in cash. With this information in hand, a warrant to search the suspect's apartment and station wagon was obtained and executed on Friday afternoon, the second day following the murder.

The search of the suspect's apartment brought forth the following:

1. A paper target with bullet holes which appeared to be about .30 caliber.
2. One fired caliber .30-'06 cartridge case (established by laboratory examination to be not connected with the stolen rifle).
3. A caliber .22 rifle, a .410 gauge shotgun, and a caliber .25 pistol.
4. An electric shaver identified as belonging to the boarder living in the victim's house and reported stolen in a burglary.
5. A pair of stained trousers (lab examination revealed no blood or human tissue on these trousers).

The search of the suspect's station wagon developed the following:

1. Cuff links identified as taken with the electric shaver found in the apartment.
2. A large "gunshot" penetration from interior to exterior at about a 45 degree angle in the right side with the entry in line with the top of the rear-seat cushion.

The "gunshot" hole in the suspect's vehicle was an unexplained event which later developed into yet another interesting speculative aspect of this case. From an examination of the penetration, powder, pattern, and lead pellets found in the vehicle, it was determined that this hole was consistent with the firing of a .410 gauge shotgun. It was found that this single shot, bolt action Mossberg, Model 173 A, .410 gauge shotgun found in the suspect's apartment would fire when dropped on its butt with the thumb safety in the "fire" position. This information at the time did little more than add mystery to the investigation. About 19 days after the murder, however, this event assumed new significance when one of the investigators in checking out the neighborhood near the scene observed what appeared to be a pellet pattern on the sidewalk next to the curb in front of the house on the corner next to the victim's residence. This was the area in which the red and white station wagon had been observed parked on previous occasions. Examination of the pattern in conjunction with the hole in the vehicle indicated that the pattern, size, shape, shot imprints, and angle were all consistent with the hypothesis that the suspect's .410 shotgun discharged through the right side while parked at the curb. No statements had been given by the suspect to the point of this evidence.

When again questioned about the items recovered in the search and his alibis, the suspect refused to answer most questions without his attorney. He did, however, attempt to explain the target with the caliber .30 bullet holes by saying that he had recently been to a local outdoor shooting ranch where he was shooting a "large caliber rifle" which he described as "more than a .22 and smaller than a cannon." This statement, which must have been an inadvertent "slip" by the suspect, provided a useful clue.

All information thus far obtained pointed to a connection between the suspect and the victim, the burglaries, and possibly the murder; but a direct link with the crime was not a matter of established fact. Based upon these tenuous developments and on the advice of the District Attorney of Santa Clara County, the suspect was arrested and charged with Burglary, Receiving Stolen Property, and Murder. After the arrest the chief detective found a key in the personal property taken from the suspect at the time of booking which appeared to be identical with the house key to the victim's residence. The suspect when questioned about the key said that it was for a prior residence in the area and gave an address. A check of this alibi address revealed that the suspect and his wife had lived at that address. The locks had not been changed after they had moved, and the key taken from the suspect and matching the victim's key did not open any of the locks at the alibi address; but it did open the entrance door to the victim's house. How or when the suspect obtained this key has never been determined, but it was known that the victim stored her wraps and purse in the cloak room at dancing periods when the suspect was present. Consequently, he had an opportunity to make a duplicate.

At this point, a service station attendant was located who tentatively identified the suspect as one who had stopped at his gas station in the vicinity of the death scene on the night of the murder.

The suspect, when faced with all of the apparent contradictions to his alibis, accused the police of lying and attempting to falsely implicate him and refused to answer further questions. When the time for an agreed polygraph examination arrived, he refused to undergo the examination. From this point on no further information was obtained directly from the suspect which would aid in the solution of the case.

Two days after the murder, the police were faced with an array of alibis, contradictions, and facts which appeared to be pieces of a puzzle, but which defied fitting together in any logical way. It was again time for reflection and contemplation before planning the next move. A review of the progress to date indicated that the next two main lines of investigation should be:

1. To contact the neighbors of the suspect who resided in the apartment adjacent to the suspect to determine whether any fired components from the caliber .30-'06 Remington Model 760 rifle were available from the period prior to the time of the burglary in which the rifle was taken.
2. To investigate the shooting range for spent bullets where the suspect indicated that he may have fired a rifle.

The neighbors were contacted first, and three fired .30-'06 cartridge cases were obtained which had been fired from the rifle before it was stolen. When asked when and where the rifle had last been fired, the neighbor replied that it had been at a pine tree during the recent fall deer hunting season in the Sierra Nevada mountains located about 150 miles from his apartment. This occurred while he was hunting with a friend and a nephew. The neighbor had his .30-'06 Remington Model 760 rifle; the friend had a .30-'06 Springfield Model 1903 rifle; and his nephew had a .30-30 Winchester Model 94 rifle. He said that he and his nephew had sighted in their rifles with targets placed against a large pine tree at a distance of about 150 feet from a clearing near a road. Several shots were fired. He thought that he could locate the tree. Four days after the murder, the neighbor guided investigators to a pine tree approximately 100 feet tall and about 30-in. in diameter. A small section surrounding one apparent bullet hole was cut out, and a jacketed bullet was recovered and returned to the laboratory in San Jose for examination. This bullet was found to be from a caliber .30 weapon of six right-hand riflings with a land width consistent with the Model 94 Winchester used by the neighbor's nephew. A second trip to the pine tree was made; and with permission and assistance of the U.S. Forest Service, the tree was felled. A five-foot section of the trunk was returned to Santa Clara County where it was split and dissected. With the aid of X-ray equipment, a second bullet was recovered. The bullet was fully mushroomed, leading to a cover over the rifling marks which had preserved the class and individual characteristics on the base portion of the metal jacket. The bullet proved to be a soft point fired from a caliber .30 weapon with class characteristics consistent with a Remington Model 760 rifle. These class characteristics were the same as those of the fatal bullet. Further study revealed a significant similarity of individual characteristics between the fatal bullet and the bullet from the tree indicating that both had been fired by the neighbor's stolen rifle (Figs. II-1 and II-2).

The next phase of the investigation proceeded to the shooting range where it was believed that the suspect may have fired a rifle prior to the murder. Nine days after the murder the range master of the Sunnyvale Rod and Gun Club was contacted, and it was determined that the range had opened about a month prior to the murder after renovating the sandstone-shale embankment which served as a backstop at 100 yards from the firing point. The range had been closed for about three months while the embankment was scraped and cleared. When shown a photo of the suspect and asked if he recognized the person, the range master stated that the photo resembled a person using the range during the past month who was shooting a .30-'06 Remington Model Gamemaster "pump-action" rifle. Entries on the sign-in register required for all persons using the range were hastily searched for the name and address of the suspect. None being found, the list was submitted to the Laboratory of Criminalistics for a handwriting examination to determine whether or not the suspect could have signed the register using an assumed name.

When the register was examined at the Laboratory, the only immediately available authentic specimen of handwriting of the suspect was his endorsement of a $140 check which he had earlier mentioned in connection with the purported sale of a painting to the victim. An examination of the complete range record revealed the name of the suspect one week later than the date first indicated by the range master. This name was identified with the writing on the check endorsement. There was further examination of the check which will be discussed separately. The signature on the range record was dated three days prior to the murder. The register indicated that he was assigned to firing Point #29. Point #30 was the last firing position. A man and his son assigned lanes 27 and 28 and another person assigned lane 30 were immediately contacted and questioned. Lanes 29 and 30 were customarily the only targets used for high velocity weapons.

Figure II-1.   Bullets used to link the FATAL bullet with the missing murder rifle. The FATAL bullet and the two RANGE bullets are metal-jacketed, spitzer, 150 grain M2 ball (U.S. Army) military type. The bullet from the TREE is a 180 grain soft point corresponding to ammunition possessed by the owner of the stolen rifle. The two tests were *not* fired by the murder weapon and are included solely for the purpose of illustrating bullet type and class characteristics of rifling marks.

Figure II-2. Comparison photomicrographs demonstrating the identification between the bullets shown in Figure II-1.

The man and his son from shooting lanes 27 and 28 identified the suspect from a photograph and said he was firing a .30-'06 Remington Model 742 or 760 in lane 29. Also that he was firing military type ammunition and when asked if they could have his brass, the suspect replied that he was saving it for a friend. They further noted that a girl, about 5, and a boy, about 3, accompanied the suspect at the range. Based upon this information the embankment covering targets #28, 29, and 30 was searched with the aid of a screen. Several buckets of metal jacket fragments were recovered. The buckets of projectiles were taken to the laboratory where rapid sorting based on gross class characteristics eliminated all but a few jackets and jacket fragments with class characteristics similar to the fatal bullet (Fig. II-1).

A detailed comparison microscope examination was now begun which revealed that two bullet jackets from the range had class and individual characteristics that established an identity between the .30 caliber bullet from the tree and the fatal bullet (Fig. II-1 and II-2). Thus, about three weeks after the murder, the two bullets from the range provided the needed missing link between the stolen rifle and the fatal bullet. Without this evidence a connection between the stolen rifle and the fatal bullet would never have been established because the rifle had not been found. The physical evidence had now provided a link between the murder weapon and the suspect and the fatal bullet. To strengthen this link further, a third trip was made to the area from which the neighbor had fired at the pine tree. With the aid of a metal detector, three fired .30-'06 cartridge cases were found. Microscopic comparisons of breech bolt marks on these cases led to an identification with the three fired cases previously obtained from the neighbor (Fig. II-3).

Returning to the subject of the $140 check, the endorsement was of interest as an exemplar of the defendant's signature for the purpose of comparison with the range record. Much to the surprise of the investigators during the preliminary examination of this document at the laboratory, it was discovered that the entire face of the check was traced. It was further determined that the payer signature was traced from an authentic victim's signature and the remainder of the check was traced from authentic writing of the suspect, including his own name as payee.

The document examiner, upon this finding, asked the detectives to obtain the victim's check stubs for the period involved with the $140 check.

Figure II-3. Comparison photomicrographs demonstrating the identification between cartridge cases recovered near tree to cases from the owner of stolen rifle.

It was found that the traced check was numbered in a sequence different from those covering the period of her stubs. The traced check was number 330. A new group of five personalized checkbooks had recently been received from the bank by mail. Four of these were found by the detectives in an opened bank envelope on the victim's desk. The fifth book containing checks No. 325 through 349 was missing. Speculate now as to the reason that check No. 330 was cashed by the defendant rather than Nos. 325, 326, 327, 328 and 329.

The prosecutor charged first degree murder. The defendant was found guilty and was sentenced to life. The prosecutor used the following lines of argument following the presentation of all the evidence:

1. The victim was a lonely woman who had spent several thousand dollars for dancing lessons over a period of years as a form of recreation.

2. The defendant gained a knowledge of the victim's habits, address, and situation through frequent association as a dance instructor.

3. Through access to the defendant's wraps and purse while at dancing sessions, the defendant gained possession of a key by either replication or theft.

4. Using this illicit key, the defendant had made visits to the victim's home while she was attending dance sessions in other areas. He had taken property from this home on several occasions. This included the furniture, boarder's cuff links, and checkbook.

5. The defendant had burglarized his neighbor's apartment and had taken the .30-'06 rifle. When entering the victim's home, he was armed, first with the .410 gauge shotgun, later with the .30-'06 rifle. The long-barreled weapons were concealed by placing them on the floor behind the driver's seat of the vehicle. On one of these occasions, while the vehicle was parked near the victim's home, the shotgun was accidentally discharged while in the act of placing or removing it from this position.

6. The defendant traced the victim's signature on check No. 325, using the technique of carbon paper; however, when he covered the tracing with ink, it was a different color than his freehand writing on the remainder of the check face. He continued practicing the forgery until he learned that tracing the entire check face was the only method of avoiding a difference in appearance of the ink color between the payer line and remaining entries. In this way he used up checks Nos. 325, 326, 327, 328, and 329, and finally perfected the forgery on check No. 330.

7. After cashing the check, the defendant waited until the day that he thought cancelled checks through the mail would arrive at the victim's house, at which time he again entered the home armed with the rifle intending to remove the cancelled check No. 330 and destroy it in

order to conceal the forgery; he unexpectedly encountered the victim and killed her.

The case is bizarre for several reasons:

1. The connection of the fatal bullet with the suspect without the rifle is exceptionally uncommon.
2. The fact of a defendant tracing his own name is very peculiar.
3. The good fortune of finding exemplar bullets in examinable condition from the tree and range under the circumstances described is unlikely.

It is to the credit of the investigators, examiners, and prosecutors that they recognized the value and significance of all of the facets of the evidence and were able to communicate with each other in a manner which made the most effective use of all of it.

Glossary

Acid	A compound capable of donating a hydrogen ion (H^+) to another compound.
Agglutination	The clumping together of red blood cells by the action of an antibody.
Allele	Any of several alternative forms of a gene located at the same point on a particular pair of chromosomes. For example, the genes determining the blood types A and B are alleles.
Alpha Ray	A type of radiation emitted by a radioactive element. The radiation is composed of helium atoms minus their orbiting electrons.
Alveolus	A small sac in the lungs through whose walls air and other vapors are exchanged between the breath and the blood.
Amorphous Solid	A solid in which the constituent atoms or molecules are arranged in random or disordered positions. There is no regular order in amorphous solids.
Analgesic	A drug or substance that lessens or eliminates pain.
Anthropometry	A system of identification of individuals by measurements of parts of the body, developed by Alphonse Bertillon.
Antibody	A protein that destroys or inactivates a specific antigen. Antibodies are found in the blood serum.

461

Anticoagulant	A substance that prevents coagulation or clotting of the blood.
Antigen	A substance, usually a protein, that stimulates the body to produce antibodies against it.
Antiserum	Blood serum in which there are specific antibodies.
Artery	A blood vessel that carries blood away from the heart.
Aspermia	The absence of sperm; sterility in males.
Atom	The smallest unit of an element; not divisible by ordinary chemical means. Atoms are made up of electrons, protons, and neutrons plus other subatomic particles.
Atomic Mass Number	The sum of the number of protons and neutrons in the nucleus of an atom.
Atomic Number	The number of protons in the nucleus of the atom. Each element has its own unique atomic number.
Base	A compound capable of accepting a hydrogen ion (H^+).
Becke Line	A bright halo that is observed near the border of a particle immersed in a liquid of a different refractive index.
Beta Ray	A type of radiation emitted by a radioactive element. The radiation consists of electrons.
Birefringence	A difference in the two indices of refraction exhibited by some crystalline materials.
Black Powder	Normally, a mixture of potassium nitrate, carbon, and sulfur in the ratio 75/16/10.
Caliber	The diameter of the bore of a rifled firearm. The caliber is usually expressed in hundredths of an inch, or millimeters, e.g., .22 caliber, and 9 mm.
Capillary	A tiny blood vessel across whose walls exchange of materials between the blood and the tissues takes place; receives blood from arteries and carries it to veins.
Catalyst	A substance that accelerates the rates of chemical reactions but is not itself permanently changed by the reaction.
Celsius Scale	The temperature scale using the melting point of ice as 0 and the boiling point of water as 100, with 100 equal divisions or degrees between.
Chemical Property	Describes the behavior of a substance when it reacts or combines with another substance.

Chromosome	A rodlike structure in the cell nucleus, along which the genes are located.
Class Characteristics	Properties of evidence that can only be associated with a group and never with a single source.
Combustion	The rapid combination of oxygen with another substance accompanied by the production of noticeable heat and light.
Compound	A pure substance composed of two or more elements.
Continuous Spectrum	A type of emission spectrum showing a continuous band of colors all blending into one another.
Crystalline Solid	A solid in which the constituent atoms have a regular arrangement.
Density	A physical property of matter that is equivalent to the mass per unit volume of a substance.
Depressant	A substance used to depress the functions of the central nervous system. Depressants calm irritability and anxiety, and may induce sleep.
Depth of Focus	The thickness of a specimen entirely in focus under a microscope.
Detonating Cord	A cordlike explosive containing a core of high-explosive material, usually PETN. Also called *primacord*.
Dispersion	The separation of light into its component wavelengths.
Egg	The female reproductive cell.
Ejector	The mechanism in a firearm that throws the cartridge or fired case from the firearm.
Electron	A very light, negatively charged particle that is one of the fundamental structural units of the atom.
Electron Orbitals	The pathway of electrons as they move around the nuclei of atoms. Each orbital is associated with a particular electronic energy level.
Electrophoresis	A technique for the separation of molecules through their migration on a support medium while under the influence of an electrical potential.
Element	A collection of atoms all having the same atomic number. An element cannot be broken down into simpler substances by chemical means.
Emission Spectrum	Light emitted from a source and separated into its component colors or frequencies.

Endothermic Reaction	A chemical transformation in which heat energy is absorbed from the surroundings.
Energy	The combined ability or potential of a system or material to do work. Some forms of energy are heat energy, chemical energy, and electrical energy.
Enzyme	A type of protein that acts as a catalyst for certain specific reactions.
Erythrocyte	A red blood cell.
Exothermic Reaction	A chemical transformation in which heat energy is liberated.
Explosion	A chemical or mechanical action resulting in the rapid expansion of gases.
Extractor	The mechanism in a firearm by which a cartridge of a fired case is withdrawn from the chamber.
Fahrenheit Scale	The temperature scale using the melting point of ice as 32° and the boiling point of water as 212°, with 180 equal divisions or degrees between.
Flash Point	The minimum temperature at which a liquid fuel will produce enough vapor to burn.
Fluoresce	To emit visible light when exposed to light of a shorter wavelength—i.e., ultraviolet light.
Frequency	The number of waves that pass a given point per second.
Gamma Ray	A high-energy form of electromagnetic radiation emitted by a radioactive element.
Gas	A state of matter in which the attractive forces between molecules is small enough to permit them to move with complete freedom.
Gauge	Size designation of a shotgun, originally the number of lead balls with the same diameter as the barrel that would make a pound. For example, a 12-gauge shotgun would have a bore diameter of a lead ball 1/12 of a pound in weight. The only exception is the .410 shotgun, in which bore size is .41 inch.
Gene	A unit of inheritance located on a chromosome.
Genotype	The particular combination of genes present in the cells of an individual.
Glowing Combustion	Burning at the fuel air interface. Examples are a red-hot charcoal or a burning cigarette.

Hallucinogen	A substance that induces changes in mood, attitude, thought, or perception.
Heat of Combustion	The heat evolved when a substance is burned in oxygen.
Hemoglobin	A red blood cell protein responsible for transporting oxygen in the bloodstream and the red coloring of blood.
Heterozygous	Having two different allelic genes on two corresponding positions of a pair of chromosomes.
High Explosive	Explosive with a velocity of detonation greater than 1000 meters per second. For example, dynamite and RDX.
Homozygous	Having two identical allelic genes on two corresponding positions of a pair of chromosomes.
Hydrocarbon	Any compound consisting only of carbon and hydrogen.
Ignition Temperature	The minimum temperature at which a fuel will spontaneously ignite.
Individual Characteristics	Properties of evidence that can be attributed to a common source with an extremely high degree of certainty.
Inorganic Compound	A chemical compound not based on carbon.
Ion	An atom or molecule bearing a positive or negative charge.
Iso-enzymes	Multiple molecular forms of an enzyme, each having the same or very similar enzyme activities.
Isotope	An atom differing from another atom of the same element in the number of neutrons it has in its nucleus.
Laser	Light Amplification by the Simulated Emission of Radiation. Light that has all its waves pulsating in unison.
Latent Fingerprint	A fingerprint made by the deposit of oils and/or perspiration. It is invisible to the naked eye.
Line Spectrum	A type of emission spectrum showing a series of lines separated by black areas. Each line represents a definite wavelength or frequency.
Liquid	A state of matter in which molecules are in contact with one another but are not rigidly held in place.
Low Explosive	Explosive with a velocity of detonation less than 1000 meters per second. For example, black powder and smokeless powder.
Mass	A constant property of matter that reflects the amount of material present.

Matter	All things of substance. Matter is composed of atoms or molecules.
Microcrystalline Tests	Tests to identify specific substances by the color and morphology of the crystals formed when the substance is mixed with specific reagents.
Mineral	A naturally occurring crystalline solid.
Molecule	Two or more atoms held together by chemical bonds.
Monochromatic Light	Light having a single wavelength or frequency.
Monomer	The basic unit of structure from which a polymer is constructed.
Narcotic	Analgesic or pain-killing substance that depresses vital body functions such as blood pressure, pulse rate, and breathing rate. The regular administration of narcotics will produce physical dependence.
Neutron	A particle having no electrical charge, which along with the proton is a basic unit in the structure of the nucleus of an atom.
Nucleus	The core of an atom in which the protons and neutrons exist.
Oligospermia	A condition describing an abnormally low sperm count.
Organic Compound	Substance composed of carbon and hydrogen, and, often, smaller amounts of oxygen, nitrogen, chlorine, phosphorus, or other elements.
Oxidation	The combination of oxygen with other substances to produce new products.
Oxidizing Agent	A substance that supplies oxygen to a chemical reaction.
Parfocal	Construction of a microscope such that when an image is focused with one objective in position, the other objective can be rotated into place and the field will remain in focus.
Periodic Table	Chart of elements arranged according to their atomic numbers. Vertical rows are called *groups* or *families*; horizontal rows are called *series*.
pH	A symbol used to express the basicity or acidity of a substance. A pH of 7 is neutral; lower values are acidic, higher values basic.
Phase	A uniform piece of matter. Different phases are separated by definite visible boundaries.
Phenotype	The physical manifestation of a genetic trait such as shape, color, and blood type.

Photon	A small packet of electromagnetic radiation energy. Each photon contains a unit of energy equal to the product of Plank's constant and the frequency of radiation: $E = hf$.
Physical Dependence	Physiological need for a drug that has been brought about by its regular use. Dependence is characterized by withdrawal sickness when administration of the drug is abruptly stopped.
Physical Evidence	Any object that can establish that a crime has been committed or can provide a link between a crime and its victim or between a crime and its perpetrator.
Physical Property	Describes the behavior of a substance without reference to any other substance.
Plane-Polarized Light	Light confined to a single plane of vibration.
Plasma	The fluid portion of unclotted blood.
Plastic Fingerprint	A fingerprint impressed in a soft surface.
Polymer	A substance composed of a large number of atoms. These atoms are usually arranged in repeating units or monomers.
Polymorphism	The occurrence in a population of two or more common alleles producing a variety of phenotypes. For example, blood types are examples of polymorphism. Similarly, some enzymes exist in different forms and are therefore polymorphic.
Precipitin	An antibody that reacts with its corresponding antigen to form a precipitate.
Preservative	A substance added to blood in order to inhibit the growth of micro-organisms. Sodium fluoride is a common preservative.
Proteins	Polymers of amino acids that play basic roles in the structures and functions of living things.
Proton	A positively charged particle that is one of the basic structures in the nucleus of an atom.
Psychological Dependence	The conditioned use of a drug caused by underlying emotional needs.
Pyrolysis	The decomposition of organic matter by heat.
Radioactivity	The particle and/or gamma ray radiation emitted by the unstable nucleus of some isotopes.
Real Image	An image formed by the actual convergence of light rays upon a screen.

Refraction	The bending of a light wave as it passes from one medium to another.
Refractive Index	The ratio of the speed of light in a vacuum to its speed in a given substance.
Ridge Characteristics	Ridge endings, bifurcations, enclosures, and other ridge details, which must match in two fingerprints in order for their common origin to be established. Also called *minutiae*.
Safety Fuse	A cord containing a core of black powder. It is used to carry a flame at a uniform rate to an explosive charge.
Secretor	An individual who secretes his/her blood-type antigen(s) in body fluids. Approximately 80 percent of the population are secretors.
Serology	The study of antigen-antibody reactions.
Serum	The liquid that separates from the blood when a clot is formed.
Smokeless Powder (double-base)	An explosive consisting of a mixture of nitrocellulose and nitroglycerin.
Smokeless Powder (single-base)	An explosive consisting of nitrocellulose.
Solid	A state of matter in which the molecules are held closely together in a rigid state.
Sperm	The male reproductive cell.
Spontaneous Combustion	A fire caused by a natural heat-producing process in the presence of sufficient air and fuel.
Stimulant	A substance taken to increase alertness or activity.
Sublimation	A physical change from the solid directly into the gaseous state.
Titration	The analytical operation of adding a reagent until a reaction is complete, and then measuring the volume so added.
Vein	A blood vessel that transports blood toward the heart.
Virtual Image	An image that cannot be seen directly. It can only be seen by a viewer looking through a lens.
Wavelength	The distance between crests of adjacent waves.
Weight	A property of matter that depends both on the mass of a substance and the effects of gravity on that mass.

X Chromosome   The female sex chromosome.

X-ray   A high-energy, short-wavelength form of electromagnetic radiation.

Y Chromosome   The male sex chromosome.

Appendices

GUIDE TO THE COLLECTION OF PHYSICAL EVIDENCE— NEW JERSEY STATE POLICE

Specimen	Packaging	Control	Amount Required — Evidence	Collection Procedure
AMMUNITION				
Cartridges (unfired)	Place in small clasp-type envelope.		Submit separately those found in gun from all other evidence cartridges.	Initial on case near bullet end.
Discharged bullets	Same as above. (Separate envelope for each specimen.)		All found.	Initial on base or nose, never on side.
Discharged shells	Place in small clasp-type envelope. (Separate envelopes if found at different locations; mark each envelope.)		All found.	Initial on inside or outside of case near open end. (Never mark where firing pin strikes.)
Shotgun shells	Same as above.		All found.	Initial on brass near paper or plastic.
Pellets	Same as above.		All found.	Not necessary to mark pellet. Mark envelope with initials.
Wadding	Same as above; if taken from body, dry before submitting. Place in clasp-type envelope; mark outside.		All found.	Mark envelope with initials.
ARSON ACCELER-ANTS				
Gasoline, Kerosene, etc.	Metal or glass container with airtight seal.	One ounce, 30 ml	One ounce, 30 ml	Volatile liquids must be poured into clean containers and sealed. Submit original container.
Residues	Gallon, quart, or pint clean metal paint can (not coated on inside) with air-tight seal.	Identical material uncontaminated with suspect accelerant.	All; fill container to approximately one-half volume.	Collect specimens which have an odor or trace of fluid, or those which are capable of absorbing the suspect accelerant.

GUIDE TO THE COLLECTION OF PHYSICAL EVIDENCE— NEW JERSEY STATE POLICE

Specimen	Packaging	Control	Amount Required / Evidence	Collection Procedure
BLOODSTAINS*	Stained objects are separately placed in a solid container or druggist fold. Bloodstained clothing, fabrics, etc., are separately placed in clean paper bags. DO NOT Use PLASTIC BAGS.	5 cc of whole blood from suspect and like amount from victim. Anticoagulant and preservative should NOT be added to blood (use red top tube). If no control blood is available, submit the following: 1. Pulled head hairs from deceased and 2. One square inch of liver, or 3. Piece of muscle tissue, or 4. One square inch of spleen.		On small objects—send entire stained object. On large objects, moisten a sterile swab with a minimum amount of distilled water and swab stained area. A negative control must be submitted. Moisten a second swab with a minimal amount of distilled water. Swab an unstained area close to the bloodstain. Allow both swabs to air-dry. Do not handle tip of swab. Package each in an envelope individually and submit to laboratory. If evidence is wet, air-dry thoroughly. DO NOT use heat to dry.
CLOTHING	Place each item in a clean paper bag. DO NOT USE PLASTIC BAGS. Wrap or bag each item separately.		All	Leave clothing whole. DO NOT cut out suspect area. Air-dry wet clothing.

*NOTE: *All blood and/or additional controls must be kept refrigerated (not frozen).*
Transport liquid blood samples and body specimens to laboratory as soon as possible.
No blood grouping or enzyme analysis results will be reported unless whole blood controls are submitted.
In cases where victims have been transfused a sample of pre-transfusion blood is to be obtained, this is usually available at the hospital if the investigator is aware of the need for this sample. If none is available, wait 6–8 weeks from date of last transfusion, to draw a blood control sample.

DOCUMENTS Anonymous letters, extortion letters, bank robbery notes.	Plastic sheet protector.	Original documents in document cases, reproductions are acceptable in certain cases. (See *Notes* at end of table on p. 479.)	All original documents.	**DO NOT** handle with bare hands. Place in proper enclosure envelope and seal with cellophane tape. Specify if evidence is to be treated for latent prints.
Charred or burned paper.	Solid container		All	**DO NOT** handle with bare hands.
Checks	Envelopes.	See *Notes* at end of table on p. 479.	All	Advise what parts questioned or known. Furnish physical description of suspect.
Check protector, rubber stamp and dater stamp sets, known standards.	Plastic sheet protectors.	Obtain several in full (complete series of numbers).	All	**DO NOT** disturb inking mechanisms on printing devices. **SEND ACTUAL DEVICE WHEN POSSIBLE.**
Handwriting and hand-printing, known standards.	Same as above.	See *Notes* at end of table on p. 479.	All	See Anonymous letters under *Documents*.
Obliterated, eradicated, or indented writing.	Same as above. **DO NOT** fold.		All	Advise if bleach or staining method may be useful.
Typewriting, known standards.	Same as above.	Obtain minimum of one copy in full word-for-word order of questioned typewriting. Include partial copies in light, medium, heavy touch. Also carbon samples of each character on keyboard.	All	Examine ribbon for evidence of questioned message thereon. For carbon paper samples, either remove ribbon or place in stencil position and type directly on carbon paper placed over bond paper.
EXPLOSIVE RESIDUES	Solid sealed container	All	All	Collected debris and bomb fragments around suspected origin or explosion. The laboratory **WILL NOT** accept potentially explosive bombs or chemicals. These items should be deac-

473

GUIDE TO THE COLLECTION OF PHYSICAL EVIDENCE— NEW JERSEY STATE POLICE

Specimen	Packaging	Control	Amount Required Evidence	Collection Procedure
FIBERS	Individual fibers are packaged in a druggist fold, pillbox, or vial. DO NOT place loose in an envelope.	Entire garment or other cloth items.	All	tivated by the nearest bomb disposal unit. Package separately, fibers collected from different sources; whenever possible submit the entire article on which the fibers have been observed.
FINGERNAIL SCRAPINGS	Druggist fold or plastic vial.		All available.	A blunt object should be used to scrape under each fingernail. A separate druggist fold or vial should be used for each finger and clearly marked identifying the finger or fingers.
FIREARMS Automatic pistols	Unload weapon unless the presence of other evidence prohibits handling i.e., blood, hair, fibers, prints, etc. Weapons not involving other types of physical evidence may be placed in a heavy-duty envelope or carried by hand. Weapons requiring examination of other physical evidence— blood, hair, fibers,		All found.	Attach a tag indicating the name, caliber, and serial number of the weapon along with the investigators initials. Special care should be exercised to preserve other evidence on the weapon, i.e., blood, hair, fibers, latent prints. Should these items be present, the weapon should be carefully packaged in a cardboard box. Exterior of the carton or box marked "LOADED" or "UNLOADED." Request for examination should specify the weapon is to be examined for other types of evidence—blood, hairs, fibers, latent prints.

Type	Amount Desired	Packing and Handling	Identification / Remarks
(Automatic pistols, continued)		prints—must be carefully packed in a cardboard box or carton to preserve the evidence. Indicate whether "LOADED" or "UNLOADED."	Initials of the investigator should be placed in the magazine well and under the slide.
Revolvers	All found.	Same as for automatic pistols. Unload weapon unless the presence of other evidence prohibits handling; i.e., blood, hairs, fibers, prints.	Procedure same as automatic pistols. Initial under top strap.
Rifles and Shotguns	All found.	Weapons not involving other types of physical evidence may be hand-carried. Weapons requiring examination of other physical evidence—blood, hair, fiber, prints—must be carefully packed in a cardboard box or carton to preserve the evidence. Indicate whether "LOADED" or "UNLOADED."	Attach a tag indicating the name, caliber, and serial number of the weapon along with the investigator's initials. Initials of the investigator should be placed inside the trigger guard.
GLASS	One square inch of broken item. / All	Place questioned and known fragments in solid containers. DO NOT place loose in envelope. Avoid breakage.	Foreps can be used to collect glass particles. Whenever possible, submit the entire article on which the particles have been observed. Plate glass samples: If direction of break is desired, mark each piece as to inside or outside surface.

GUIDE TO THE COLLECTION OF PHYSICAL EVIDENCE—NEW JERSEY STATE POLICE

Specimen	Packaging	Amount Required			Collection Procedure
		Control	Evidence		
HAIR	Druggist fold, pillbox, or vial. **DO NOT** place loose in envelope.	Twenty or more full-length hairs pulled, not clipped, from different part of the body or head. Pubic 12 or more.	All		Package separately, hairs collected from different sources. Label location from which taken. Whenever possible, submit the entire article on which the hairs have been observed.
NARCOTICS AND DANGEROUS DRUGS					
Liquids	Solid container.	All	All		Separate drugs and package individually.
Powders, tablets, and capsules.	Druggist fold, pillbox, vial, or glassine envelope (aluminum foil is acceptable for powders).	All	All		Same as above.
Vegetation	Plastic or paper bag.	All	All		Package vegetation separately. If wet, air-dry thoroughly before submission. Smoking instruments are packaged individually to prevent contamination.
Plants	Paper bags or wrapped in paper.		Representative sample plants.		
PAINT (paint chips or scrapings)	Druggist fold, pillbox, or vial. **DO NOT** place loose in envelope or in plastic bag.	At least ½ square inch of solid, with all layers represented. Taken adjacent to damaged area.	Recover all the layers.		Whenever possible, submit the entire article on which the paint has been observed. Otherwise, use a clean knife blade to remove all the layers of paint from the object. **DO NOT** use tape to collect paint.

SEMINAL STAINS	Wrap each stained item separately in clean paper bags.	Obtain saliva moistened onto a paper towel. Also obtain blood from parties involved.	All	If wet, air-dry evidence thoroughly.
SOIL	Solid container or druggist fold. DO NOT place loose in envelope.	Collect a quantity approximating 1-2 teaspoons of soil at crime scene (top layer only) as representative samples in a 200-foot radius of the crime scene.	All	Package separately soil collected at different areas. Whenever possible, submit the entire article on which the soil has been observed. Label all samples with proper location (approximately 8 to 10 representative samples).
TOXICOLOGY (*Living*) Blood	Whenever possible, obtain two 10 cc grey top vials of blood. These vials contain both a preservative and anticoagulant. They are vacuum sealed and provide the best guard against contamination. There are commercially available blood collection kits manufactured for the convenience of law enforcement agencies.		20 cc of blood for drug determination. 10 cc of blood for alcohol.	Physicians taking blood samples should add anticoagulant (*e.g.*, sodium oxalate) and preservative (*e.g.*, sodium floride). Refrigerate until delivery to laboratory. The vials should be properly labeled with such information as the patient's name, the date, the time samples were drawn, and by whom. The law enforcement officer witnessing the procedure should also include some identifying marks on the vials. The vials should then be sealed and placed in a separate container with the appropriate identification on the container. This information is necessary to provide legally acceptable specimen identification, integrity, and chain of custody. The vials should then be submitted IMMEDIATELY to the laboratory. If this is not possible, they should be stored under refrigeration. It is recommended that the police agency storing the vials obtain a separate refrigerator that
Urine	Urine specimens should be submitted in clean containers. There are plastic specimen cups with screw-on or snap-on caps.		AT LEAST 50 ml or 2 oz (minimum 50 cc).	

GUIDE TO THE COLLECTION OF PHYSICAL EVIDENCE—
NEW JERSEY STATE POLICE

Specimen	Packaging	Control	Evidence	Collection Procedure
			Amount Required	
Stomach washing	Same as above.		All	can be locked and used only for the storage of forensic evidence. If this is not feasible, a locked strong box placed in the refrigerator would also guarantee security of the evidence. A log sheet documenting the personnel having access to the box would maintain the chain of custody. After analysis has been performed by the Toxicological Unit, the vials and/or specimen cups will be rinsed out and returned to the submitting agency. It is then the responsibility of the submitting agency to safeguard that evidence until the trial date. The containers should be made available as evidence if required by the courts.
TOXICOLOGY *(Dead)* Blood	Clean test tube or vial.		20 cc for drugs. 10 cc for alcohol.	Add anticoagulant and preservative. Refrigerate until delivery to the laboratory.
Brain	Plastic container.		300 grams.	Keep refrigerated until delivery to laboratory.
Bile	Same as above.		All	Same as above.
Liver	Same as above.		300 grams.	Same as above.
Kidney	Same as above.		All	Same as above.
Urine	Same as above.		All in bladder.	Same as above.
Skin around puncture marks	Same as above.		All	Same as above.

478

TOOL MARKS

Solid container package in order to prevent damage to area of tool mark.

Submit suspect tool. Package in separate container. Whenever possible, submit entire object containing the tool mark.

DO NOT attempt to reproduce marking by casting a mold unless that is the only method by which the evidence can be preserved.

VOICEPRINT
Magnetic ¼" recording tape and cassette recordings.

Suspect(s) must repeat identical words appearing in questioned tape.

Use containers that original tape came in. Properly marked and initialed.

All original recording or best copy available.

Obtain best recording by eliminating background noise (typewriters, telephones, air conditioners, conversation, etc.). In hand-printing cases, both upper-case (capital) and lower-case (small) samples should be obtained. Have writer prepare some specimens with hand not habitually used. Obtain undictated handwriting when feasible. In certain investigations, it may not be possible to have suspect prepare specimen writings. For this purpose a list has been prepared giving the investigative sources for obtaining standards for comparison.

Notes: *Duplicate the original writing conditions as to text, speed, slant, size of paper, size of writing, type of writing instrument, etc. Do not allow suspect to see questioned writing. Give no instructions as to spelling, punctuation, etc. Remove each sample from sight as soon as completed. Suspect should fill out blank check forms. In forgery cases, obtain sample signatures of the person whose name is forged.*

Sources of Handwriting Specimens

1. Account books
2. Affidavits
3. Application forms
4. Assignments
5. Autographs
6. Automobile insurance applications
7. Automobile license applications
8. Automobile title certificates
9. Bank deposit slips
10. Bank safe deposit entry slips
11. Bank savings withdrawal slips
12. Bank signature cards
13. Bank statements, receipts for
14. Bible entries
15. Bills of sale
16. Bonds
17. Books, signatures of owner in
18. Building "after hours" registers
19. Business license application
20. Charity pledges
21. Checkbook stubs
22. Checks, including endorsements
23. Church pledges
24. Convention registration books
25. Contracts
26. Cooking recipes
27. Corporation papers
28. Criminal records
29. Credit applications
30. Credit cards
31. Deeds
32. Deeds of trust
33. Depositions
34. Diaries
35. Dog license applications
36. Drafts
37. Drive-it-yourself applications
38. Drivers' licenses and applications
39. Druggists' poison registers
40. Employment applications
41. Envelopes
42. Fishing licenses
43. Funeral attendance registers
44. Gas service applications
45. Gasoline mileage records
46. Gate records at defense plants
47. Greeting cards, Christmas cards, etc.
48. Hospital entry applications etc.
49. Hotel and motel guest registers
50. Hunting licenses
51. Identification cards
52. Inventories

(continued next page)

Appendix I, continued

GUIDE TO THE COLLECTION OF PHYSICAL EVIDENCE—
NEW JERSEY STATE POLICE

53. Jail records
54. Leases, real property
55. Letters
56. Library card applications
57. Light company applications
58. Life insurance applications
59. Loan applications
60. Mail orders
61. Manuscripts
62. Marriage records
63. Membership cards
64. Memoranda of all kinds
65. Military papers
66. Mortgages
67. Motor vehicle records
68. Newspaper advertisement copy

69. Occupational writings
70. Package receipts
71. Parents' signatures on report cards
72. Partnership papers
73. Pawn tickets
74. Passports
75. Payroll receipts
76. Pension applications
77. Permit applications
78. Petitions, referenda, etc.
79. Photograph albums
80. Pleadings
81. Postal cards
82. Probate court papers
83. Promissory notes
84. Property damage reports

85. Recipes
86. Receipts for rent, etc.
87. Registered mail return receipts
88. Release of mortgages
89. Rental contracts for equipment
90. Reports
91. Retail store sales slips
92. School and college papers
93. Social security cards and papers
94. Sport and game score cards
95. Stock certificates, endorsements

96. Surety bond applications
97. Tax estimates and returns
98. Telegram copy
99. Telephone service applications
100. Time sheets
101. Traffic tickets
102. Vehicle rental forms
103. Voting registration records
104. Water company service applications
105. Wills
106. Workmans' compensation papers

Appendix II

THE COLLECTION OF EVIDENCE FOR DETERMINING
GUNSHOT RESIDUES ON THE HANDS

INFORMATION ON GUNSHOT
RESIDUE

The presence of two chemical elements, barium and antimony, in sufficient amounts on test swabs is considered indicative of gunshot residue (GSR). The two elements are present in most cartridge primers, and antimony is often found in the bullet lead as well.

It has been found that cotton swabs are quite useful for collecting GSR, but because the amounts of these elements deposited on the firing hand is quite small, contamination of the swab by either barium or antimony from other sources may prevent GSR detection. Of particular concern is the quality of the collection materials themselves. Only plastic-shafted cotton swabs packaged after use in plastic containers such as vials or self-sealing bags are suitable.

There are situations in which a laboratory will not accept hand swabs for analysis because the analysis would not be meaningful. A list of these reasons is given below:

1. A .22 caliber weapon was used, but not with Federal Brand ammunition.
2. Six or more hours elapsed between the weapon firing and the hand swabbing.
3. The subject's hands were washed or fingerprinted between the time the weapon was fired and the hands were swabbed.
4. The swabs are obviously contaminated (e.g., by blood), have been exposed to contamination by container breakage, or have had prolonged contact with foreign materials such as paper labels.
5. Unsuitable collection materials were used (e.g., gauze, swabs with wooden shafts).
6. Specimens are not labeled.
7. Specimens are packaged in other than plastic containers.
8. Transmittal letter is missing or inadequate.

COLLECTION AND PACKAGING

1. When **not** to collect residues:
   (a) If more than six (6) hours have elapsed since the weapon was fired. (**Exception:** Suicide victims whose hands have been protected with plastic or paper bags.)
   (b) If the suspect's hands have recently been washed or fingerprinted.
   (c) If .22 caliber ammunition (other than Federal Brand) was used.
2. What materials to use? (**Do not substitute!**)
   (a) **Single-tipped** cotton swabs on **plastic** shafts.
   (b) A 5% solution of nitric acid ("reagent" grade) using distilled or demineralized water.
   (c) Plastic (polyethylene, polypropylene, or polystyrene) vials with tight-fitting plastic caps, or plastic evidence bags (with interlocking closure), preferably not larger than 3" × 4".
3. How to collect and package?
   (a) Put on disposable plastic gloves before handling materials.
   (b) Remove one swab from package, being careful not to touch the cotton tip. Using eyedropper, moisten cotton tip of swab with 2-3 drops of 5% nitric acid solution. (Don't overmoisten swab.)

(c) Thoroughly swab a portion of the thumb, forefinger and connecting web area of the right hand. Swab the remaining portion of this area using a second swab moistened as in step 3 (b). Place both swabs in a plastic bag labeled "Back of Right Hand of (**person's full name**)." Seal bag to make it airtight.

NOTE: Thorough swabbing is accomplished by swabbing for approximately 30 seconds with each swab and rotating the swab so as to utilize all surfaces of the cotton tip. **Do not swab the fingerprint pattern area.**

(d) Repeat steps 2 and 3 on left hand. Place both swabs in a plastic bag labeled "Back of Left Hand of (**person's full name**)."

(e) Prepare two swabs as in step 3 (b). Place in a plastic bag labeled "Control Swabs."

(f) If available and practical, any fired cartridge cases should be submitted with the swabs.

TRANSMITTAL OF EVIDENCE

1. Prepare a transmittal letter containing **as much** of the following information as is available to you at time of writing. Please acknowledge all requested items of information. For example, if the gun type, or caliber, or brand of ammunition is not known, include in your letter a statement of that fact.

(a) Date of your letter.

(b) Your case number.

(c) Subject's full name.

(d) Date and time of shooting.

(e) Date and time of swabbing.

(f) Type and caliber of gun.

(g) Brand of ammunition.

(h) Subject's occupation.

(i) Subject's hobbies.

(j) Is subject right-handed or left-handed?

(k) Brief description of incident.

Appendix III

CHROMATOGRAPHIC AND SPECTROPHOTOMETRIC PARAMETERS FOR FIGURES CONTAINED WITHIN THE TEXT

1. *Figures 5-6 (a) and (b)*
   3' X 1/4" glass column; 3% OV-17 on Varaport 30, 80/100 mesh.
   T(injection port) = 280°C, T(defector) = 280°C, T(column) = 200°C
   Carrier Gas: Nitrogen at 50 ml/min

2. *Figure 5-7*
   8' X 1/8" stainless steel, 15% carbowax 20M, AW-DMCS treated 80/100 mesh chromosorb W plus 3' X 1/8" stainless steel, 10% silicone D.C. 200 in series.
   Temperature unknown
   Carrier Gas: Nitrogen

3. *Figure 5-8*
   Absorbent: Silica Gel G
   Developing Solvent: Benzene
   Visualizer: Fast Blue B Salt

4. *Figure 5-9*
   Absorbent: Silica Gel G
   Developing Solvent: Chloroform-Diethylamine (9:1)
   Visualizer: Iodoplatinate

5. *Figure 5-14*
   Solvent: 0.1N HCL

6. *Figure 5-15 (a)*
   Heroin hydrochloride in KBr

7. *Figure 5-15 (b)*
   Secobarbital (free acid) in KBr

8. *Figure 8-13*
   Acrylic fibers ground in KBr

9. *Figure 8-15*
   1.83 m X 0.32 cm stainless steel column, 20% carbowax 1540 on 60/80 mesh chromosorb W.
   Pyrolysis temperature unknown
   T(injection port) = 250°C, T(detector) = 250°C, T(column) − programmed at 2 minutes initial hold at 50°C, then 10°C/minute to 180°C, hold for 25 minutes
   Carrier Gas: Argon at 50 ml/min.

10. *Figure 8-18 (a) and (b)*
    Same as Figure 5-7.

11. *Figure 9-8*
    Solvent: 0.1N HCL

12. *Figure 10-9*
    Ethanol in whole blood analyzed by "head space" technique.
    A porous polymer column was used.
    T(injection port) = 132°C, T(detector) = 132°C, T(column) = 132°C
    Carrier Gas: Helium (thermal conductivity detector was used).

13. *Figure 11-5*
    30 m X 0.75 mm I.D. glass capillary column, SPB-1, bonded phase with a 1.00 um film thickness. Column oven temperature program: 40°C. for 3 min., 12°C. up to

250°C. FID temperature 280°C. Injection port temperature 250°C. Helium carrier and make-up gas.

14. *Figure 11-9*
    RDX in KBr

15. *Figure 15-8*
    Absorbent: Silica Gel
    Developing Solvent: Ethyl acetate, absolute ethanol, water (70:35:30)

Answers

CHAPTER 1

1. forensic science
3. Alphonse Bertillon
5. Leone Lattes
7. Albert Osborn
9. Edmond Locard
11. California
13. drug
15. federal, state, county, and municipal
17. biology
19. toxicology
21. *Frye* v. *United States*
23. *Coppolino* v. *Florida*
25. True
27. training

CHAPTER 2

1. physical evidence
3. False
5. photography, sketching, notes
7. close-ups
9. systematic
11. clothing, fingernail scrapings, head and pubic hairs, blood, vaginal, anal and oral swabs, bullets, and hand swabs
13. separate
15. is not
17. False
19. control
21. arson or fire

CHAPTER 3

1. identification
3. comparative
5. individual
7. True
9. weight
11. False

CHAPTER 4

1. physical
3. metric
5. 1/100
7. 200
9. True
11. True
13. 180
15. mass
17. density
19. refraction

21. True
23. birefringence
25. glass
27. density, refractive index
29. Becke line
31. radial
33. False
35. will
37. minerals
39. True

CHAPTER 5

1. matter
3. 107
5. atom
7. molecule
9. has no
11. less
13. organic
15. qualitative, quantitative
17. chromatography
19. higher
21. gas chromatography

23. pyrolyzed
25. thin-layer chromatography
27. R_f
29. electrophoresis
31. wavelength
33. electromagnetic
35. laser
37. True
39. can
41. spectrophotometer
43. infrared

CHAPTER 6

1. oxygen, silicon
3. trace
5. emission spectrum
7. line
9. False
11. laser beam
13. does
15. proton, neutron, electron
17. positive

19. protons
21. True
23. light
25. isotopes
27. alpha rays, beta rays, gamma rays
29. gamma rays
31. neutron activation analysis
33. crystalline

CHAPTER 7

1. lenses
3. compound
5. eyepiece or ocular lens
7. True
9. vertical or reflected
11. parfocal
13. magnifying power
15. numerical aperture

17. decreases
19. decreases
21. True
23. False
25. plane-polarized
27. polarizing
29. microspectrophotometer
31. X-rays

CHAPTER 8

1. hair follicle
3. True
5. medulla
7. 1/3, 1/2
9. animal
11. comparison
13. is
15. often
17. 24
19. Natural
21. True
23. False
25. monomer
27. True
29. double refraction or birefringence
31. class
33. color
35. acrylic lacquers
37. False
39. inorganic

CHAPTER 9

1. True
3. physical
5. False
7. analgesics, depressive
9. morphine
11. True
13. Hashish
15. True
17. lysergic acid
19. depresses
21. long
23. Tranquilizers
25. Amphetamines
27. clandestine
29. sniffed
31. five
33. four
35. Marquis
37. marijuana
39. Microcrystalline
41. infrared
43. chain of custody

CHAPTER 10

1. ethyl alcohol
3. is
5. faster
7. watery
9. oxidized
11. breath
13. stomach, small intestine
15. pulmonary
17. 2100
19. potassium dichromate
21. catalyst
23. infrared
25. nonalcoholic
27. 0.10
29. morphine
31. acids, bases
33. acidic
35. immunoassay
37. percent saturation
39. synergistic
41. corroborate

CHAPTER 11

1. False
3. False
5. chemical, mechanical
7. absorb, liberate
9. exothermic
11. endothermic
13. ignition
15. flash point
17. Glowing combustion or smouldering
19. Spontaneous combustion
21. potassium nitrate, charcoal, sulfur
23. origin
25. porous
27. gas chromatograph
29. thin-layer chromatography
31. low
33. black powder, smokeless powder
35. False
37. is not
39. PETN
41. crater
43. microscopic
45. color spot tests, thin-layer chromatography, high-performance liquid chromatography
47. X-ray diffraction

CHAPTER 12
1. type
3. Plasma
5. Red blood cells
7. A
9. A,B
11. antibodies
13. True
15. neither
17. serology
19. A
21. radioimmunoassay (RIA)
23. three
25. benzidine
27. precipitin
29. absorption-elution
31. Enzymes
33. electrophoresis
35. dry
37. gene
39. 23
41. alleles
43. phenotype
45. will
47. AA, BB, AB
49. acid phosphatase
51. oligospermia
53. can
55. True

CHAPTER 13
1. Alphonse Bertillon
3. Sir Edward Richard Henry
5. is not
7. Fingerprints
9. Dermal papillae
11. loop, whorls, arches
13. arch
15. type lines
17. one
19. plain whorl
21. have no
23. 1/1
25. True
27. Plastic
29. powder
31. Iodine
33. silver nitrate
35. Super Glue® fuming
37. photography

CHAPTER 14
1. land
3. class
5. comparison microscope
7. sometimes
9. gauge
11. can
13. True
15. 12, 18
17. True
19. primer
21. False
23. is not
25. False
27. tool mark
29. individual

CHAPTER 15
1. questioned document
3. known, questioned
5. False
7. *Gilbert* v. *California*
9. individual
11. infrared
13. indented
15. sound spectrograph
17. False

Index